Manual of Geriatric Anesthesia

Sheila Ryan Barnett
Editor

Manual of Geriatric Anesthesia

Springer

Editor
Sheila Ryan Barnett, MD
Harvard Medical School
Department of Anesthesia, Critical Care, and Pain Medicine
Beth Israel Deaconess Medical Center
Boston, MA, USA

ISBN 978-1-4614-3887-8 ISBN 978-1-4614-3888-5 (eBook)
DOI 10.1007/978-1-4614-3888-5
Springer New York Heidelberg Dordrecht London

Library of Congress Control Number: 2012943387

Printed on acid-free paper

Springer is part of Springer Science+Business Media (www.springer.com)

To my wonderful husband John—for his humor, support, and encouragement—and to Elizabeth and Gannon: two truly great kids!

Preface

Old and older: ready or not, here they come!

It is common knowledge that the population is aging—in 2011, the 78 million baby boomers born between 1946 and 1964 began to turn 65, marking the beginning of a new and considerably greyer America. By 2030, 20% of the US population will be over 65 years—up from 12% in 2005. The shift in the demographics is going to significantly challenge our healthcare system. The question is, are we ready? In the field of anesthesiology—especially in our role as leaders in perioperative medicine—we need to address the aging problem aggressively—by educating and engaging our residents and peers. By putting together a manual of geriatric anesthesiology, I have attempted to combine a mix of geriatric anesthesia "must knows" and some more general discussions on some very "elderly" topics—such as ethics, dementia, polypharmacy, and the role of the geriatric consultant. Many thanks to all the authors who participated so enthusiastically on this important mission!

Boston, MA, USA — Sheila Ryan Barnett

Acknowledgments

I would like to acknowledge the unique role of the Society for the Advancement of Geriatric Anesthesiology (SAGA) in my personal and professional life, and especially Alec and Jeff, who have provided unbelievable encouragement, mentorship, and friendship.

I'd also like to thank Fritz, Deb, Xie, Chris, Sham, Terri, Mike, Jackie, Jacques any other SAGA supporters I may have missed – you have all made it possible to have fun being a geriatric anesthesiologist!

Contents

Contributors

Suresh Agarwal, MD, FACS, FCCM Chief, Trauma, Acute Care Surgery, Burn, and Surgical Critical Care, University of Wisconsin Hospital and Clinics, Madison, WI, USA

Shamsuddin Akhtar, MBBS Department of Anesthesiology, Yale University School of Medicine, New Haven, CT, USA

Ruben J. Azocar, MD Department of Anesthesiology, Boston Medical Center, Boston University School of Medicine, Boston, MA, USA

Sheila Ryan Barnett, MD Harvard Medical School, Department of Anesthesia, Critical Care, and Pain Medicine, Beth Israel Deaconess Medical Center, Boston, MA, USA

Ruma Bose, MD Department of Anesthesiology, Beth Israel Deaconess Medical Center, Boston, MA, USA

Asokumar Buvanendran, MD Department of Anesthesiology, Rush University Medical Center, Chicago, IL, USA

Angela Georgia Catic, MD Division of Gerontology, Department of Internal Medicine, Beth Israel Deaconess Medical Center, Harvard Medical School, Boston, MA, USA

Jacques E. Chelly, MD, PhD, MBA University of Pittsburgh Medical Center Shadyside-Presbyterian Hospitals, Posner Pain Center, Pittsburgh, PA, USA

Stacie Deiner, MD Department of Anesthesiology, Mount Sinai School of Medicine, New York, NY, USA

Adrienne N. Dixon, JD, MS, PA-C Legal Department, Johns Hopkins Health System Corporation, Johns Hopkins Bayview Medical Center, Baltimore, MD, USA

Kevin B. Gerold, DO, JD, FCCM, FCCP Department of Anesthesiology and Critical Care Medicine, Johns Hopkins School of Medicine, Baltimore, MD, USA

Jadelis Giquel, MD Department of Anesthesiology, University of Miami Miller School of Medicine, Miami, FL, USA

Yulia Ivashkov, MD Department of Anesthesiology and Pain Medicine, Harborview Medical Center, University of Washington, Seattle, WA, USA

Aaron LacKamp, MD Department of Anesthesiology and Critical Care Medicine, The Johns Hopkins Hospital and Johns Hopkins Bayview Medical Center, Baltimore, MD, USA

Steve Lee, MD, MA Department of Anesthesia, Critical Care, and Pain Medicine, Beth Israel Deaconess Medical Center, Harvard Medical School, Boston, MA, USA

Keith P. Lewis, RPh, MD Department of Anesthesiology, Boston Medical Center, Boston University School of Medicine, Boston, MA, USA

Michael C. Lewis, MD Department of Anesthesiology, Jackson Memorial Hospital, Miller School of Medicine, University of Miami, Miami, FL, USA

Cynthia A. Lien, MD Department of Anesthesiology, Weill Cornell Medical College, New York, NY, USA

Qing Liu, MD, PhD Department of Anesthesiology, UPMC Presbyterian-Montefior Hospital, Pittsburgh, PA, USA

Christina M. Matadial, MD Department of Anesthesiology, University of Miami Miller School of Medicine, Miami, FL, USA

Samir Mehta, MD Department of Orthopedic Surgery, University of Pennsylvania, Philadelphia, PA, USA

Julia I. Metzner, MD Department of Anesthesiology and Pain Medicine, University of Washington Medical Center, Seattle, WA, USA

John D. Mitchell, MD Department of Anesthesia, Critical Care and Pain Medicine, Beth Israel Deaconess Medical Center, Harvard Medical School, Boston, MA, USA

Mark D. Neuman, MD, MS Department of Anesthesiology, Hospital of the University of Pennsylvania, Philadelphia, PA, USA

Lale E. Odekon, MD, PhD Anesthesiology and Critical Care Medicine, Johns Hopkins Bayview Medical Center, Baltimore, MD, USA

Anup Pamnani, MD Department of Anesthesiology, New York Hospital, Weill Cornell Medical Center, New York, NY, USA

Gerardo Rodriguez, MD Department of Anesthesiology, Boston Medical Center, Boston University School of Medicine, Boston, MA, USA

G. Alec Rooke, MD, PhD Department of Anesthesiology and Pain Medicine, University of Washington Medical Center, Seattle, WA, USA

Steven J. Schwartz, MD Department of Anesthesiology and Adult Critical Care, Johns Hopkins Hospital, Baltimore, MD, USA

Frederick Sieber, MD Department of Anesthesiology and Adult Critical Care, Johns Hopkins Bayview Medical Center, Baltimore, MD, USA

Jeffrey H. Silverstein, MD Department of Anesthesiology, Mount Sinai School of Medicine, New York, NY, USA

Jason Strauss, MD Department of Psychiatry, Division of Geriatric Psychiatry, Cambridge Health Alliance, Harvard Medical School, Everett, MA, USA

Vijay Thillainathan, MD Department of Anesthesiology, Rush University Medical Center, Chicago, IL, USA

Punita Tripathi, MD Department of Anesthesia and Critical Care Medicine, Johns Hopkins Medical Center, Baltimore, MD, USA

Uchenna O. Umeh, MD Department of Anesthesiology, New York University Hospital for Joint Diseases, New York, NY, USA

Anna Uskova, MD Department of Anesthesiology, Shadyside Presbyterian University of Pittsburgh Medical Center, Pittsburgh, PA, USA

Mary Ann Vann, MD Department of Anesthesia, Pain, and Critical Care, Harvard Medical School, Beth Israel Deaconess Medical Center, Boston, MA, USA

Alexander A. Vitin, MD, PhD Department of Anesthesiology and Pain Medicine, University of Washington Medical Center, Seattle, WA, USA

Richa Wardhan, MD Department of Anesthesiology, Yale New Haven Hospital, New Haven, CT, USA

Adam Young, BS, MD Department of Anesthesiology, Rush University Medical Center, Chicago, IL, USA

Part I
General Issues

Chapter 1
Aging Demographics and Anesthesia

Michael C. Lewis

Introduction

Over the last century, life expectancy in the USA has increased dramatically. Only 100 years ago, it was common for people to die prior to their 50th birthday. The average age of the US population increased by as much as 14 years between 1900 and 1940. Of children born today, 95% will exceed 50 years of age with many living well into their 80s.

Improvements in social conditions paired with advances in medical science have resulted in remarkable reductions in morbidity and death from diseases that had previously been fatal. The time an American can expect to live has nearly doubled over the last 100 years and tripled over the course of human history. The latter half of the twentieth century, as well as the start of the twenty-first, is noted for an increased geriatric population size; Americans are living longer lives than ever. This "aging of America" has important implications for funding the nation's health, social, and economic institutions.

This chapter describes the demographics of the aging US population. While some might consider the contents of this section as dry, I would suggest that the demography of aging has developed into one of the most exciting fields of population study. Aging demography is a discipline with strong mathematical underpinnings and is of interest to a wide body of social and biological policymakers. Consequently, this chapter will examine how demographic data change and its relevance to the practice of medicine at large, with a particular focus on geriatric anesthesiology. The vital importance of this data in allocating health care resources for the elderly surgical population is emphasized (Fig. 1.1).

M.C. Lewis, MD (✉)
Department of Anesthesiology, Jackson Memorial Hospital, Miller School of Medicine, University of Miami, 1611 NW 12th Avenue, Miami, FL 33136, USA
e-mail: mclewis@med.miami.edu

S.R. Barnett (ed.), *Manual of Geriatric Anesthesia*, DOI 10.1007/978-1-4614-3888-5_1,

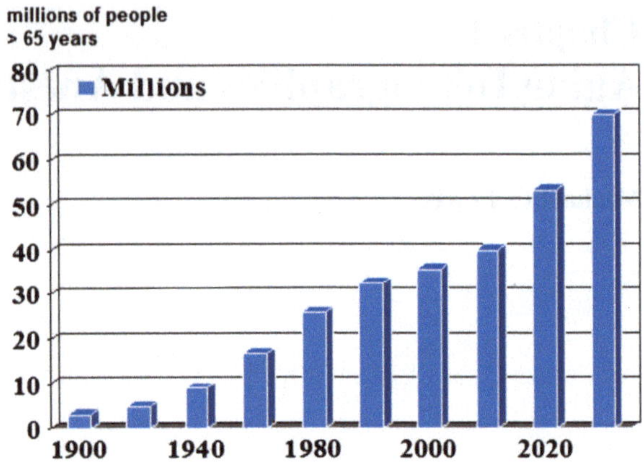

Fig. 1.1 Increased number of elderly in the population in the last 100 years. *Source*: Data from AARP and US Dept of Health and Social Services. A Profile of Older Americans, 1994

What Is Aging?

The common definition today of "elderly" is an age >65 years. It is interesting to examine the arbitrary origins of this definition. When Otto Von Bismarck (1815–1898) was chancellor of Germany, 1870–1890s, he strived to stave off a perceived threat of socialism. His plan: adopt some of the socialist's own tools. One mechanism Bismarck implemented was the introduction of a state pension system. The age chosen at that time for an individual to qualify for this pension was 65 years of age. In the late nineteenth century, only 4% of the population fell into this group, making this model economically sustainable. Now, with the potential of 20% of all Americans being over the age of 65 years, the applicability of this model has been called into question. Furthermore, the definition is rooted within social policy with no allowance given to biological, psychological, or other factors, such as socioeconomic class and education. Thus, although our present day definition of aging is somewhat arbitrary, until researchers develop a better definition of aging, we will continue to use ">65 years of age" as the reference group.

What Are Demographics?

The term demography describes the statistical study of human populations; data derived from such studies are termed demographics. Utilization of such data allows us to organize populations on the basis of a number of characteristics including age and gender. Distributions of values inside a given demographic, across populations and trends over time, provide essential information for health care planners. Understanding the demographic structure of a target population allows for rational planning and appropriate allocation of limited resources.

How Do We Describe the Distribution of Ages Within a Population?

The standard tool for describing the age distribution within a given population is termed the population pyramid (age–sex pyramid) (Fig. 1.2). This graphic illustrates the distribution of various age groups across a human population. Characteristically, this pyramid is made up of bar graphs, orientated back-to-back. In these graphs, the population is plotted on the *X*-axis, with age plotted on the *Y*-axis. They can represent the percentage or the absolute number of people in each age group. Each graph is sex–gender specific and arranged to show 5-year cohorts. Unlike classical bar graphs, these pyramidal graphs are oriented on their sides with the axis in the middle. Females are usually shown on the right, males on the left. These graphs yield much information about the development of population groups. Normally, there tends to be more females than males in the older age groups due to females' longer life expectancy.

The distribution of a population normally follows a "pyramidal" shape as illustrated in Fig. 1.2. This structure demonstrates that the proportion of a population that is made up of older individuals is less than younger people. It allows comparison of the age groups that constitute a population at a glance. The morphology of this pyramid will vary according to the type of society (Fig. 1.2).

Changes in the pyramid's morphology are accounted for in terms of the idea of demographic transition (DT). This model is used to characterize the evolution from high birth and death rates to low birth and death rates as a country develops from a preindustrial to industrialized economic system. As societies progress, fertility rates decline and mortality rates of all ages decrease. Consequently, the overall population age structure will lose its classical upright triangular form.

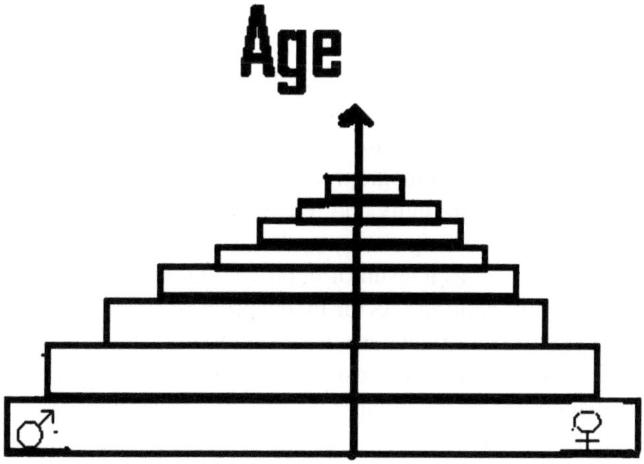

Fig. 1.2 The population triangle. This distribution is named for the *pyramidal shape* of its graph

Population pyramids are useful tools for social policy planners. They are utilized to find the number of economic dependents being supported in a particular population. Dependents are broadly defined as individuals who cannot work (children, retirees). In industrialized societies, utilization of government services is often used to calculate dependency ratios that are used in planning services.

During the evolution of a society, four distinct stages or demographic transitions have been described:

1. Stage one: preindustrial society, death rates and birth rates are high and roughly in balance. This is represented by the classical triangular distribution of the population.
2. Stage two: this usually applies to developing countries. Death rates drop rapidly due to improvements in social circumstances. During this stage, the population triangle develops a broader base consistent with a reduction in early mortality.
3. Stage three: birth rates fall further with improvements in social and medical conditions. Population growth levels off and the triangle starts developing a bulge. When societies undergo such a period of intense social expansion, they develop what has been called a "youth bulge." There is an expansion of the triangle in the middle as a result of the increasing number of young adults.
4. Stage four: this stage is characterized by low birth and death rates. During this stage, birth rates drop to below replacement levels, possibly leading to a decreasing population. This has profound social consequences resulting in an excess of older age groups, a bulge in the middle, with fewer children being born. Therefore, the triangle reverses itself. As the group born during stage two gets older because of superior medical and social factors, it results in an expansion of the expanded elderly population. The elderly are not active in the workforce and therefore represent an increasing social and economic dependency, economic burden, and a decreasing workforce. This is exactly the situation the USA now faces.

Although the original demographic transition model had only four stages, it has been recently suggested that a fifth stage may be necessary to characterize societies that have sub-replacement fertility. This is the case in many European countries with greater death rates than birth rates.

As one moves through the demographic transition model, the implication is that there is a reduction in both mortality and fertility resulting in a fundamental alteration of the age structure. During the second stage, as mortality falls, population increases in size. Moreover, as a result of improved infant survival rates, there is an increase in the number of children. As the model progresses, superior survival means the population ages. There is an underlying assumption that fertile populations will maintain high reproductive rates, increasing the number of children born. The overall effect of these changes is that the triangular structure observed in Fig. 1.2 develops a bulge in the middle and starts to reverse. This is illustrated in Fig. 1.3.

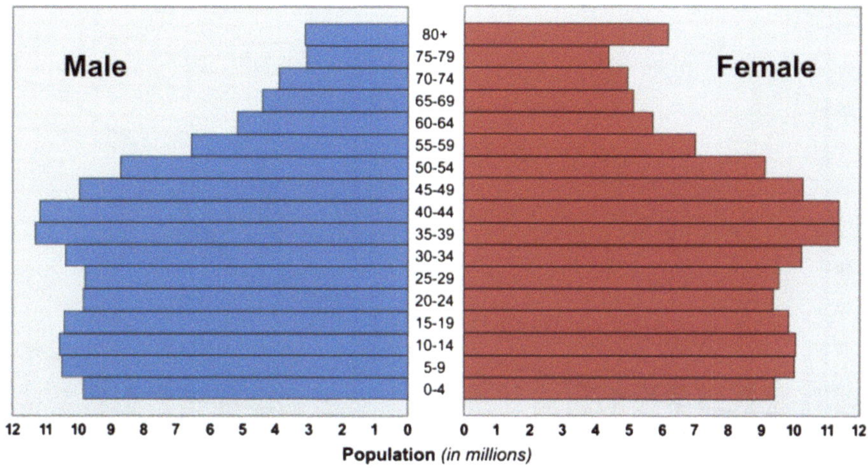

Fig. 1.3 United States Population (2000). Data source US Census Bureau. International Data Base (IDB). http//www.census.gov/ipc/www/idbnew.html

The Graying of America

It has been estimated that if the rate of increase in life expectancy in industrialized societies continues through the twenty-first century, most babies born after 2000 in these nations will celebrate their 100th birthdays! The World Health Organization (WHO) estimates that, globally, there were 600 million people aged 60 years and over in 2000 and that there will be 1.2 billion by 2025 and 2 billion by 2050. Furthermore, it estimates that there are about 492 million people aged 65 and over globally: 117 million in Europe, 43 million in North America, and 258 million in the much greater total population of Asia.

Population aging is clearly a universal phenomenon. Gary S. Becker, Nobel Laureate in Economics at the University of Chicago (1992), wrote in the January 31, 2000, issue of *Business Week*, "Longer life was the twentieth century's greatest gift." The twentieth century significantly increased the general population of the USA, and the twenty-first century will be recorded as the century of aging.

As Fig. 1.4 reveals, the growth of the US population was not uniform. Whereas the overall US population increased approximately threefold, the elderly population increased by an approximate factor of 10. It has been estimated by the US Census Bureau that at the end of the century individuals over the age of 65 will comprise ~13% of the total population. The marked increase of the population at the extreme of the elderly age group is truly remarkable, especially for the "oldest old" demonstrated in Fig. 1.5. In 1900, <125,000 persons were 85 years and older, comprising 4% of the elderly; this increased to around 12% of all elderly people in 2000. By 2030, the number of persons aged 85 and over is projected to double to 8.9 million. This increase can be most appreciated when considering those people over 100 years of age. In the USA,

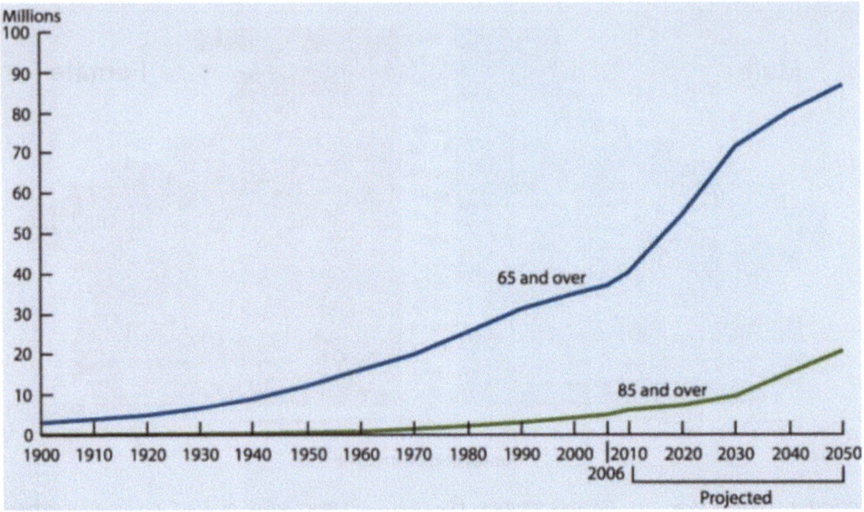

Fig. 1.4 The number of older Americans. *Source*: US Census Bureau. Populations estimates and projections

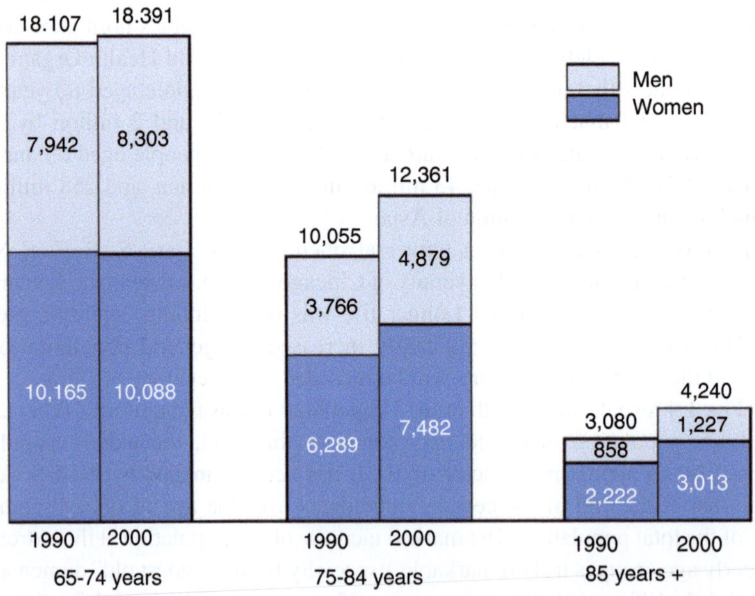

Fig. 1.5 Increases in sizes of various age groups. *Source*: US Census Bureau. Census 2000 Summary File 1; 1990 Census of Population, General Population Characteristics, United States (1990 CP-1-1)

individuals reaching retirement age are entitled to receive during 2000, there were 50,000 such people; the number is expected to rise ten–tenfold over the next 50 years. It is projected that in 2030 there will be over 130,000 Americans over the age of 100 years (Fig. 1.5).

Life expectancy has steadily increased over the last 100 years; however, there are significant economic, regional, and gender differences in life expectancy. Furthermore the increases in the elderly population have not been geographically uniform across the USA. Going forward, it is predicted that northern states will lose elderly citizens while the southern and western states will gain people.

Surprisingly, US life expectancy (~78 years) is lower than Western Europe (>80 years). The increase in life expectancy is more significant for females; women aged 65 years old can expect to live about 6 years longer than a comparable male. However, by 85 years of age, the gender difference in life expectancy has largely disappeared.

The increase in size of the elderly population has been more significant in developing countries and has a significant impact on health care providers in general including anesthesiologists. When the older population was relatively small, an extended social welfare system was financially viable. However, as the proportion of older to younger adults increases, the amount of financial and social support available for the elderly decreases.

Why Is the Age Structure of a Population Important?

The significance of the age structure for health care providers is based on the fact that people of different ages have different requirements, abilities, and social entitlements. Many of these characteristics are biologically determined alterations that are associated with chronological age. From the health care perspective, age-related changes impact not only the resources that need to be expended towards surgical care but also a patient's response to anesthesia.

In the USA, individuals over the age of 67 are entitled to receive medical care under the government-sponsored program Medicare and may also be enrolled in the Social Security system. As we have seen in recent years, these programs are already experiencing significant financial pressure, and that is likely to get worse with the continuing elderly population growth and the explosion of health care costs in the USA. As a result of the recently enacted health care reform legislation, the challenge of maintaining such a social policy is likely to be increased.

As we have seen, society defines "dependency," whether social or medical, based on an arbitrary social cutoff point. This cutoff age when elderly dependency starts is largely dependent on the ability of the country to afford entitlement programs and is in part a social decision. Data from population pyramids can assist in the decision-making process.

Population pyramids provide information that government agencies can use to recommend a set of social policies. These graphs are not deterministic; they merely illustrate the natural increase of the median age, birth, and death rate. These models can help in estimating the number of economic dependents in a specific populace. For social planning purposes, economic dependents are defined as those children who are in full-time school, not capable of working, and those over 65 (choice of being retirees). Therefore, the definition provides an approximation. This number can be further used to calculate the dependency ratio in that population.

Implication for Health Care Providers

This graying of America is often regarded as a major cause of upward pressure on health care costs. One of the natural consequences of aging is the increased incidence of disease and disability. Among those aged over the 85-year-old age group, the incidence of disease sharply increases. This is not uniform across all races, and older African Americans and Hispanics have a greater incidence of disease than Caucasians.

It is important to keep in perspective that although the aging population is an important factor in rising health care costs, analyses of health care spending suggest that other factors, particularly the growing complexity of equipment, have a considerably greater bearing. Fortunately, even though population aging will bring a number of added costs, these may be decreased by the application of appropriate and well-coordinated health policies aimed at slowing the rate of health decline associated with aging and thus the amount of health care services required. Thus both the increasing number of elderly patients as well as the higher costs of technologies used in their medical care continue to strain an already overstretched health care system.

Older Americans utilize about 50% of all federal health expenditures on medical needs. Older patients occupy about 40% of all hospital beds in the USA, and their hospital admissions tend to be longer. When an acute illness occurs in the most aged, the cost associated can often be greater than for a younger adult because of the coexisting morbidities associated with aging. The elderly also have a greater incidence of residual disability reflected in higher, long-term nursing costs. These sociological changes have had a significant impact on US health care costs. They have also led to major stresses on the Medicare system and have been one of the major accelerators of health care reform.

Aging and Surgical Procedures

As described, increased life expectancy and reduced mortality from chronic age-related diseases continue to enlarge that fraction of the surgical patient population considered elderly. As they age, adult patients also exhibit an increasingly complex array of unique physical responses to environmental and socioeconomic conditions as well as to concurrent disease states. Survival to adulthood and beyond permits the full expression of even the most subtle genetic differences between individuals, differences that might not be fully apparent over shorter life span intervals. People are never more alike than they are not at birth nor more different or unique than when they enter the geriatric era. Precise assessment and appropriate perioperative management of the elderly surgical patient represents a great challenge to all medical health care providers.

Although they represent only 12% of the United States population, individuals 65 years of age or older undergo almost one-third of the 25 million surgical procedures performed annually. They consume about one-third of all health expenditures and fully one-half of the $140 billion annual US federal health care budget. Therefore, every anesthesiologist in contemporary practice eventually becomes a subspecialist in geriatric medicine, with a special responsibility for delivering cost-effective health care to older adults.

Impact on Anesthesiology

Surgical procedures in the elderly will continue to require a disproportionately large share of societal and institutional health care resources. Increasing morbidity with aging, and a number of advances in surgical, anesthetic, and intensive care techniques, has led to a larger proportion of the elderly population undergoing surgical procedures. One striking paradigm shift in anesthesiology over the last several decades has been the increasing size of the elderly surgical population. It is estimated that the percentage of anesthetics given in the USA will increased about 50% overall, significantly enhancing the anesthesia workload.

Routine postoperative hospitalization and intensive care, especially after major trauma, are frequently protracted and may be further complicated by infection, by poor wound healing, and by multiple organ system failure for critically ill elderly patients. Of equal concern are recent findings that postoperative cognitive dysfunction may persist at least 3 months after an otherwise uncomplicated surgery. Additional time and effort will need to be spent on caring for the geriatric patient and therefore impact the work of most anesthesiologists.

Morbidity and mortality among this group are different from other cohorts. Special education in geriatric anesthesiology is essential to prepare the trainee in anesthesiology for the future. Pediatric anesthesiology has developed during the lifetime of the baby boomers, a cohort that has now become elderly. It is now the era of geriatric anesthesiology.

Summary

The last 100 years have seen an explosive increase in the number of elderly Americans. Improvements in medical care, as well as improved social conditions, have led to a decrease in death rates. This decrease is especially marked in the oldest segments of the population. Description and analysis of these population changes are aided by the discipline of demographics in general as well as a specific tool developed from this discipline, the population pyramid.

Aging is associated with increased morbidity that often requires surgery. Increased health care resources will therefore have to be directed towards this growing population. Furthermore, this new workload will significantly impact the provision of anesthesiology well into the twenty-first century and is a salient issue for the current and future generations of anesthesia providers.

Key Points

- The elderly population of the USA is growing. This is especially true of the cohort of individuals over the age of 85 years.
- There is a significant impact on health care delivery from this "graying" of America. Health care costs are different in the elderly as compared to younger adults. These are significantly increased if one considers care required at the end of life.
- Surgical procedures in the elderly will continue to require a disproportionately large share of societal and institutional health care resources; therefore, an increased workload strain will be placed on the anesthesiologist of the early to mid-twenty-first century.

Suggested Reading

Administration on Aging. A Profile of Older Americans in 2002: Washington DC: US Department of Health and Human Services 2003.

Christensen K, Doblhammer G, Rau R, Vaupel JW. Aging populations: the challenges ahead. Lancet. 2009;374:1196–1208.

Christensen K, Doblhammer G, Rau R, Vaupel JW. Ageing populations: the challenges ahead. Lancet. 2009;374:1196–1208.

Haaga JG, et al. What's next for the demography of aging? Popul. Dev. Rev. 2009;35:323–365.

Klopfenstein CE, Herrman FR, Michel JP, Clergue F, Forster A. The Influence of an Aging Surgical Population on the Anesthesia Workload: A Ten-Year Survey. Anesth. Analg. 1998; 86:1165–70.

Manton G. Demographic trends for the aging female population. J Amer Womens Medical Association. 1997;52:95–105.

Owens WD. Overview of anesthesia for the geriatric patient. Int Anesthesiol Clin. Summer. 1988;26:96–97.

Rice DP, Fineman N. Economic implications of increased longevity in the United State07/Table02. pdfs. Annu Rev Publ Health. 2004;25:457–473.

United Nations Statistics Division, Demographic yearbook, Table 2 http://unstats.un.org/unsd/demographic/products/dyb/dyb20.

United States Census Bureau State and County Quickfacts. http://quickfacts.census.gov/qfd/states/00000.html.

US Census Bureau 1990. Current Population Reports. Special Studies, Centenarians in the United States.

US Census Bureau. The 65 Years and Over Population: 2000, October 2001.
Veering BT. Management of anaesthesia in elderly patients. Curr Opin Anaesthesiol. Jun 1999;12:333–336.
Wilmouth JR. Demography of Longevity: past, present and future trends. Exp Gerontol. 2000;35:1111–1119.
World health Organization, Ageing and lifecourse http://www.who.int/ageing/en/.

Chapter 2
Ethical and Legal Considerations

Kevin B. Gerold and Adrienne N. Dixon

Introduction

Ethics are the standards that societies, organizations, and professions establish to define expectations for behavior among members of that group. They broadly define right from wrong and create expectations of appropriate behavior. Laws, regulations, and policies are used to more clearly define ethical behavior and to impose sanctions for wrongful actions. This chapter will describe established ethical and legal principles that anesthetists should consider when acting appropriately and professionally within their practice. Because laws, regulations, and policies differ among states and within institutions, anesthetists must familiarize themselves with the proper policies where they practice.

The ethical principles and laws that apply when caring for the elderly are the same as those applying for the care all patients. Ethical and legal issues arise more frequently among the elderly and present frequent challenges for health care providers because the number of elderly is increasing as a percentage of the population. Twelve percent of the US population is now over the age of 65, and this percentage is expected to grow to more than 20% by the year 2050. Many of these patients will have diminished decision-making capacity due to chronic infirmary or acute illness, and many will outlive or lose touch with traditional surrogate decision-makers such as spouses, siblings, and other family members. Ethical and legal issues that confront anesthesiologists when caring for elderly patients include obtaining informed

K.B. Gerold, DO, JD, FCCM, FCCP (✉)
Department of Anesthesiology and Critical Care Medicine, A5W-588,
Johns Hopkins School of Medicine, 4940 Eastern Avenue, Baltimore, MD 21224, USA
e-mail: kgerold1@jhmi.edu

A.N. Dixon, JD, MS, PA-C
Legal Department, Johns Hopkins Health System Corporation,
Johns Hopkins Bayview Medical Center, 4940 Eastern Avenue,
ASC Building, Room 247, Baltimore, MD 21224, USA

S.R. Barnett (ed.), *Manual of Geriatric Anesthesia*, DOI 10.1007/978-1-4614-3888-5_2,

consent, determining whether a patient has the capacity to make an informed choice and provide consent, the selection of a surrogate decision-maker for patients who lack decisional capacity, the effect orders to forego resuscitation ["do not resuscitate (DNR)"] affects a decision to undergo surgery and anesthesia, and medical futility.

Informed Consent

The need to obtain informed consent arises from a physician's ethical obligation to assist patients in making a choice from among therapeutic alternatives consistent with good medical practice. Informed consent, as we interpret it today, did not emerge until in the early 1900s when doctors reluctantly abandoned a long-held authoritarian doctor relationship and gradually accepted a growing social expectation that they disclose matters relating to a patient's care and treatment, even if this included the disclosure of a dire prognosis.

The legal approach to informed consent is rooted within the ethical principle of autonomy. Justice Cardozo clarified this principle in law when he stated in 1914, "Every human being of adult years and sound mind has the right to determine what shall be done with his own body…." The need to obtain consent arises because society believes that legally competent patients have the right of self-determination and it prohibits physicians from substituting his or her judgment for that of the patient in matters relating to care and treatment. Subordinate ethical principles that further define a practitioner's obligations to patients include beneficence, the obligation to act in a helpful or therapeutic manner ("do what is right"); nonmaleficence, an obligation to act in ways that avoid harm ("do no harm"); and social welfare, an obligation to act in ways that benefit the community welfare ("the social good").

Informed consent is the discussion that takes place between physician and patient prior to engaging in a proposed plan, treatment, or procedure and results in the patient's giving permission to go forward. This discussion must include the material aspects of the patient's diagnosis and proposed treatment sufficient to enable a reasonable patient to consider his or her options, including having no treatment, and enable the making of an educated decision in the context of his or her needs and values. While signing a consent form creates a legal presumption that the consent was informed, signing a consent form alone is inadequate to meet the obligation for a proper consent.

Until recently, it was generally assumed that consent for surgery implied consent for anesthesia; making it was for anesthesiologists to obtain a separate consent. With the increasing complexity of surgery and the division of care among specialists, each with control over their portion of the overall treatment plan, courts have abandoned "Captain of the Ship" doctrines in favor or holding each practitioner liable for the care rendered under her control. The anesthetic plan is outside of the surgeon's direct control making the anesthesiologist separately liable for care rendered under that plan. As such, anesthesiologists are obligate to develop an anesthetic plan in discussion with the patient and obtain consent before providing care.

Table 2.1 Elements for breach of informed consent under the negligence standard

Legal elements associated with negligent informed consent
Failure to disclose the patient's diagnosis or condition
Failure to disclose adequately the nature of the proposed treatment plan
Failure to provide probabilities that the proposed therapy will succeed
Failure to provide the patient with reasonable alternatives to the proposed treatment plan
Failure to disclose the material risks and burdens associated with reasonable treatment options enabling a reasonable patient to make an informed choice, including the choice to refuse care

Physicians may delegate the process of obtaining consent to others, but they maintain responsibility for the adequacy of that consent. Once consent is obtained, practitioners should document the discussion that took place in the medical record. Hospital policies often require patients and practitioners to complete and sign a consent form. The utility of a signed consent form is that it creates a legal presumption that informed consent was obtained, making it difficult for a plaintiff–patient to allege that they were not informed of the risks and alternatives of a procedure or treatment plan. A signed consent form never excuses a physician of his or her obligation to inform the patient, personally or through others, about the plan of treatment or a proposed procedure.

The essential steps to fulfilling informed consent requirements are outlined in Table 2.1. Information generally considered material and necessary for a patient to make an informed decision includes (1) providing the diagnosis; (2) present the nature and purpose of the proposed treatment or procedure, the probability and severity of its risks, and whether those risks would be temporary or permanent; and (3) provide reasonable treatment alternatives including general anesthesia, local anesthesia with or without moderate sedation, and axial or regional nerve block. When describing the proposed treatment, it is unnecessary to describe specific details and the technical or mechanical means of performing an operation or procedure, and it is unnecessary to inform the patient of what he or she already knows. The discussion should occur in the patient's preferred language, and plain language terms are preferable to medical terms. If the patient requires an interpreter, the physician is obligated to obtain one who is credentialed as fluent in the language and culture sufficient to express the subtleties necessary for a patient to understand their medical condition and proposed treatment. There is an increasing expectation that informed consent should also include material information relating to the probability of success for a proposed treatment or procedure as well as the risks and benefits of reasonable alternative(s), including those procedures not performed by the practitioner.

Other emerging aspects relating to informed consent include whether physicians are required to include his or her own experiences or outcomes with a proposed treatment or procedure and whether they should disclose information about their own health status that may affect the treatment plan or affect the patient's risk. As studies increasingly demonstrate reductions in morbidity and mortality are achievable when treatment such as cardiac surgery or cancer treatments are performed in specialized centers, it is anticipated that disclosing success rates with a proposed treatment as benchmarked against other physicians or centers will become an additional element of the informed consent discussion. A Maryland court held that a physician had a duty to disclose to patients that he was infected with the human immunodeficiency virus (HIV+), even though the risk of transmitting the infection was small.

Legal liability for practitioners who fail to properly obtain consent arose originally under the tort of battery. Battery is a civil wrong arising from an intentional and wrongful physical contact with a person without his or her consent and entails some injury or offensive touching. A physician–surgeon in Minnesota was the first physician sued successfully for failing to obtain consent under battery in 1095. In Mohr v. Williams, a patient consented to surgery for a diseased condition of the right ear. While the patient was under anesthesia, the surgeon determined that the condition of the right ear was not serious enough to require surgery and determined that the left ear was more seriously diseased and required surgical treatment. Without stopping the surgery, waking the patient, and obtaining permission to operate on the left ear, the surgeon proceeded to with the necessary operation. The operation was performed skillfully, and the outcome was successful. Following surgery, the patient sued the surgeon for failing to obtain proper consent and was awarded monetary compensation. When reviewed on appeal by the Supreme Court of Minnesota, the court acknowledged that the left ear was diseased, that the ear required surgery, that the operation was performed skillfully, and that the physician–surgeon acted in good faith and without evil intent. Nonetheless, the court concluded that performing an operation without the patient's consent was wrong and, as such, was unlawful. This legal remedy for a lack of informed consent persisted until the 1960s when courts began to view battery as too strong a legal remedy for failures of informed consent and now reserve it for limited cases where a physician fails to obtain any consent. Today, nearly all states regard the failure to obtain a proper informed consent as a breach of the doctor's professional duty to his or her patient and apply a negligence test.

Under a negligence theory, the legal obligation to obtain informed consent arises from a duty of every physician to exercise due care in his or her conduct toward others from which injury may result. The duty to obtain informed consent is excused only when (1) an emergency condition exists, the patient is unconscious or is otherwise incapable of consenting, and the failure to treat poses an imminent harm; or (2) in rare circumstances when the risk of disclosure would pose such a serious psychological threat of detriment to the patient as to be medically contraindicated.

Some states define negligent informed consent narrowly, requiring the plaintiff–patient to show a violation of physical integrity before asserting a claim. Others apply a broader test for negligence. These states require plaintiff–patients to show only that the physician was negligent in his or her failing to obtain adequate consent (see also Table 2.1). When attempting to determine whether a physician or other medical providers' care was negligent, courts will examine the conduct in the context of the standard of care viewed in the context of a reasonable practitioner and patient. A reasonable patient or practitioner at law is someone who exercises the qualities of attention, knowledge, intelligence, and judgment which society requires of its members for the protection of their own interests and the interests of others. The reasonable person is a fictitious person, who is never negligent and whose conduct is always up to standard. By applying a reasonable person test, the courts insulate physicians from individuals who may claim negligence through an unreasonable expectation about the adequacy of consent in a specific instance.

The legal threshold for a plaintiff–patient to assert successfully the failure of informed consent is generally high, and it is unusual for plaintiffs to sue for negligent consent alone. When appropriate to do so legally, lawyers may incorporate negligent consent to a lawsuit alleging other claims of medical malpractice.

The best strategy to insure the adequacy of consent is to adhere to the standards of good medical practice. Prior to initiating an anesthetic plan or beginning a procedure, anesthesiologists should invest the time to inform the patient of their diagnosis and prognosis, offer reasonable therapeutic options including no treatment, and make recommendations as to what the physician believes to be the best plan of care. The patient should be provided the opportunity to have their questions answered to their satisfaction and then be permitted to choose among the options available, including the option to request another anesthesia provider or to forego a surgical procedure. If the physician chooses to forego obtaining consent because (1) an emergency condition exists, the patient is incapable of consenting, and the failure to treat poses an imminent harm; or (2) the risk of disclosure poses such a serious psychological threat of detriment to the patient as to be medically contraindicated, then the physician should document these special circumstances in the medical record.

If a patient has diminished capacity or is unable to provide an informed consent, then the physician is obligated to obtain informed consent from the patient's legal health care agent, guardian, or surrogate decision-maker. In cases where the patient has diminished decision-making capacity, it is reasonable to enlist the support of surrogate decision-makers, family members, and friends in the discussion to assist the patient with making an informed decision. In nonemergency circumstances where a patient lacks the capacity to make an informed decision and a legally authorized surrogate decision-maker is unavailable, physicians must seek the appointment of a court-appointed guardian to decide on the patient's behalf.

Evaluating Capacity to Make an Informed Choice

Inherent in a patient's right of self-determination and a physician's obligation to obtain consent prior to initiating medical treatment or invasive procedure is the assumption that the patient has the mental capacity to make an autonomous choice. An autonomous choice is one that is intentional, made with understanding and without controlling influences. While increasing age does not reduce the right to make autonomous choices, there is a relationship between advanced age and impaired decision-making capacity. The incidence of dementia increases with age, especially among those older than 85 years of age. Together with an increasing incidence of chronic illness, susceptibility to medication side effects and other risk factors combine to increase the incidence of impaired decision-making capacity among the elderly. Impaired decision-making capacity may be temporary or permanent and has legal and medical implications.

Competency is a legal term that describes a person's right to manage his or her own affairs and be held legally accountable for their actions and decisions. The law presumes generally that adult patients are competent unless a court declares them incompetent. Previously competent persons may be found incompetent by court order (de facto incompetence) after a formal inquiry into their actual mental capacities and the presenting of evidence showing that they lack the requisite functional abilities to make decisions on their own behalf. De facto incompetents include patients in coma, the severely mentally impaired, and those with severe mental illness. When a court finds a person incompetent, it acts to protect his or her welfare and appoints a guardian to act on the person's behalf. Declaring a patient incompetent as a matter of law is a serious matter that can be more intrusive and liberty depriving than a criminal conviction. Courts viewed competence traditionally in broad terms; the person was either competent or not competent. More recently, some courts have begun to consider competency in contextual terms. For example, a person in the early stages of dementia may remain competent to make all or some of their own health care decisions but may be deemed incompetent to manage his financial affairs.

In contrast to the legal determination of competency made by courts, physicians and other practitioners are often asked to make determinations of a patient's capacity to make a reasoned choice. In clinical practice, a determination that a patient lacks decision-making capacity has nearly the same consequences as a legal determination of incompetence. The degree of medical capacity to make an informed decision is not a bright-line matter but is instead nuanced, often making such determinations difficult. As a general rule, patients must have high degrees of capacity to consent or refuse treatment involving complex or nuanced decisions, when treatments will result in significant burdens or disability, to forego treatments that most reasonable patients would accept under the circumstances or consent to treatments that most patients under the circumstances would refuse. Low levels of decisional capacity are required when consenting to care associated with simple decisions, small burdens, or is in agreement with care that reasonable patients in same or similar circumstances would consent. Further, a patient's cognitive ability to understand and reason may change during the course of their condition or illness, or as a consequence of medications or treatment. As a result, a patient's capacity to make informed decisions may change from hour to hour or from day to day.

While it is important that physicians protect patients' right to autonomy and obtain their consent, they are also obligated to identify patients unable to make a reasoned choice and find a suitable surrogate decision-maker. The process of obtaining consent should include an examination sufficient to dermine a patient's abilty to communicate a choice without outside influence or coercion, their capacity for insight, reasoning, and judgment required to understand the risks and benefits of the proposed treatment in the context of other options, the capacity for reasoning

Table 2.2 Elements of competence

Functional cognitive abilities required to make an informed choice
The ability to communicate and express a choice
The insight, judgment, and memory, necessary to evaluate information relevant to treatment decision-making
The ability to understand the significance of treatment within the context of the patient's own values—especially the significance of their condition and the potential benefits and burdens associated with treatment, including no treatment
The ability to arrive at a reasoned decision and select a treatment among available treatment options

Table 2.3 Capacity assessment instruments

Instruments used to assess mental capacity
Mini-Mental Status Examination (MMSE)
MacArthur Competence Assessment Tool (MacCAT-T)
Edelstein's Hopemont Capacity Assessment Inventory
Neurobehavioral Cognitive Status Examination
Dementia Rating Scale
Wechsler Adult Intelligence Scale
Geriatric Depression Scale
Center for Epidemiological Studies Depression Scale
Short Psychiatric Evaluation Schedule
Global Deterioration Scale
Alzheimer's Disease Assessment Scale
Brief Cognitive Rating Score
Cambridge Mental Disorders of the Elderly Examination
Dementia of the Alzheimer's Type Inventory
Dementia Diagnostic Screening Questionnaire
Mental Status Questionnaire
AARP Executive Cognitive Function Measure (ECF)

required to make a rationale decision among choices, and whether their decisions are consistent with their beliefs and values and with his or her prior expressed wishes (Tables 2.2 and 2.3).

If during a patient interview, the physician develops a suspicion that a patient may lack the capacity to make an informed decision, then the physician should request and obtain a formal evaluation of the patient's competency prior to obtaining consent. In the absence of an emergency condition, patients who appear to lack the functional abilities to make an informed decision should have a formal evaluation of competency before undertaking a treatment plan. When confronted with a questionably competent patient, practitioners should also avoid the inclination to turn immediately to the patient's surrogate decision-maker to make decisions on the patient's behalf.

For patients lacking capacity, the physician has an obligation to obtain informed consent from the patient's designated health care agent, or if unavailable, the patient's surrogate decision-maker. In cases where the patient has diminished capacity yet retains the ability to make informed decisions, it may also be proper to obtain the patients permission to engage family members or friends in the discussion to aid the patient in arriving at an informed decision. In nonemergency circumstances where a patient lacks capacity to make an informed decision and a legally authorized surrogate decision-maker is unavailable, physicians must seek the appointment of a court-appointed guardian to decide on the patient's behalf.

Advanced Health Care Directives

Historical and scientific developments have complicated medical decision-making for seriously ill patients. A culture of medical paternalism has given way to one of patient's rights, autonomy, and informed consent. At the same time, complex technologies now enable us to extend the lives of elderly patients using artificial means but are often unable to restore these patients to their prior level of function or independence. Determining the best plan of care for individual patients requires that health care practitioners make sound medical judgments and offer reasonable choices that consider each patient's values and preferences in decisions that will affect the quality and quantity of his or her life. The complexity of these decisions becomes complicated further when patients lose the capacity to make their own decisions and someone else must make decisions on their behalf. The medical, legal, and ethical communities continue to advocate for the use of advance directives to minimize the uncertainty in these circumstances.

Advance health care directives enable agents, surrogates, and families to act on the patient's behalf at times of incapacity. They are legal documents used more commonly in medical settings than in courts. "This is what we should do"—medical decisions are private matters best left to patients, assisted by their physicians. There is a widely held belief in medicine and in law that courts should remain the place of last resort to resolve disputes between patients and care providers. The emotional toll upon all parties can be enormous and the delays significant and legal remedies are often "clumsy, intrusive, overbearing, and counterproductive. Doctors don't want to litigate health care. Patients don't want it to litigate it, and lawyers and judges probably don't want it either."

In 1992, in an effort to encourage hospitalized patients to express advance directives, Congress enacted the Patient Self-Determination Act. The act requires hospitals, nursing homes, home health agencies, and hospice programs to provide written information concerning their rights under state law as to medical decisions, including the right to formulate advance directives. Despite this mandated effort directed at encouraging the execution of advance directives, only 10–25% of patients complete an advance directive, and these documents are regularly disregarded by health care practitioners. Of those who create advance directives, ~5% exist for adults under age 40, while 70% are elderly. Interestingly, physicians are no more likely to execute advance directives for themselves than occurs is the general population. However, when physicians are surveyed, they describe a preference for limiting medical interventions for themselves in the event of a serious or life-threatening illness.

In the spring of 2005, the end-of-life decision-making for Terri Schiavo, a Florida woman in a persistent vegetative state, played out as a public spectacle and a tragedy for her and her husband. Mr. Schiavo's private feud with his wife's parents over his continued attempts to discontinue the administration of fluids and nutrition delivered artificially through a feeding tube was taken to the media, the courts, the Florida legislature, Florida Governor Jeb Bush, the US Congress, and President George Bush. After more than 7 years of litigation involving nearly 20 judges, Ms. Schiavo's case caused a reexamination of issues that most physicians, lawyers, and bioethicists considered well settled since the 1976 New Jersey Supreme Court decision in the case of Karen Quinlan and later by the 1990 US Supreme Court decision in the case of Nancy Cruzan.

Although the majority of Americans believed the Terri Schiavo case represented an intrusion of politics into medical decision-making and well-defined law, it highlights the reality that most people do not wish to remain in a persistent vegetative state kept alive by artificial means. The publicity generated by this case called attention to the need for families to discuss openly their medical wishes among each other and hopefully create an advanced directive and designate a health care agent.

Following the Schiavo case, the law remains clear; incompetent patients retain an interest in self-determination. Physicians should encourage health care agents to act on the patient's best interest and assist them with making treatment decisions consistent with what they believe the patient would request if they were expressing a choice for themselves.

Early forms of advanced directives took the form of a living will. Living wills, or declarations, are death with dignity directives recognized in law in 47 states. Living wills are documents providing specific instructions to attending physicians, stating the patient's desires for treatment in the event they become incapacitated in a terminal or end-stage condition. Treatment choices usually relate to the limits to which a patient wishes to be kept alive by artificial life-support measures. Living wills become effective of a loss of decisional capacity in the context of the diagnosis of terminal illness, end-stage condition, or a persistent vegetative state as diagnosed by two physicians. Often living wills instruct physicians to provide or withhold death-delaying procedures such as artificial nutrition, mechanical ventilation, renal dialysis, and when to implement comfort only care. The advantage of a living will is that it permits patients to communicate directly with their care providers and does not require the presence of a third party to act on the patient's behalf. The limitation, however, is living wills do not provide instructions for unforeseen circumstances. For this reason, lawyers increasingly encourage persons to identify a durable power of attorney for health care or designate a health care agent. In the event of incapacity, a durable power of attorney for health care has advantages over a living will in that it permits a person to delegate any or all medical decisions, routine and end-of-life care, to a health care agent, proxy, or surrogate. The durable power of attorney normally terminates if the patient regains the ability to express informed choices.

Under this form of advance directive, the designated health care agents are permitted to confer with treating physicians, review medical records, and act on the patient's behalf. If those wishes are unknown or unclear, the agent can act in what they believe is the patient's best interest. Physicians who disagree with a patient's advance health care directive or decisions made by a health care agent should avoid the temptation to substitute his or her own values and make judgments about a patient's care. Physicians or other practitioners who do so expose themselves to assertions of battery, negligence, or the intentional infliction of emotional harm. In the rare circumstances when a physician or other members of the care team are genuinely concerned by choices exercised by the patient's agent, then an ethics committee review or seeking the advice of the hospital risk management office is warranted.

Although most advance directives are made in writing, some states permit the creation of an oral advance directive made by a patient with capacity to their treating physician or statutorily defined licensed independent professional. In these circumstances, the physician should document the oral directive in the medical record and should consider having the patient and a witness sign the entry.

Only a competent individual may create or revoke an advance directive, and a certification of incapacity usually implies that the patient may no longer create or change an advance directive. However, in some states, the law permits patients to revoke an advance directive at any time, irrespective of their mental state. In these states, once revoked, the durable power is terminated no matter how implausible or inopportune the revocation.

Surrogate Decision-Making

In the absence of an advance directive or a living will, some states have enacted laws permitting family members, close friends, and domestic partners to serve as surrogates able to make medical decisions on the patient's behalf. These laws generally establish hierarchy defining in law who is authorized to serve as a surrogate. Surrogates differ from health care agents in they are limited in their authority to make decisions that are reasonably in the patient's best interest. While the use of legal surrogates to consent on a patient's behalf are accepted widely, in one third of all cases, they fail to accurately reflect a patient's end-of-life treatment preferences and more commonly err by providing interventions that differ from what patients want. Further, disagreements among surrogates, for example among adult children or among siblings, may complicate decision-making on the patient's behalf.

Perioperative DNR Orders

One area relating to advanced directive that anesthesiologists will encounter, particularly when caring for the elderly patients, is a DNR order. Whereas these orders have been accepted widely in general medical practice since the 1970s, they were

Table 2.4 Assessment of capacity

When to consider impaired decision-making capacity
Patients presenting with abrupt change(s) in mental status
Patients who refuse reasonable treatments and who are unable to provide rational or reasonable explanations for doing so
Whenever consent is required for treatments that are especially invasive, experimental, or burdensome
Patients with an unstable or untreated neurologic or psychiatric diagnoses (i.e., anxiety, depression, psychosis)
Patients with situational factors associated with impaired decision-making such as sleep deprivation, sepsis, delirium, prolonged inpatient hospitalization, mild dementia, recent surgery, or the extreme of age

discouraged or ignored by surgeons and anesthesiologists, and some hospital operating rooms had policies suspending a patient's DNR order perioperatively.

Advocates for suspending DNR orders during the operative and postoperative period argue that surgery and anesthesia often induce physiologic instability requiring interventions considered acts of resuscitation and that foregoing resuscitation unfairly limited the treatment options of the operative team. Such acts of resuscitation include procedures such as tracheal intubation, mechanical ventilation, the administration of blood products and intravenous fluids, and administering medications to treat arrhythmias or to support blood pressure; interventions typically withheld in a DNR order. Other reasons to forego a DNR order perioperatively is to protect the staff from feeling responsible for possibly precipitating a patient's death or to avoid the unfounded legal concerns that the surgical team would become liable for acting in a negligent manner.

Arguments for continuing to honor a patient's DNR request in the operating room acknowledge the need to balance the benefits of a procedure against the associated burdens (Table 2.4). At the end of life, surgery may offer palliative benefits to patients who will not survive long-term, or in whom resuscitation will not benefit. For example, a patient with obstructing esophageal cancer may benefit from a gastrostomy to permit feeding and improve the quality of life, but may not wish the surgical team to resuscitate him in the event a cardiac arrest occurred during or soon after the procedure.

In response to changing social values, the American Society of Anesthesiologists published statements in 1993 and 1994 advocating the reevaluation of a surgical patient's DNR order rather than its automatic revocation. These position statements encourage members of the surgical team to meet with patients before surgery and negotiate a resuscitation care plan in the event such care becomes necessary. When terminally ill patients were asked about how they wanted their DNR interpreted during the perioperative period, nearly all wanted to participate in a discussion about what would occur. The options available to the surgical team include (Table 2.5) (1) suspending the DNR for a prescribed period during the perioperative period; (2) initiate a procedure-directed order that permits or forbids specific interventions such as tracheal intubation, postoperative mechanical ventilation, chest compressions,

Table 2.5 Criteria for various do-not-resuscitate orders in the perioperative period

Options for modifying the do-not-resuscitate orders during the perioperative period
Full resuscitation—suspend the DNR during the perioperative period
Procedure-directed, limited resuscitation—determine in advance a mutually agreeable list of specific resuscitative interventions that can be used, if necessary, during the perioperative period
Goal-directed, limited resuscitation for temporary and reversible conditions—provide resuscitative measures for temporary and reversible events that may occur during the perioperative period
Goal-directed, limited resuscitation consistent with the patient's expressed goals and values—provide general resuscitative measures that promote the patient's goals and values

defibrillation or blood transfusion, the administration of vasoactive medications, or the insertion of invasive hemodynamic monitors; and (3) initiate a goal-directed order set that prioritizes outcomes rather than procedures. Goal-directed outcomes recognize that patients consider treatments in terms of their ability to affect outcomes. By consenting to expected outcomes, the surgical care team can exercise their clinical judgment to direct specific interventions to achieve the patient's goals. A goal-directed approach addresses the benefits the patient hopes to gain from the procedure against the burdens the patient is willing to endure and in the context of the probability for success.

Since the goal of medical therapy and surgical procedures is to provide benefits meaningful to the patient, it is important to discuss DNR orders in the context of the proposed surgery. Anesthesiologists recognize that up to 46% of patients may be unaware a DNR order exists in their medical record, even when they are competent. The approach to discussing how to modify a DNR order for the perioperative period will depend on the type of surgery, the patient's condition and personal values, and the beliefs held by the surgical care team. Discussions should include pertinent caregivers such as surgeons, intensivists, primary care practitioners, and nurses, and when finalized, the patient's right to autonomy is respected, and all members of the care team are able to abide by the agreement.

Anesthesiologists unable to abide by a patient's request or the request of their surrogate on medical or moral grounds should withdraw in a nonjudgmental manner and provide for an alternative anesthesiologist in a timely manner. If proposed modifications of the DNR conflict with "generally accepted standards of care, ethical practice, or institutional policies, then the anesthesiologist should voice such concerns and then present the situation to the ethics committee or other appropriate institutional body." Under circumstances where an alternative practitioner is unavailable within a time necessary to prevent further morbidity or to limit suffering, the conflicted practitioner should proceed with providing care with reasonable adherence to the patient's directives while being mindful of the patient's treatment goals and personal values. Doing so is in accordance with the American Medical Association's principles of medical ethics.

An exception to an anesthesiologist's obligation to clarify a patient's wishes regarding their care is an emergency situation requiring immediate intervention. In the absence of a clear instruction to limit treatment options, the surgical care team should reach a consensus as to the medical benefit or futility of different treatment alternatives and initiate care. In times of uncertainty, it is reasonable to err on the side of continuing care until a patient's preferences are known. Legally and ethically, physicians should consider withholding and withdrawing medically ineffective treatments as the same.

Medical Futility in Perioperative Period

Medical futility refers to interventions that no longer provide any significant benefit to the patient. In contrast to informed consent and advanced health care directives which emphasize a patient's right to choose from among medically acceptable treatment options, including the right to refuse further treatment, medical futility concerns itself with a physician's right and obligation to withhold care that is determined to be without therapeutic benefit.

Futility may be viewed as quantitative, where the likelihood of benefit to the patient is exceedingly small, or qualitative, where the quality of benefit from the intervention is exceedingly small. In both instances, futility considers the prospect of whether a particular medical intervention or treatment will serve the patient's interest. Concerns about medical futility arise, in part, from the conflict between the ability of the technological advances in medicine to permit physicians to keep critically ill patients alive longer and the reality that such treatment is often unable to cure or resolve the patient's underlying condition. Interventions that support blood pressure, provide respiration, provide nutrition, or treat infection may prolong life but may not succeed in restoring patients to a condition that permits them a meaningful and dignified existence and may prolong suffering.

Determinations of medical futility do not attempt to address the issue of rationing patient care because it does not include an analysis of cost or consider the allocation of available resources. The analysis of futility asks the question, "What is the likelihood that a specific intervention will benefit the patient," without contemplating "How much does this treatment cost" or "Who else might benefit from this treatment." Medical futility determinations are also unable to contemplate experimental interventions because an analysis of futility requires the evaluation of evidence to arrive at a conclusion that a proposed treatment provides no significant likelihood of conferring a reasonable benefit. Experimental treatments, by their nature, are considered experimental because the effects of the intervention are unknown.

Medical futility is an issue that is well-developed in the ethics of medicine and the medical profession instructs its physicians on how to proceed when such circumstances arise. The American Medical Association's Code of Medical Ethics provides specific guidance as to a physician's obligation in matters of futility. It instructs physicians that when "further intervention to prolong the life of a patient becomes futile, [they] have an obligation to shift the intent of care toward comfort and closure." It recognizes that the process of arriving at a determination of futility

Table 2.6 Declaration of futility

Six steps to determining medical futility
Make earnest attempts in advance to deliberate and negotiate prior understandings between patient or proxy and the physician on what constitutes futile care for the patient and what falls within acceptable limits for the physician, the family, and possibly, the institution
To the extent possible, the patient or proxy and the physician should agree that further care is futile
If disagreements arise about the futility of continuing care, parties should enlist the assistance of ethics committees or other consultants in an effort to reach an agreement about ongoing care
If the institutional review process supports the patient's position and the physician remains unpersuaded, then the physician should arrange for a timely transfer of care to another physician
If the review process supports the physician's position and the patient or proxy remains unpersuaded, then the family should be provided the assistance needed to transfer the patient to another institution
If the patient cannot be transferred, then the physician and the institution are not obligated to continue futile care, and the physician should notify the hospital risk management and/or legal department for further advice and/or instruction on how to proceed

requires making value judgments; that such decision-making should consider the "patient's or proxy's assessments of worthwhile outcome"; and, take "into account the physician's or other provider's perception of intent in treatment, which should not be to prolong the dying process without benefit to the patient or to others with legitimate interests." Determinations of futility must "also take into account community and institutional standards, which in turn may have used physiological or functional outcome measures." When disagreements arise between physician and the patient or proxy about whether care is futile, efforts to resolve the disagreement should occur using a process that affords the patient a form of due process (see Table 2.6).

In some circumstances, it may be medically appropriate to continue interventions deemed futile temporarily in order to assist a patient or his or her family to come to terms with the gravity of their situation or to provide time to reach a point of personal closure. For example, it may be appropriate to continue mechanical ventilation or renal dialysis in a terminally ill patient in order for family members to consult with members of the clergy or to allow a family member to arrive from another state so that they may visit the patient one last time. At all times it is important to reassure the patient or proxy that everything possible is being done to ensure the patient's comfort and dignity.

Although ethics and medical communities have achieved a clear consensus on how to proceed in matters relating to medical futility, the issue remains unexplored in law. Experience demonstrates that nearly all disagreements between patients or proxies and physicians are resolved successfully using the due process approach described above. In rare cases, physicians' attempts at withholding medical care have been challenged in the courts with unpredictable results.

Recent efforts by state legislators in Virginia and Maryland have attempted to balance the patients' right to make their own health care decisions weighed against a physician's obligation to forego futile care. In 1992, Virginia amended its Health Care Decisions Act to include the following provision, "Nothing in this article shall be construed to require a physician to prescribe or render medical treatment to a patient that the physician determines to be medically or ethically inappropriate." While the statute does not define what constitutes what is medically or ethically appropriate, it serves to acknowledge the concept of physician autonomy. A statute similar to Virginia's appears in Maryland's Health Care Decisions Act. Enacted in 1993, the act includes specific language that codifies a physician's right to decline treating patients when doing so would be contrary to his or her medical judgment. Section 5-611 provides: "Nothing in this subtitle may be construed to require a physician to prescribe or render medical treatment to a patient that the physician determines to be ethically inappropriate… or… medically ineffective." It provides further that a physician may withhold or withdraw medically ineffective treatment if the physician and a second physician certify in writing that the treatment is medically ineffective, and the patient or surrogate is informed of the decision. The Maryland law goes further than Virginia's law by providing a definition of medically ineffective treatment under the statute: "'Medically ineffective treatment' means that, to a reasonable degree of certainty, a medical procedure will not (1) prevent or reduce the deterioration of the health of an individual; or (2) prevent the impending death of an individual." It remains uncertain as to how state courts will interpret these laws if challenged and whether federal laws such as EMTALA will preempt states' efforts to address this important issue.

Until future court challenges define more clearly the legal limits of a physician's obligation to withhold futile care, physicians and hospitals should continue to work within existing ethical and professional guidelines to balance medical obligations with a patient's right of self-determination.

Key Points

- Ethical and legal principles are the same for elderly and young patients. However issues may arise more commonly in elderly patients due to the increased frequency of diminished mental capacity, acute and chronic illness and disability.
- Informed consent should include a discussion about the proposed procedure and reasonable anesthetic alternatives, for example, the benefits and drawbacks of general versus regional anesthesia.
- In the event of an emergent procedure the duty to obtain informed consent may be excused.
- If a patient has diminished capacity or is unable to provide an informed consent, the physician is obligated to obtain informed consent from the patient's legal health care agent, guardian, or surrogate decision-maker.
- Competency is a legal term that describes a patient's right to manage their own affairs and make decisions. In general a patient is deemed competent unless found incompetent in a court of law.

- An advanced directive allows patient agents to act on the patient's behalf at the time of incapacity; an early example is the living will.
- DNR orders should be discussed in the context of the proposed procedures; this should include discussion with all appropriate caregivers.
- Medical futility refers to interventions that no longer provide any significant benefit to the patient.

Suggested Reading

American Medical Association. Code of Medical Ethics Current Opinions with Annotations, Chicago: American Medical Association. http://www.ama-assn.org/ama/pub/physician-resources/medical-ethics.page and www.ASAhq.org.

American Society of Anesthesiologists: Perioperative DNR Orders to Limit Resuscitation. Syllabus on Ethics, American Society of Anesthesiologists. http://www.ama-assn.org/ama/pub/physician-resources/medical-ethics.page and http://www.ASAhq.org.

Annas GJ, Densberger, JE. Competence to refuse medical treatment: Autonomy versus Paternalism, 15 Toledo L. Rev. 1984; 561 at 568.

Appelbaum P, Grisso T. Assessing Patients' Capacities to Consent to Treatment. N Engl J Med. 1988; 319:1635–8.

Chow G, Czarny M, et al. CURVES: A Mnemonic for Determining Medical Decision-Making Capacity and Providing Emergency Treatment in the Acute Setting. CHEST. 2010; 137:421–427.

Gorman WF. Testamentary Capacity in Alzheimer's Disease. 4 Elder L. Rev. 1996; 225.

Grisso T, Applebaum PS. Assessing Competence to Consent to Treatment, A Guide for Physicians and Other Health Professionals. New York: Oxford University Press. 1998.

Hoehner P. Ethical Management of the Elderly Patient. Chapter 4. Geriatric Anesthesiology. 2nd Edition. 2008.

Kapp MB, Mossman D. Measuring Decisional Capacity: Cautions on the Construction of a "Capacitometer." 2 Psych. Pub. Pol. and L. 1996; 73.

Norman GV. Do-not-resuscitate Orders During Anesthesia and Urgent Procedures. Ethics in Medicine. Seattle Washington: University of Washington School of Medicine 1998.

Pollock, SG. Life and Death Decisions: Who Makes Them and by What Standards? 47 Rutgers L. Rev. 1989; 505.

Post LF, Blustein J, Dubler NN. 1999. The doctor-proxy relationship: An untapped resource Journal ofLaw, Medicine & Ethics 27(1):5–12. Prendergast TJ. 2001.

Simon J. Refusal of Care: The Physician-Patient Relationship and Decisionmaking Capacity. Ann Emerg Medicine. 2007; 50:456–461.

Shalowitz DI, Garrett-Mayer E, Wendler D. The Accuracy of Surrogate Decision Makers, Arch Intern Med. 2006; 166:493–497.

Relevant Statutes and Case Law

Patient Self-Determination Act, 42 USCA §1395cc(f), 1992.

Health Care Decisions Act; Section 5, Subtitle 6, Maryland Annotated Code; Health General

Faya v. Almaraz, 329 Md. 435; 620 A.2d 327 (1993).

Mohr v. Williams, 95 Minn. 261, 104 N.W. 12 (Minn. 1905).

McQuitty v. Spangler, et al., 410 Md. 1; 976 A.2d 1020 (2009).

Chapter 3
The Anesthetic Regimen for the Elderly Patient

Sheila Ryan Barnett

Why is Anesthetic Choice Important for Elderly Patients?

Older patients carry a higher risk of postoperative morbidity and mortality compared to younger counterparts. Although much of the increased risk cannot be influenced by the choice of the anesthetic alone, avoiding even minor complications may improve outcomes. A postoperative complication in an older patient can be devastating. A study examining data from the Veterans Administration demonstrated that the development of a postoperative complication was associated with a 25% increase in 30-day mortality in patients over the age of 80 years. Clearly the oldest old patients represent one of the most vulnerable patient groups during the surgical period, and meticulous attention to detail is required during the administration of the anesthetic.

Older patients presenting for surgery with complex medical histories and limited physiologic reserve may exhibit unpredictable responses to anesthetic and analgesic agents, even when undergoing elective or nonemergent surgery. In general, elderly frail patients with underlying chronic diseases are less tolerant of brief episodes of hemodynamic instability such as hypotension or desaturation that may not be preventable during the course of a surgery. While these events and other similar minor physiologic perturbations may be insignificant in the young patient, in the frail elder, they may lead to serious consequences, such as cardiac ischemia and arrhythmias.

As healthcare costs continue to rise, it will be increasingly important for all healthcare providers to function in an efficient and fiscally sound manner. Avoiding complications during anesthesia and the immediate postoperative period is one way

S.R. Barnett, MD (✉)
Harvard Medical School, Department of Anesthesia, Critical Care, and Pain Medicine,
Beth Israel Deaconess Medical Center, 330 Brookline Avenue, Boston, MA 02215, USA
e-mail: sbarnett@bidmc.harvard.edu

S.R. Barnett (ed.), *Manual of Geriatric Anesthesia*, DOI 10.1007/978-1-4614-3888-5_3,

anesthesiologists can contribute to a more viable health system. Preoperatively anesthesiologists can contribute by advising on preoperative testing guidelines and reducing the request for needless and repetitive preoperative laboratory tests.

Choosing the Anesthetic Regimen

The choice of anesthetic regimen is primarily dictated by the needs of the surgeon or the proceduralist. Several factors are important to consider, including the patient's medical and psychological condition, the type and duration of the procedure or surgery, and the requirements of the surgery itself. However even within one category of anesthesia—for example, a general anesthetic—there are multiple decisions made by the anesthesiologist that may influence a patient's response to the surgery. For example an elderly patient presenting with a perforated bowel for an exploratory laparotomy will require a general anesthesia with endotracheal intubation. In this example there are no viable alternatives for the anesthetic type. However there will be decisions to be made that require an understanding and appreciation of basic age-related physiologic changes. The choice of induction agent is important; etomidate is preferred over propofol, thus avoiding the exaggerated hypotension observed following a propofol bolus in an older patient. Blood pressure lability may be an issue, and the decision to proceed with invasive monitoring with an arterial line may be needed. Pain control in the setting of a large abdominal incision may be challenging, yet appropriate pain control in this instance may reduce the risk of a pulmonary complication.

General Considerations for the Elderly Patient

Mortality and risk of an adverse event associated with surgery increase with advanced age. This is due to multiple factors including age-related reductions in physiologic reserve, the increase in comorbid conditions, and the magnitude and type of the surgery itself. Complex emergency cases in the elderly carry the highest mortality, with a suggested threefold increase in mortality. The risk of cardiac complications in geriatric patients following emergency surgery increases 3–5 times, and the chance of postoperative intubation and ventilation is five times that of a young patient undergoing a major emergency surgery. The magnitude and size of surgery is very relevant: thoracotomy mortality in patients over 70 years has been reported as high as 17%, and emergency abdominal surgery in patients over the age 80 years carries a mortality rate of 10–25%.

As stated, the occurrence of any complications appears to be a major factor influencing outcomes in the elderly surgical patient. Several studies have shown a significant increase in 30-day mortality in patients who experienced complications following noncardiac surgery. In addition, patients experiencing a cardiac or noncardiac complication had a threefold increase in length of stay. Thus, avoiding complications—even minor ones—and conducting a careful review of the patients' physical and medical status prior to anesthesia must be a primary focus for all anesthesiologists taking care of older patients.

The increased morbidity experienced by older patients largely reflects the burden of disease encountered in this age group. Data from a study examining preoperative health status in elderly patients found that over 84% of 544 patients had at least one comorbid condition, 30% of patients had three or more preoperative health conditions, and 27% had two and 28% had one preexisting disease. Common conditions include hypertension, diabetes mellitus, cardiac dysrhythmias, pulmonary disease, neurologic disease, arthritis, and ischemic heart disease, including congestive failure. Despite a long list of diseases, functional status and clinical evidence of congestive heart failure are two of the most important predictors of an adverse postoperative event. Functional status is particularly important, yet in the oldest patients—over 80 years—74% have a disability and 35% of the group requires assistance with daily activities.

Atypical and Delayed Presentations

The presentation of common diseases in the older patient can be different, frequently the elderly present with more subtle symptoms; this can result in a missed or delayed diagnosis. This can lead to devastating consequences. A study comparing autopsy results to the immediate premortem diagnosis in elderly patients found a discrepancy in over one-third of autopsy cases. Significant missed diagnoses included unrecognized ruptured aortic aneurysm, the existence of a pulmonary embolus, and tracheal obstruction. In another group, myocardial infarction in older male patients was unrecognized in patients that presented with nonspecific symptoms including nausea, cough, fatigue, and syncope. Similarly, elderly patients sustaining a pulmonary embolus tend to present with vague symptoms. These atypical presentations may lead to an underestimation of a preoperative condition and potentially resulting in an intraoperative catastrophic event. The preoperative evaluation of the elderly patient should take into account the potential for an unusual presentation of a significant cardiac or pulmonary event.

The initial presentation of a surgical condition may also be different in the older patient. In over 50% of elderly patients undergoing surgery for appendicitis; the appendix had already ruptured. The delayed care in these cases means the older patient may require a more complex and extensive surgery and be hemodynamically compromised. This is in sharp contrast to the classic presentation of the 20-year-old college student with localizing abdominal pain who presents and is in the operating room undergoing a laparoscopic appendectomy just a few hours from the original symptoms. Similar late presentations have been described in patients with colon cancer undergoing colorectal surgery. The oldest patients tended to present later, have more comorbidities, and emergency surgery is more common. Not surprisingly, ultimate survival for these patients is lower. The constellation of presenting later with more advanced disease and complicated medical histories probably accounts in part for the increased mortality and morbidity in the elderly patient.

Anesthetic Choices

Aspiration

The geriatric patient is at increased risk of aspirating due to physiologic changes and common disease conditions. A reduction in pharyngeal sensitivity has been demonstrated and common comorbidities such as a previous cerebrovascular accident, swallowing disorders, and diseases such as Parkinson's disease lead to the increased possibility of aspiration. The development of aspiration pneumonia can be devastating in the in older patient with reduced functional reserve. Thus, regardless of the anesthetic regimen, protection of the airway is paramount, and sedation should be administered cautiously in elderly patients with an unprotected airway.

General Anesthesia

A general endotracheal anesthesia with paralysis allows maximal exposure for abdominal surgery and is necessary for abdominal and laparoscopic surgeries. When paralysis is not required, provided the patient is fasting and not significantly obese with a low risk of aspiration and the surgery site and positioning is appropriate, the laryngeal mask airway (LMA) has largely replaced the traditional mask anesthetic. For certain very brief surgeries, a mask anesthetic is still desirable. Advantages of intubation compared to the LMA include the ability to protect the airway from aspiration and possible reduction in the risk of development of intraoperative atelectasis through the use of positive pressure volume ventilation with or without additional positive end-expiratory pressure. Mucociliary dysfunction occurs after using an LMA or an endotracheal tube, but is worse following intubation.

The prevalence of dementia increases with age, and depending on the ability to cooperate, these patients may require a general anesthesia or deeper sedation than would normally be indicated by the procedure itself. Examples include a brain MRI during which a patient must lie still or a simple breast biopsy. The patient's safety must come first, and sometimes a general anesthetic may provide the least traumatizing experience for the patient, even for a simple procedure.

Regional Anesthesia

Regional anesthesia includes both neuraxial techniques such as spinal and epidural anesthesia and peripheral nerve blocks. Regional anesthesia may be administered as the primary anesthetic or as an adjuvant for pain relief during or after the surgery. When utilized to treat postoperative pain as well, epidural analgesia and peripheral nerve blocks improve pain relief and functional outcomes and have been shown to reduce hospital stay in selected patient groups. Advantages of a pure regional anesthesia include a reduction in the requirement for sedatives, preservation of spontaneous ventilation, the absence of airway instrumentation, and potential decrease in the incidence of postoperative thrombosis and blood loss following orthopedic surgery.

Monitored Anesthesia Care

Monitored anesthesia care (MAC) is the most common type of anesthesia administered. This can range from the administration of minimal anxiolysis to deep sedation. In older patients continuous supplemental oxygen is recommended in all cases. Physiologic changes with aging result in a lower arterial oxygen tension on room air, even before the administration of sedation. Patients undergoing a MAC frequently need to be at least partially cooperative and able to lie still without significant pain. For the older patient with agitation, dementia, uncontrollable tremors, chronic cough, or chronic pain, this can be difficult, and a lower threshold for recommending a general anesthesia may be needed.

Medications

Elderly patients are on average taking three medications, and patients should receive clear instructions on which medications should be held or continued on the day of surgery. As a general rule most medications should be continued until the morning of surgery, especially cardiac and antihypertensive medications. Angiotensin-converting-enzyme inhibitors (ACEIs) and angiotensin receptor blockers (ARBs) have been associated with profound and prolonged hypotension following the induction of anesthesia, and provided they are not being administered for congestive heart failure, these should be held prior to surgery. Similarly, diuretics can be continued in the presence of significant fluid overload; however, for the most part, thiazide diuretics can be held for patient convenience.

Special Consideration

Cardiac Adverse Events and Risk Reduction

In general, the risk of a cardiac event following a noncardiac surgery is 1–2%, and advanced age (over 65 years) is associated with an almost 2½-fold increase in risk of a significant event. In a prospective observational study of over 8,000 patients undergoing general, urological, and vascular surgery, Kheterpal et al. identified nine risk predictors for a cardiac adverse event. These predictors were age >65 years, BMI >30, emergent surgery, prior cardiac intervention or surgery, active congestive heart failure, cerebrovascular disease, hypertension, operative duration >3.8 h, and administration of packed red blood cells intraoperatively. They also found that high-risk patients experiencing hypotension or tachycardia were more likely to experience a cardiac adverse event.

Beta Blockers

Early data on perioperative beta-blocker use resulted in widespread perioperative administration of beta blockers to low- and moderate-risk as well as high-risk patients. Data from more recent randomized control trials including over 8,000 patients found a reduction in myocardial infarction, coronary revascularization, and atrial fibrillation within 30 days of surgery in the metoprolol vs. placebo group. However, they also found a significant increase in death, stroke, hypotension, and bradycardia. These data and others have resulted in a reevaluation of the beta-blockade recommendations. The most recent guidelines recommend (class 1 evidence) that beta blockers should be continued in patients who are currently receiving beta blockers during the perioperative period. There is class 2a evidence to suggest that beta blockers should be administered to patients with inducible ischemia on testing prior to high-risk vascular surgery. There is also some evidence to recommend beta blockers for high-risk patients, defined as more than one clinical risk factor, undergoing vascular or intermediate surgery, with careful titration of heart rate and blood pressure. In contrast to the earlier guidelines, beta blockers are not recommended in patients undergoing low-risk surgery. These recommendations are not specific to the elderly but clearly will impact a large percentage of vascular patients.

Statins

Statins have been shown to reduce lipid levels, decrease vascular inflammation, and stabilize atherosclerotic plaques. Several trials have demonstrated significant benefits in patients with coronary artery disease demonstrating a reduction in myocardial infarction, stroke, and death. Recommendations for perioperative statin use are based on observational data, and there are limited randomized trials. Current guidelines recommend that patients undergoing vascular surgery be started on statins in advance of surgery, preferably 30 days. Abrupt discontinuation of statins has been associated with increased risk of myocardial infarction and death, and continuing statin therapy in the perioperative period is recommended. Statins are not available intravenously. However, there are extended-release formulations (e.g., fluvastatin) available that may be used to bridge the NPO status over surgery.

The Intraoperative Course

Monitoring

Basic monitoring standards for all patients, including the elderly, undergoing anesthesia have been established by the American Society of Anesthesiology (ASA). The first standard requires the continuous presence of qualified anesthesia personnel in the operating room. The second standard requires a continuous assessment of the patient's oxygenation, ventilation, circulation, and temperature. Although these standards are not different for older patients, aging patients may have associated comorbid conditions that influence monitoring choices.

A fall in oxygenation may actually be a late indicator of hypoventilation, and ventilation should be monitored using end-tidal carbon dioxide to provide early identification of hypoventilation and possible hypercapnia. The decision to use additional invasive monitoring depends on the patient and the procedure. In the older patient, labile blood pressure is commonly encountered, and a low threshold for continuous arterial blood pressure monitoring should be maintained. An arterial line can assist in both the precise titration of medications as well as access for blood sampling during the case.

Aging cardiac changes render the older patient more susceptible to congestive heart failure in the event of excessive fluid administration or significant shifts in volume. Central monitoring of the central venous pressure or pulmonary artery catheter may be useful to manage the fluid administration during a case. Interpretation of the central pressure requires a careful consideration of the aging patient's underlying physiologic condition. For instance, an older hypertensive patient with a "normal" CVP may actually be modestly hypovolemic. In general, elderly patients benefit from higher preloads and are very dependent on the atrial contraction during diastole.

The Surgery

Laparoscopic surgery carries significant advantages in the elderly patient including a more rapid recovery, less pain following surgery, and reduced fluid requirements. Laparoscopic cholecystectomy has been associated with improved postoperative pulmonary function vs. open cholecystectomy, and that may be advantageous for the frail elder with reduced pulmonary reserve. General anesthesia with controlled ventilation is preferred to allow adequate abdominal insufflation. During the surgery, absorption of CO_2 can result in hypercapnia and acidosis. The rise in intra-abdominal pressure accompanying the insufflation can lead to reduced venous return and increased peripheral resistance and intrathoracic pressure leading to a diminished cardiac output and hypotension. In the frail elderly patient with reduced cardiac function, these cardiovascular challenges can be significant, requiring increased monitoring and adjustment of the anesthetic medications to optimize cardiac function.

Medications

Neuromuscular Blocking Agents and Risk Reduction

Muscle relaxation during surgery is critical for exposure and to prevent patient movement and is generally achieved through the administration of nondepolarizing drugs such as vecuronium and cisatracurium. These drugs are competitive antagonists of acetylcholine at the nicotinic receptor and act at the postjunctional membrane of the neuromuscular junction. The most important anesthetic concern for the elderly patients is the complete reversal of these agents at the end of the surgery. Results from a randomized controlled trial found that 26% of patients receiving pancuronium vs. 5% ($p<0.001$) receiving atracurium or vecuronium had residual block. In patients with residual blockade, patients that received pancuronium also had a higher rate of pulmonary complications 17% vs. 5% ($p<0.02$). Although this trial was not designed to address age risk factors per se, their conclusions are highly relevant to the elderly patient for several reasons. Advanced age is associated with a gradual decrease in chest wall compliance and decreased respiratory muscle strength, so any diminution in strength may lead to hypoventilation and postoperative pulmonary complications. In addition, older patients have blunted responses to hypoxia and hypercapnia; thus, respiratory drive is also impacted. In general, it is reasonable to conclude that the evidence supports that long-acting neuromuscular blockers such as pancuronium should be avoided in elderly patients.

Ambulatory Surgery

Older age is not a contraindication to ambulatory surgery. Indeed, some studies have suggested elderly patients may be more able to be fast tracked through the recovery area and discharged, possibly due to a reduction in medications and a lighter level of sedation administered compared to young healthy patients. In general, there is limited data on outcomes in older patients following surgery; however, there is the suggestion that intraoperative arrhythmias and hypertension are more common in older patients vs. younger and that the incidence of postoperative nausea may be diminished with age. Postoperative urinary retention can lead to significant morbidity, for instance, in older males following hernia repair. In general, urinary retention has been associated with the administration of opioids, regional anesthesia (spinal or epidural anesthetics), male sex, older age, and anticholinergic medications.

Positioning

The elderly patient may have particular characteristics that predispose them to accidental injury from seemingly benign positions. Predisposing features include bony prominences that are accentuated by the age-related loss of subcutaneous and intramuscular fat. Atrophy of elasticized tissues such as the skin makes the skin more likely to tear, and older patients tend to heal slower as well, so skin abrasions may be more significant. Demineralized long bones and osteoporosis result in fragile bones that are susceptible to fracture in the event of a relatively minor accident and/or fall. Vertebrobasilar insufficiency may predispose the vasculopathic patient to unexpected cerebral ischemia during positioning that involves neck extension. Cardiopulmonary compromise secondary to positioning, for example, in the prone position, may be less well tolerated in the elderly patient. Malnutrition is more common especially in the very old as evidenced by a high number of older patients presenting with reduced albumin levels. This contributes to poor wound healing, and in general a preoperative low albumin is associated with increased mortality.

Temperature Control

In general, exposure of a nonanesthetized patient to a cold environment such as the operating room will result in activation of receptors peripherally and centrally that lead to vasoconstriction and an increase in heat production and basal metabolic rate. Usually, the core temperature is maintained a few degrees higher than the peripheral tissues through tonic vasoconstriction. Unfortunately, normal aging results in the deterioration in thermoregulation both peripherally and centrally leading to an increased risk of hypothermia. The age-related physiologic changes blunt vasoconstriction and heat production; shivering is less effective and induced at lower temperatures compared to younger subjects. Furthermore, older patients have less lean body mass and lower basal metabolic rates at the outset, and they lose heat more quickly compared to younger patients.

The issues with temperature regulation are further exacerbated in the anesthetized elderly patient, and the ability to withstand cold temperatures is inhibited in the presence of all anesthetic agents. Disordered temperature regulation has been observed following both general and regional anesthetics. The risks of hypothermia to an older patient are substantial and include myocardial ischemia, surgical infection, coagulopathy, bleeding, delayed drug metabolism, and arousal.

Since older patients may not respond appropriately to a drop in core temperature, the anesthetic plan should include the ability to actively warm older patients in and outside of the operating room. Intraoperative heat loss may be minimized by prewarming surfaces and maintaining room temperatures high until the patient is fully draped. Warmed forced-air blankets have been associated with improved maintenance of temperature.

Quality Measures

Despite the growing popularity of quality measurements in healthcare, there are few recognized quality measures directed at the elderly surgical population. Standard quality assessment performance measures for surgery (myocardial infarction, surgical site infection, and deep venous thrombosis) are not specific to the elderly. Although older patients do have a higher incidence of cardiac complications, the same has not been shown for deep venous thrombosis and surgical site infection. It seems clear that the development of more relevant quality improvement methods and markers for elderly surgical patients are needed especially for postoperative pulmonary and urological complications. In contrast to quality measures, process measures assess multiple aspects of care such as interpersonal communication and diagnostic and treatment strategies. These more global markers may provide more valuable methods of assessing the quality of care in complex elderly patients. So far, 96 perioperative quality candidate indicators of care in eight domains for elderly surgical patients have been identified. The eight domains identified are comorbidity assessment, medication usage, patient's provider discussion, postoperative management, discharge planning, and ambulatory surgery. Within each domain, a number of quality indicators were identified. In many instances, these are quite specific to the elderly, for example, an assessment of an elderly patient's decision-making capacity and specific discussions about expected functional outcome. This approach provides an opportunity to investigate in more elder-specific issues. However, there are significant difficulties in implementing follow-up on such a vast number of both objective and subjective indicators. Despite these challenges, measuring quality of care is especially important given the excess morbidity and mortality in this growing population.

Guidelines for Treating Geriatric Patients

As stated, elderly patients can be challenging to take care of, as there is tremendous heterogeneity within this age group. However, a few common themes arise when taking care of older patients which can help guide the care of the elderly patient.

- Clinical presentation of disease is frequently atypical, leading to delays and errors in diagnosis. This may result in a later presentation to the operating room and more advanced disease condition and instability.
- Individuals over age 65 years have on average three or four medical diseases, often limiting function and increasing morbidity.
- Polypharmacy is a major issue in this population, and many older patients are on multiple medications that may impact the administration of anesthesia.
- Diminished organ reserve can be unpredictable, and even significant limitations may only become apparent during stressful events.
- The impact of extrinsic factors—smoking, environment, and socioeconomic—on physiologic age is difficult to quantify.
- Significant interindividual variability and heterogeneity exists in the aged population making responses difficult to predict based on age alone.
- A disproportionate increase in perioperative risk may occur without adequate preoperative optimization, and adverse events are more frequent when cases are done on an emergent basis.

- Meticulous attention to detail can help avoid minor complications—which in elderly patients can rapidly escalate into major adverse events.

Summary

In summary, "choosing the best anesthetic" for the geriatric patient requires meticulous attention to detail, knowledge of the physiologic changes that can be expected to occur during aging, and an understanding of common comorbidities found in the elderly population. The risk of anesthesia and surgery is increased in frail older patients, and anesthetics should be designed to avoid side effects and eliminate the occurrence of even small complications.

Key Points

- Elderly represent a heterogeneous group of patients.
- Functional capacity is one of the most important makers of outcome in the elderly patients.
- Atypical disease presentation can predispose to missed diagnoses and a more advanced stage of disease at the time of surgery.
- Aspiration risk is increased in older patients.
- Even minor complications can lead to increase in morbidity and mortality.
- Positioning in the older patient can be more complex.
- Risk reduction strategies, for example, through beta-blocker administration and avoidance of long-acting muscle relaxants, can improve outcomes select patients.
- Elderly patients are predisposed to developing hypothermia, and management should include active warming whenever possible.

Suggested Reading

Cook, DJ, Rooke GA. Priorities in Perioperative Geriatrics. Anesth Analg. 2003; 96:1823–1836.
Chung F, Mezei G, Tong D. Adverse events in ambulatory surgery. A comparison between elderly and younger patients. Can J Anesth. 1999; 46(4):309–21.
Gibb J, Cull W, Henderson W, et al. Preoperative serum albumin level as a predictor of operative mortality and morbidity. Arch Surg. 1999; 134:36–42.
Hasuke S, Mesic D, Dizdarevic E, Keser D, Hadziselimovic S, Bazardzanovic M. Pulmonary Function after laparoscopic and open cholecystectomy. Surg Endosc. 2002; 16:163–165.
Hosking MP, Warner MA, Lobdel CM, et al. Outcomes of surgery in patients 90 years of age and older. JAMA. 1989; 261:1909–1915.
Karayiannakis AJ, Makri GG, Mantzioka A, Karousos D, Karatzas G. Postoperative pulmonary function after laparoscopic and open cholecystectomy. Br J Anaesthesia. 1996; 77:448–452.

Kheterpal S, O'Reilly M, Englesbe, MJ, Rosenberg AL, Shamks AM, Zhang L, Rothman ED, Campbell DA, Tremper KK. Preoperative and intraoperative predictors of cardiac adverse events after general, vascular and urological surgery. Anesthesiology. 2009; 110-58–66.

Leung JM, Dzankic S. Relative importance of Preoperative Health Status Versus Intraoperative Factors in Predicting Postoperative Adverse outcomes in Surgical Patients. JAGS. 2001; 49: 1080–1085.

Manku K, Bacchetti P, Leung JM. Prognostic significance of postoperative in-hospital complications in elderly patients. I. Long-term survival. Anesth Analg. 2003; 96:583–589.

Marick PE, Kaplan D. Aspiration pneumonia and dysphagia in the elderly Chest. 2003; 124: 328–336.

Pedersen T, Eliasen K, Henriksen E. A prospective study of mortality associated with anaesthesia and surgery: risk indicators of mortality in hospital. Acta Anaesthesiol Scand. 1990; 34(3):176–182.

Phillip B, Pastor D, Bellows W, Leung JM The prevalence of preoperative diastolic filling abnormalities in geriatric surgical patients. Anesth Analg. 2003; 97:1214–1221.

Power LM, Thackray NM. Reduction of preoperative investigations with the introduction of an anesthetist led preoperative assessment clinic. Anaesth Intensive care. 1999; 27:481–488.

Reich DL, Hossain S, Krol M, et al. Predictors of hypotension after induction of general anesthesia Anesth Analg. 2005; 101:622–628.

Sessler DI. Perioperative thermoregulation, Geriatric Anesthesiology. 2nd Edition. Edited by Silverstein JH, Rooke GA, Reves JG, McLeskey, CH. New York: Springer; 2008: 107–122.

Turrentine FE, Wang H, Simpson VB, Jones RS. Surgical Risk factors, morbidity, and mortality in elderly patients. J Am Coll Surg. 2006; 203:865–877.

White PF, Kehlet H, Neal JM, Schricker T, Carr DB, et al. The role of the anesthesiologist in fast-track surgery: from multimodal analgesia to perioperative medical care. Anesth Analg. 2007; 104:1380–1396.

Chapter 4
The Perioperative Geriatric Consultation

Angela Georgia Catic

Introduction

With the recent aging of America and prediction that the number of individuals aged 65 years or older will skyrocket to 87 million by 2050, the number of geriatric patients undergoing surgical procedures will continue to increase over the next several decades. Currently, more than half of all surgeries occur in elders. The most common procedures in this population include percutaneous coronary intervention with stenting, coronary artery bypass graft surgery, and open reduction internal fixation for hip fractures. Preparation for surgery and the postoperative course are impacted by many conditions common in elders including dementia, frailty, poor nutrition, and inability to care for oneself. In addition, postoperative cognitive dysfunction (POCD) and delirium are more common among geriatric patients. Geriatric consultation can improve outcomes in elders undergoing surgical procedures through assessment of risk prior to surgery and management of complications during the postoperative period.

Geriatric Perioperative Consultation

Optimizing the care of complex patients through effective consultation has long been a topic of academic consideration. In 1983, Goldman and colleagues established guidelines for medical consultation entitled "Ten Commandments for

A.G. Catic, MD (✉)
Division of Gerontology, Department of Internal Medicine,
Beth Israel Deaconess Medical Center, Harvard Medical School,
110 Francis Street, Suite 1B, Boston, MA 02215, USA
e-mail: acatic@bidmc.harvard.edu

S.R. Barnett (ed.), *Manual of Geriatric Anesthesia*, DOI 10.1007/978-1-4614-3888-5_4,

Effective Consultations." These included the following: determine the question asked, establish the urgency of the consultation, gather primary data, communicate as briefly as appropriate, make specific recommendations, provide contingency plans, understand one's role in the process, offer educational information, communicate recommendations directly to the requesting physician, and provide appropriate follow-up. Although these tenants remain relevant, the relationship between geriatricians and consulting surgical subspecialists has shifted significantly since publication of the guidelines. The number of elderly, medically complex surgical patients has increased, and there has been a significant growth in available pharmacology, laboratory tests, and surgical technology. Surgeons are now spending an increased amount of time in the operating room secondary to financial and productivity demands. Salerno et al. surveyed surgical subspecialists regarding their consult preferences and found several differences compared to nonsurgical providers. Surgeons were more likely to prefer a comanagement relationship, to not want consultants to restrict themselves to a narrowly defined question, and to desire formal input as opposed to informal verbal input. In addition, 63% of surgeons wanted the consulting physician to write orders. Only 18% of surgeons valued literature references as part of the consult as compared to 41% of nonsurgeons. Based on these findings, Salerno and colleagues recommended the following modifications to the "Ten Commandments for Effective Consultations" when consultative services are requested by surgeons: focus less on defining a specific question and more on how the consultant can be of help, establish if a comanagement relationship is desired, clarify order-writing authority, and do not hesitate to offer multiple recommendations if salient to patient care.

In concordance with the consultative preferences of surgical subspecialists, comanagement or geriatrician-led consultative models are becoming increasingly common and resulting in improved patient outcomes. Among patients aged 60 years and older admitted to a community teaching hospital with a hip fracture, comanagement by a geriatrician and orthopedic surgeon resulted in improved outcomes. Although subjects were significantly older (84.7 versus 81.6 years), less likely to live in the community, had more comorbid conditions, and were more likely to have dementia (53.9% versus 21.5%) than controls, they had shorter times to surgery (24.1 versus 37.4 h), fewer postoperative infections (2.3% versus 19.8%), fewer overall complications (30.6% versus 46.3%), and shorter length of stay (4.6 versus 8.3 days). There was no difference in in-hospital mortality or 30-day readmission rate. Another geriatric consult model which has been evaluated is a geriatrician-led hip fracture service in which the orthopedic surgeon acts as the consulting physician. Compared to historical controls, improved outcomes were demonstrated in the 91 patients aged 55 years and older admitted to this service including a reduction in length of stay, time to surgery, and total costs. Including geriatric consultation as standard of care in high-acuity surgeries such as pancreatic resection has also been shown to mitigate complications and improve outcomes in elders.

Preoperative Assessment

Comprehensive preoperative assessment is crucial to accurately determining risk and optimizing outcomes among elders. Additional preoperative geriatric consultation including a review of medications, nutrition, functional status, frailty, cognition, and goals of care should be included for patients aged 65 years and older.

Medication Review

Although individuals aged 65 years and older account for 12% of the population, they consume 25% of prescription medications with 57% of elders taking >5 medications weekly and 19% taking >10 medications weekly. Evidence shows that the risk of adverse drug events during hospitalization increases with the number of medications a patient is taking. Compared to an individual on one medication, the risk of an adverse drug event is double in patients on four medications and 14-fold higher among those on seven medications. Adverse drug events are more common among elderly patients as compared to younger individuals (Table 4.1). Gurwitz and colleagues found an adverse drug event rate of 50.1 per 1,000 person-years among Medicare enrollees aged 65 years and older. Of the 38.0% considered to be serious, life threatening, or fatal, 42.2% was deemed preventable. The most common errors associated with preventable adverse drug events occurred during prescribing (58.4%) and monitoring (60.8%). The most common medications associated with preventable adverse drug events were cardiovascular medications, diuretics, nonopioid analgesics, hypoglycemics, and anticoagulants.

Physiologic changes related to aging can also affect the impact of medications in elders. The Crockroft–Gault equation is recommended to calculate the creatinine clearance and to avoid the risk of overdosing renally cleared medications in the face of seemingly normal BUN and creatinine values (Table 4.2).

Table 4.1 Risk factors for adverse drug events in elders

Polypharmacy
Age-related physiologic changes
Multiple comorbidities
Errors in medication reconciliation during transitions of care
Multiple providers
Drug–drug interactions

Table 4.2 Crockroft–Gault equation

Estimated Creatinine Clearance = [[140 – age (year)] × weight(kg)]/[72 × serum Cr(mg/dL)] (multiply by 0.85 for women)

Preoperative geriatric consultation is an ideal time to review medications. Anticholinergic medications should be discontinued if possible since they are associated with significant adverse effects during the perioperative period including delirium and gait instability. Common anticholinergic medications include diphenhydramine, promethazine, metoclopramide, and paroxetine. Benzodiazepine use is common with 16–23% of adults aged 65 years and older using these medications on a chronic basis. However, they can result in a variety of adverse events including confusion, gait instability, and withdrawal when patients are made NPO for surgery. If possible, tapering patients off of benzodiazepines prior to surgery is recommended. In general, it is recommended that patients continue on their cardiovascular medications including beta blockers and calcium channel blockers in the perioperative period. Holding diuretics for 24–48 h prior to surgery can be considered if they are not needed to treat excess volume associated with congestive heart failure. Oral hypoglycemics are usually held the night prior to surgery to prevent hypoglycemia, and insulin-dependent patients are typically administered half of their standing dose on the morning of surgery.

It is particularly important to review over-the-counter and herbal medications with patients during preoperative consultation. In a survey by Qato and colleagues, almost 50% of elders were taking alternative medications. As many herbs and supplements can alter the metabolism and impact of other medications, the American Society of Anesthesiologists has recommended that they be discontinued at least 2 weeks prior to surgery whenever possible. Ginkgo biloba and garlic are of particular concern due to possible increased bleeding risk.

Nutrition

The decrease in appetite and calorie consumption associated with aging coupled with medical and social issues such as depression, isolation, poor dentition, and alcohol abuse makes malnutrition a significant concern in the elderly. Estimates suggest that ~25% of patients aged 65 years and older meet the criteria for malnutrition. Preoperative geriatric consultation provides an opportunity to evaluate for and intervene upon malnutrition if present. Initial assessment of nutritional status should include evaluation of body mass index (BMI) and measurement of serum albumin or prealbumin. A BMI of $<18.5\ kg/m^2$ is indicative of low body weight and possible malnutrition. If there is a concern for malnutrition due to alcohol consumption, preoperative testing should include vitamin B_{12} and folate levels.

Despite consensus that nutritional status should be reviewed during preoperative geriatric consultation, there is mixed evidence regarding the impact of nutritional repletion in the perioperative period. Multiple studies have shown that although preoperative oral dietary supplements result in increased protein levels among elders, they do not improve outcomes including morbidity, measurements of nutritional status, duration of hospitalization, or activity level 6 months postdischarge. Smedley et al. did demonstrate improved outcomes among patients undergoing lower gastrointestinal tract surgery who received oral dietary supplements for 15 days preoperatively and 4 weeks following discharge including less postoperative weight loss and fewer minor complications. Beattie and colleagues demonstrated improved nutritional status, quality of life, and decreased morbidity among malnourished surgical patients who received nutritional supplements for 10 weeks postoperatively. Preoperative consultation provides an ideal opportunity to discuss postoperative nutritional supplementation with nutritionally at-risk elders.

Functional Status

Assessing physical functional status in preoperative geriatric consultation can identify elders at increased risk of postoperative complications who might benefit from targeted interventions or avoiding surgical procedures. Typical evaluation of physical functional assessment includes a timed up-and-go test of mobility and review of activities of daily living (ADLs) and independent activities of daily living (IADLs) (Table 4.3). Studies have shown that elders with impaired mobility and dependency in performing ADLs have increased postoperative complications including delirium. Aggressive physical therapy and discussion of rehabilitation options prior to surgical intervention are indicated in these patients.

Poor functional status has also been identified as a risk factor for postoperative surgical site infection due to methicillin-resistant *Staphylococcus aureus* (MRSA). Anderson and colleagues evaluated subjects with surgical site infections due to MRSA compared to matched uninfected surgical patients and patients with surgical site infections due to methicillin-susceptible *Staphylococcus aureus* (MMSA).

Table 4.3 Activities of daily living and instrumental activities of daily living

Activities of daily living
Toileting
Feeding
Dressing
Grooming
Bathing
Ambulation
Instrumental activities of daily living
Ability to use the telephone
Shopping
Food preparation
Housekeeping
Laundry
Transportation
Medication management
Finances

Following adjustment for age, the need for assistance with three or more (ADLs) was determined to be independently associated with development of surgical site MRSA infections. Since surgical site infection in elders is associated with a four times greater mortality, understanding the increased risk for MRSA surgical site infections in those with impaired functional status and implementing targeted preventative interventions are crucial to improving outcomes.

Frailty

The importance of identifying and managing frailty has long been recognized as vital to improving surgical outcomes among elders. Frailty is defined as a state of reduced physiologic reserve associated with increased susceptibility to disability. It is probably secondary to inflammation, chronic disease, and normal changes of aging that lead to a reduced ability of the system to successfully withstand additional stressors such as surgical intervention. In preoperative consultation, frailty can be assessed using a variety of methods. Robinson et al. evaluated for frailty in subjects aged 65 years and older undergoing major surgical procedures requiring a postoperative intensive care unit admission through the following preoperative assessments: Mini-Cog test (cognition), albumin, having fallen in the previous 6 months, hematocrit, Katz score (function), and the Charlson Index (comorbidities). Among the 110 subjects, 6-month mortality was 15%, and the incidence of postdischarge institutionalization was 26%. Cognitive dysfunction, low albumin, falling within the prior 6 months, lower hematocrit, functional dependence, and increased comorbidities were closely related to 6-month mortality and institutionalization. Lee and colleagues assessed the effects of frailty, defined as deficiencies in the Katz Index of ADLs, in ambulation, or with a prior diagnosis of dementia, in patients undergoing cardiac surgery. Patients who met the criteria for frailty were older (median age of 71 years compared to 66 years), more likely to be female, and had a greater comorbidity burden. Frailty was an independent predictor of in-hospital mortality, institutional discharge, and reduced midterm survival.

Cognition

Delirium, an acute disorder of attention and cognition, and POCD are common and costly in elders undergoing surgical procedures. Cognitive evaluation should be performed during preoperative geriatric consultation to delineate a cognitive baseline and detect any deficits. Possible evaluation tools include the Mini-Mental State Exam, Saint Louis University Mental Status (SLUMS) Examination, or the Mini-Cog test. If cognitive deficits are identified, patients and families should be counseled regarding the increased risk of delirium and POCD following surgery. Aggressive prevention measures including geriatric consultation should be implemented at the time of hospitalization to minimize cognitive dysfunction in these patients.

Goals of Care

Ninety-two percent of patients report wanting to discuss advanced directives with their physician but only 2–14% of elders have actually completed any documents. Advanced directives, legal documents which convey the type of medical care patients would wish to receive if they were unable to make medical decisions, include living wills, healthcare proxy/durable power of attorney documentation, and DNR/DNI paperwork. Preoperative geriatric consultation is an ideal opportunity to discuss goals of care including advanced directives. Grimaldo and colleagues randomized patients aged 65 years and older who were scheduled for elective surgery to receive a short information session regarding the importance of communicating about end-of-life care with their proxy versus receiving the standard preoperative anesthesia screening. 87% of patients had discussions with their proxies compared to 66% of the control group. In addition, 27% of intervention subjects completed durable power of attorney documentation as compared to 10% of controls.

Postoperative Assessment

Geriatric consultation during the postoperative period can be instrumental in preventing complications and improving outcomes in elders. Specific areas in which geriatric input is often sought during the postoperative period include delirium, POCD, pain management, and comprehensive discharge planning.

Delirium (See Chap. 20 in Addition)

Delirium is defined as a change in mental status characterized by inattention, altered level of consciousness, and a waxing and waning course. It is difficult to determine the exact prevalence, and an incidence of 3–73% has been reported following cardiac surgery. Ansaloni and colleagues recently evaluated the incidence of postoperative delirium in patients aged 65 years and older admitted for emergency and elective operations. 17.9% of subjects operated on emergently developed delirium compared to 6–7% of those undergoing elective procedures. Delirium is almost always multifactorial in origin resulting from baseline vulnerability and precipitating factors. Predisposing factors which increase baseline vulnerability include advanced age, cognitive impairment, impaired functional status, sensory impairment, medical illness, and exposure to certain medications. Precipitating factors for delirium include neurologic disease, surgery, illness, environmental insults, pain, and medication issues including polypharmacy and the use of precipitating medications. By identifying risk factors for delirium during the preoperative period and addressing these postoperatively, geriatric consultation can reduce the incidence of delirium and associated adverse outcomes.

Prediction

Numerous studies have evaluated risk factors predictive for the development of postoperative delirium in elderly patients. Kalisvaart and colleagues tested a validated prediction model for delirium which had been developed in hospitalized, elderly medical patients. This model allocates one point to each of four criteria assessed: severe illness, visual impairment, cognitive impairment, and elevated serum urea nitrogen to creatinine ratio. When the rule was evaluated in hip-surgery patients aged 70 years and older, it was determined that the incidence of postoperative delirium increased with the number of risk factors present as had been determined in the original study. Low-risk subjects (0 points) had an incidence of delirium of 3.8% compared to an incidence of 11.1% in the intermediate-risk group (1–2 points) and 37.4% in the high-risk group (3–4 points). In addition, age and emergency admission were determined to be independent risk factors for delirium with postoperative delirium being four times more likely in acute patients compared to those admitted for elective repair. Robinson et al. investigated risk factors for the development of delirium in 144 patients aged 50 years or older undergoing major abdominal, thoracic, or vascular operations. Several preoperative variables were associated with an increased risk of delirium including older age (42% incidence in subjects aged 60–69 years, 72% incidence in subjects aged 70–79 years, and 92% incidence in patients aged 80–89 years), hypoalbuminemia, impaired functional status, preexisting dementia, and preexisting comorbidities. Cognitive dysfunction, identified by the Mini-Cog test, was found to be the strongest predictor of postoperative delirium. Marcantonio and colleagues developed a delirium prediction rule for patients aged 50 years and older undergoing major noncardiac surgery. Delirium was associated with the following independent correlates: aged 70 years or older; alcohol abuse; cognitive impairment as determined by the Telephone Interview for Cognitive Status; severe physical functional impairment as determined by the American Society of Anesthesiologists physical status class; markedly abnormal Na, K, or glucose; noncardiac thoracic surgery; and aortic aneurysm surgery. Subjects with no risk factors had less than a 1% rate of postoperative delirium, while this increased to 45% in subjects with three or more risk factors.

Specific tools which have been assessed for their validity in predicting postoperative delirium can be included in preoperative geriatric consultation to identify high-risk patients prior to hospitalization. A score of >50 on the Informant Questionnaire on Cognitive Decline in the Elderly (IQCODE) during preoperative evaluation is significantly associated with postoperative delirium. The Delirium Elderly At-Risk (DEAR) instrument is a brief tool that can be used preoperatively to evaluate the following risk factors: age, decreased hearing or vision, functional impairment, cognitive impairment (assessed using the Mini-Mental State Exam), history of delirium, and substance use. Studies have found a score of 2 or higher on this tool to be associated with an eightfold increase in the incidence of postoperative delirium.

Outcomes

Development of postoperative delirium in the elderly is associated with significant morbidity and mortality. Postoperative delirium following cardiac surgery is associated with increased mortality (12.5 versus 4.5%), more frequent hospital readmission, cognitive dysfunction, and sleep disturbances. In addition, Rudolph and colleagues determined that elders with delirium status post cardiac surgery experienced statistically significant functional decline determined by their ability to perform IADLs at 1 month following adjustment for age, cognition, comorbidity, and baseline function. A trend toward association persisted at 12 months but did not reach statistical significance. Poor functional recovery at 1 month has also been documented in elders who experience postoperative delirium following a noncardiac procedure. Persistent delirium, continued evidence of delirium at the time of hospital discharge, is common affecting ~39% of elders at hospital discharge with 32–39% who remained delirious at 1 month and 18% at 3 months. In addition, it is associated with significantly increased mortality. Kiely and colleagues determined that 1-year mortality among subjects aged 65 years and older admitted from an acute hospitalization with delirium to long-term care was 39%. Independent of age, sex, comorbidity, functional status, and dementia, elders with persistent delirium were 2.9 times as likely to die within 1 year compared to subjects whose delirium resolved.

Prevention

Given the significant morbidity and mortality associated with delirium in elders, preventing delirium is a primary focus of postoperative geriatric consultation. Marantonio et al. evaluated the impact of proactive geriatric consultation in preventing delirium among patients aged 65 years or older admitted to the hospital for hip fracture repair. Subjects in the intervention group underwent geriatric consultation preoperatively or within 24 h postoperatively and then were visited by a geriatrician daily throughout the remainder of their hospitalization. Targeted recommendations were made based on a structured protocol addressing the following content areas: adequate central nervous system oxygen delivery; fluid/electrolyte balance; analgesic treatment; elimination of unnecessary medications; regulation of bowel/bladder function; adequate nutritional intake; early mobilization; prevention, early detection, and treatment of postoperative complications; appropriate environmental stimuli; and treatment of agitated delirium. A statistically significant reduction in delirium was demonstrated in the geriatric consultation group compared to the usual care cohort with 32% of intervention subjects developing delirium compared to 50% of controls. The impact on severe delirium was even more significant with a reduction in delirium of over one-half between the intervention and control groups. It is important to note that geriatric consultation did not result in a reduced length of stay. Interdisciplinary geriatric consultation for patients aged 65 years and older involving a geriatrician, rehabilitation specialist, and social worker has also been found to result in a significant reduction in the occurrence of delirium. However, there was no significant effect on length of hospitalization or long-term functional recovery.

Of note, several medications have been evaluated to determine if they can prevent postoperative delirium. Haloperidol 1.5 mg/day started preoperatively and continued for 3 days postoperatively in subjects aged 70 years and older admitted for elective hip surgery was not effective in preventing delirium. However, it did reduce the severity and duration (5.4 versus 11.8 days) of delirium. Studies to date have determined that the acetylcholinesterase inhibitors rivastigmine and donepezil do not result in a statistically significant reduction in postoperative delirium.

Postoperative Cognitive Dysfunction

POCD, characterized by memory loss and lack of concentration, has long been recognized as common among elderly surgical patients. Studies have determined that POCD affects 30–80% of patients 1 week following cardiac surgery and ~60% several months after surgery. Among patients undergoing major noncardiac surgery, the incidence of POCD in the first postoperative week was 23% among patients aged 60–69 years and 29% in patients aged 70 years or older. It continued to affect 14% of individuals aged 70 years and older 3 months following surgery. Although generally considered a reversible condition, POCD may persist for a year or longer impacting ~1% of elders who have undergone a noncardiac surgery and between 10% and 30% of those status postcoronary bypass surgery.

Prediction

POCD is most certainly multifactorial with multiple contributing factors including age, cardiac procedures, lower educational level, prior cerebral vascular accident, history of alcohol abuse, preexisting cognitive dysfunction, and preoperative symptoms of depression. The exact mechanism through which increasing age places patients at increased risk for POCD remains unclear. It has been suggested that progressive atherosclerosis increases the risk of embolization and resultant POCD in elders.

Several studies have investigated specific anesthetic and surgical issues as causes of POCD. It has consistently been determined that patients receiving general anesthesia have no higher risk for POCD than those treated with regional anesthesia. Rasmussen et al. studied the incidence of POCD in patients aged 60 years and older undergoing major noncardiac surgery. Using the intention to treat approach, there was no significant difference in the incidence of POCD among subjects receiving general versus regional anesthesia at 1 week. However, if a per protocol approach was used, POCD was found to be more common in subjects who underwent general anesthesia at 1 week, but this difference between groups had resolved by 3 months. It has been suggested that other surgical factors contribute to the development of POCD. In patients undergoing hip replacement, POCD is associated with fat emboli that reach the brain through a patent foramen ovale. Emboli have also been implicated as a causative factor in procedures during which cardiopulmonary bypass is employed. It has been determined that cardiopulmonary bypass itself or manipulation of the aortic root can result in microemboli causing multiple small defects in the brain. Tissue injury during surgical procedures results in an inflammatory response including release of cortisol, cytokines, and other inflammatory mediators, which is associated with the development of POCD.

Outcomes

The impact of POCD on patients and caregivers has traditionally been underestimated but can result in significant adverse outcomes. Steinmetz and colleagues followed 701 elders for a median of 8.5 years following noncardiac surgery. The presence of POCD at 3 months, but not at 1 week, was associated with increased mortality following adjustment for age, sex, and malignancy. The risk of leaving the labor market prematurely was higher among subjects with POCD at 1 week compared to controls. POCD has also been associated with decreased ability to perform ADLs, longer length of hospitalization, and increased admission to long-term care facilities.

Prevention

Primary prevention strategies, including geriatric consultation, are most effective in preventing POCD in elders. Gustafson and colleagues investigated the occurrence of POCD in elders with femoral neck fractures treated with the following interventions: pre- and postoperative geriatric consultation, oxygen therapy, early surgery, prevention of perioperative hypotension, and treatment of postoperative complications. POCD was less common in the treatment group affecting 47.6% of subjects compared to 61.3% of controls. When treatment subjects did develop POCD, it was less severe and shorter in duration. In addition, postoperative complications including decubital ulcers, severe falls, and urinary retention were less common in the treatment group.

Pain Management

Pain is a common issue among geriatric patients with those aged 65 years and older experiencing a twofold increase in painful conditions compared to younger individuals. However, postoperative pain has traditionally been underestimated and undertreated in elders since they anticipate less pain, are less willing to spontaneously express discomfort, and can be difficult to assess given cognitive dysfunction. Undertreated pain results in significant adverse outcomes: direct suffering, decreased physical function, decreased socialization, depression, sleep disturbances, delirium, polypharmacy, increased health costs, increased length of hospitalization, and increased postoperative morbidity. Through careful pain assessment and analgesic adjustment, geriatric consultation can help optimize outcomes in postoperative elders.

Assessment

Accurate pain assessment is the key first step to understanding and optimally treating pain in elders. Postoperative pain assessment should include evaluation for pain with movement or palpation of the affected area as many elders do not report discomfort that is not present at rest. In clinical practice, pain rating scales are an important part of pain assessment. It is essential to understand the value, extent, and limitations of various assessment tools and to recognize that a combination of tools may need to be used in elders to obtain a full assessment. Unidimensional pain assessment tools are most often utilized in the hospital to assess pain because they are useful for evaluating the effectiveness of interventions and can be completed in a short period of time. Commonly unidimensional tools include the visual analogue scale, numerical rating scale, verbal rating scale, and faces pain rating scale (Table 4.4).

Cognitive impairment can make accurate pain assessment difficult in many elderly patients. However, the patient is always the best source of information regarding their pain no matter their degree of cognitive dysfunction. Elders with mild cognitive impairment are usually able to utilize one of the standard unidimensional assessment tools. As cognitive impairment progresses, patients often do best with verbal descriptors of pain or visual scales. It may be necessary to present several different scales before the patient is able to understand the assessment instrument and accurately describe their pain. Among nonverbal elders with advanced dementia, proxy reports and observational scales are utilized to assess pain. Healthcare provider proxy reports tend to underestimate pain among elders with advanced dementia with physicians identifying pain in 43% of communicative patients but only in 17% of noncommunicative elders. Therefore, it is preferable to use one of the many observational assessment methods: The Observed Pain Behavior Scale, Discomfort Scale for Dementia of the Alzheimer's Type (DS-DAT), Checklist of Nonverbal Pain Indicators (CNPI), Pain Assessment for the Dementing Elderly

Table 4.4 Key features of unidimensional pain assessment tools

Visual analogue scale
Quick and easy to use
Requires intact visual acuity and motor abilities
Confusing to 20% of elders
Numerical rating scale
Quick and easy to use
Easily understood by elders
Can be administered verbally
Verbal rating scale
Dependent on patient interpretation and understanding of descriptive terms
May lack accuracy and sensitivity
Preferred by some elders who can more easily describe their pain in words than numbers
Faces pain rating scale
Designed for children but has been used successfully in elders
Appropriate for patients with learning difficulties
Useful in patients with hearing impairment or poor language skills

Table 4.5 The Pain Assessment in Advanced Dementia scale

	0	1	2	Score
Breathing independent of vocalization	Normal	Occasional labored breathing. Short period of hyperventilation	Noisy labored breathing. Long period of hyperventilation. Cheyne–Stokes respirations	
Negative vocalization	None	Occasional moan or groan. Low-level speech with a negative or disapproving quality	Repeated troubled calling out. Loud moaning or groaning. Crying	
Facial expression	Smiling or inexpressive	Sad. Frightened. Frown	Facial grimacing	
Body language	Relaxed	Tense. Distressed pacing. Fidgeting	Rigid. Fists clenched, knees pulled up. Pulling or pushing away. Striking out	
Consolability	No need to console	Distracted or reassured by voice or touch	Unable to console, distract, or reassure	

Adapted from Warden V, Hurley AC, Volicer L. Development and psychometric evaluation of the Pain Assessment in Advanced Dementia (PAINAD) scale. J Am Med Dir Assoc 2003;4(1):9–15

(PADE), and Pain Assessment in Advanced Dementia (PAINAD). The PAINAD scale is one of the most common clinically utilized observational scales as it is a brief, easy-to-administer tool that provides an overall pain score and is sufficiently sensitive to detect changes over time (Table 4.5).

Management

Multiple treatment modalities including nonpharmacologic, pharmacologic, and interventional should be considered in the management of postoperative pain. Postoperative geriatric consultation can be very helpful in developing an individualized pain management plan and preventing related complications in elders. For the purposes of this chapter, the focus will be on geriatric-specific pharmacologic pain management.

The first step of the World Health Organization (WHO) ladder utilizes nonopioid analgesics such as acetaminophen and nonsteroidal anti-inflammatory agents (NSAIDS). Among elders, scheduled acetaminophen is the first-line pain treatment, and dosages of 650–1,000 mg every 6 h are recommended unless contraindicated due to hepatic dysfunction. Several studies have demonstrated improved pain control when scheduled acetaminophen is used in conjunction with an as-needed opioid analgesic. In a systematic review evaluating the opioid-sparing effect of acetaminophen combined with patient-controlled analgesia (PCA) with morphine in postoperative patients, the addition of acetaminophen to the morphine PCA was associated with a morphine-sparing effect of 20%. In addition, studies have found decreased sedation and improved pain scores in postoperative elders who were treated with acetaminophen in addition to a morphine PCA. NSAIDS are relatively contraindicated given the two times increased risk of gastrointestinal bleeding in patients over age 65 and association with renal dysfunction. In addition, indomethacin is associated with delirium.

Opioids are the analgesics of choice for step two and three of the WHO analgesic ladder. The utility of "weak" opioids (i.e., codeine, tramadol) is hindered by a ceiling effect resulting in limited analgesia and dose-related adverse effects. Since scheduled acetaminophen is standard first-line pain treatment, combination medications consisting of an opioid and acetaminophen are best avoided in elders due to risk of acetaminophen toxicity. No particular opioid regimen is most efficacious in older patients, but the analgesic should be chosen on a case-by-case basis. In general, administration intervals should be extended and dosages reduced among geriatric patients due to delayed opioid clearance. The use of short-acting formulations is recommended for initial treatment until a stable dose is established. At that time, if the elder will be using the analgesic long term, the dosage requirement can be converted to a long-acting opioid for ease of administration. In some cases, such as demented elders who cannot request as-needed pain medications, it is reasonable to start with a very low dose of a scheduled opioid (i.e., oxycodone 2.5 mg every 4–6 h) to provide baseline pain relief and then utilize additional medication for breakthrough pain as needed.

Opioid Adverse Effects

Although opioid analgesics are often necessary for the optimal management of acute and chronic pain, side effects are not uncommon including respiratory depression, constipation, and delirium. Geriatric consultation can be useful in minimizing adverse effects and treating any that do occur. Constipation, a common side effect occurring in 15–41% of patients being treated for nonmalignant pain, is often dose related, and tolerance rarely develops. Nonpharmacologic treatment measures include increasing fluid intake, encouraging ambulation, and having the patient attempt to stool at the same time every day. A pharmacologic bowel regimen including a stool softener and stimulant laxative should be initiated whenever opioids are prescribed. If constipation continues, obstruction should be ruled out, and then an osmotic agent, lubricant, or cathartic laxative can be added to the bowel regimen. Bulking agents such as psyllium should be avoided postoperatively because without adequate fluid intake and ambulation, they can worsen constipation. Approximately 25% of elders treated with opioids develop nausea and vomiting. Of note, it is important to rule out severe constipation with fecal impaction as the cause of symptoms before treating with antiemetic medication.

Comprehensive Discharge Planning

Early, intensive discharge planning including input from geriatricians addressing mobility, nutrition, and pain management issues can enhance quality of life and reduce hospital costs. Preoperative geriatric consultation is an ideal time to begin discussing postdischarge plans including rehabilitation options. Geriatricians should then monitor patients during the postoperative period for any evidence of cognitive dysfunction, poor nutrition, undertreated pain, or other adverse outcomes which may impact final discharge plans. Nikolaus et al. investigated the impact of a comprehensive geriatric assessment coupled with a postdischarge home intervention in elders admitted to the hospital from home. Outcomes among the intervention group included reduced length of hospitalization, reduced immediate nursing home admission, delay in permanent nursing home admission, and reduced medical costs.

Conclusion

The multiple benefits of perioperative geriatric consultation have become evident over the last several years as an increasing number of frail, medically complex elders are undergoing surgical procedures. During the preoperative period, geriatric consultation can be crucial to determining risk and planning ahead to minimize postoperative adverse events through review of medications, nutrition, functional status, frailty, cognition, and goals of care. Postoperative geriatric consultants can assist in the prevention or management of delirium and POCD, optimal pain assessment and management, and comprehensive discharge planning. Through thoughtful collaboration, geriatricians and surgical subspecialists can optimize outcomes in the most vulnerable surgical patients today and in the future.

Key Points

- Research indicates that many surgical subspecialists prefer geriatric consultants to assume a comanagement role. Comanagement or geriatrician-led consultative models have resulted in improved patient outcomes including decreased postoperative complications, shorter length of stay, and decreased costs.
- A majority of elders take multiple medications placing them at increased risk for adverse drug events during hospitalization. Medication review and modification during preoperative geriatric consultation can help prevent postoperative adverse drug events including delirium and gait instability.
- Preoperative geriatric consultation is an ideal time to identify and address poor physical functional status which places elders at risk for postoperative delirium and MRSA wound infections.
- Advanced directive decisions including discussing goals of medical care, healthcare proxy/durable power of attorney, and code status should be addressed during preoperative geriatric consultation.
- Postoperative geriatric consultation has been shown to significantly reduce the incidence of delirium and should be implemented in elders identified as high risk for developing delirium during preoperative evaluation.
- Geriatric consultation is useful in optimizing pain assessment and management in all elders but particularly in those with cognitive impairment. In nonverbal patients with advanced dementia, pain should be assessed using an observational tool such at the PAINAD scale. Elders with advanced dementia may be unable to request as-needed pain medication, and scheduled analgesics should be considered.

Suggested Reading

Anderson DJ, Chen LF, Schmader KE, et al. Poor functional status as a risk factor for surgical site infection due to methicillin-resistant Staphylococcus aureus. Infect Control Hosp Epidemiol. 2008;29(9):832–9.

Barnett SR. Polypharmacy and perioperative medications in the elderly. Anesthesiol Clin. 2009;27(3):377–89, table of contents.

Friedman SM, Mendelson DA, Bingham KW, Kates SL. Impact of a comanaged Geriatric Fracture Center on short-term hip fracture outcomes. Arch Intern Med. 2009;169(18):1712–7.

Goldman L, Lee T, Rudd P. Ten commandments for effective consultations. Arch Intern Med. 1983;143(9):1753–5.

Gurwitz JH, Field TS, Harrold LR, et al. Incidence and preventability of adverse drug events among older persons in the ambulatory setting. Jama. 2003;289(9):1107–16.

Kalisvaart KJ, Vreeswijk R, de Jonghe JF, van der Ploeg T, van Gool WA, Eikelenboom P. Risk factors and prediction of postoperative delirium in elderly hip-surgery patients: implementation and validation of a medical risk factor model. J Am Geriatr Soc. 2006;54(5):817–22.

Kiely DK, Marcantonio ER, Inouye SK, et al. Persistent delirium predicts greater mortality. J Am Geriatr Soc. 2009;57(1):55–61.

Koster S, Hensens AG, van der Palen J. The long-term cognitive and functional outcomes of postoperative delirium after cardiac surgery. Ann Thorac Surg. 2009;87(5):1469–74.

Malani PN. Functional status assessment in the preoperative evaluation of older adults. Jama. 2009;302(14):1582–3.
Marcantonio ER, Flacker JM, Wright RJ, Resnick NM. Reducing delirium after hip fracture: a randomized trial. J Am Geriatr Soc. 2001;49(5):516–22.
Marcantonio ER, Goldman L, Mangione CM, et al. A clinical prediction rule for delirium after elective noncardiac surgery. Jama. 1994;271(2):134–9.
McCusker J, Cole M, Abrahamowicz M, Primeau F, Belzile E. Delirium predicts 12-month mortality. Arch Intern Med. 2002;162(4):457–63.
Miura LN, DiPiero AR, Homer LD. Effects of a geriatrician-led hip fracture program: improvements in clinical and economic outcomes. J Am Geriatr Soc. 2009;57(1):159–67.
Ramaiah R, Lam AM. Postoperative cognitive dysfunction in the elderly. Anesthesiol Clin. 2009;27(3):485–96, table of contents.
Rasmussen LS, Johnson T, Kuipers HM, et al. Does anaesthesia cause postoperative cognitive dysfunction? A randomised study of regional versus general anaesthesia in 438 elderly patients. Acta Anaesthesiol Scand. 2003;47(3):260–6.
Robinson TN, Eiseman B, Wallace JI, et al. Redefining geriatric preoperative assessment using frailty, disability and co-morbidity. Ann Surg. 2009;250(3):449–55.
Robinson TN, Raeburn CD, Tran ZV, Angles EM, Brenner LA, Moss M. Postoperative delirium in the elderly: risk factors and outcomes. Ann Surg. 2009;249(1):173–8.
Rudolph JL, Inouye SK, Jones RN, et al. Delirium: An Independent Predictor of Functional Decline After Cardiac Surgery. J Am Geriatr Soc. 2010;58(4):643–9.
Salerno SM, Hurst FP, Halvorson S, Mercado DL. Principles of effective consultation: an update for the 21st-century consultant. Arch Intern Med. 2007;167(3):271–5.
Sauer AM, Kalkman C, van Dijk D. Postoperative cognitive decline. J Anesth. 2009;23(2):256–9.
Steinmetz J, Christensen KB, Lund T, Lohse N, Rasmussen LS. Long-term consequences of postoperative cognitive dysfunction. Anesthesiology. 2009;110(3):548–55.
van Venrooij LM, van Leeuwen PA, de Vos R, Borgmeijer-Hoelen MM, de Mol BA. Preoperative protein and energy intake and postoperative complications in well-nourished, non-hospitalized elderly cardiac surgery patients. Clin Nutr. 2009;28(2):117–21.
Vidan M, Serra JA, Moreno C, Riquelme G, Ortiz J. Efficacy of a comprehensive geriatric intervention in older patients hospitalized for hip fracture: a randomized, controlled trial. J Am Geriatr Soc. 2005;53(9):1476–82.

Part II
Anesthesia Delivery

Chapter 5
Preoperative Assessment of the Elderly Patient

Ruma Bose and Sheila Ryan Barnett

Introduction

Aging is an inevitable process producing changes in the structure and function of tissues and organ systems. The term "elderly" is generally reserved for individuals 65 years and older; this definition includes a heterogenous group of people with a wide range of physical and mental abilities. In contrast, "age-related illnesses" are conditions that occur with increasing frequency in the aged individual but are not inevitable or proportional to chronological aging. One of the main preoperative issues encountered by anesthesiologists is distinguishing the impact of age vs. the effect of disease processes on organ function. The challenge includes performing an accurate estimate of the functional reserve of organ systems, providing a realistic risk assessment associated with the procedure and making appropriate recommendations regarding optimization of the patient's condition.

Anesthesia and Surgery-Related Morbidity and Mortality

Among the steadily increasing population of surgical patients aged 65 years and older, the fastest growing sector is individuals 85 years or older. It is estimated that 50% of all Americans over 65 years will undergo a surgery before death, thus a working knowledge of geriatric physiology is essential to all practicing anesthesiologists.

R. Bose, MD (✉)
Department of Anesthesiology, Beth Israel Deaconess Medical Center,
330 Brookline Avenue, Boston, MA 02215, USA
e-mail: rbose@bidmc.harvard.edu

S.R. Barnett, MD
Harvard Medical School, Department of Anesthesia, Critical Care, and Pain Medicine,
Beth Israel Deaconess Medical Center, 330 Brookline Avenue, Boston, MA 02215, USA

S.R. Barnett (ed.), *Manual of Geriatric Anesthesia*, DOI 10.1007/978-1-4614-3888-5_5,

Table 5.1 The goals of the preoperative assessment

Obtain a thorough history and physical examination
Provide a risk assessment
Recognize high-risk patients
Implement risk reduction strategies
Perform selected laboratory and cardiac testing
Improve control of perioperative diseases
Formulate and discuss the anesthetic plan
Obtain informed consent
Formulate a postoperative plan
Reduce anxiety through education

Major perioperative complications and in-hospital mortality are high in the elderly population. Age has been stated an independent risk factor for postoperative complications per the American Heart Association 2007 guidelines. The rate of perioperative morbidity increases progressively with each decade of life (4.3% of patients 59 years of age or younger, 5.7% in patients 60–69 years of age, 9.6% in patients 70–79 years of age, and 12.5% in patients 80 years of age or older). In-hospital mortality is also significantly higher in patients 80 years or older compared to those younger than 80 years (2.6 vs. 0.7%, respectively). Major and emergent surgeries carry the highest morbidity and mortality rates especially in the elderly; for example, emergency abdominal surgery results in a 9.7% mortality for patients over 80 years of age, and thoracotomy has a 17% mortality for those over 70 years.

Surgical interventions for abdominal disease carry a higher risk for complications and death in older compared to younger patients. The most common complications are hypotension and respiratory depression within the first day. The highest incidence of respiratory failure, pulmonary embolism, myocardial infarction and congestive heart failure (CHF) occur between 1 and 3 days. Pneumonia is more common between 4 and 7 days. Renal failure had a bimodal distribution with increased frequency in the early postoperative period between 1 and 3 days and later in the postoperative period between 8 and 30 days of surgery. One of the goals of the preoperative assessment is to identify high-risk individuals and suggest treatment strategies that may reduce morbidity and mortality (Table 5.1).

Risk Assessment in the Elderly

Assessment of perioperative risk includes an assessment of baseline physical status, functional reserve of organ systems, comorbid conditions, including their severity and optimization, and the surgery-specific risk. This composite risk profile should be shared with all the physicians involved in the care of the individual as well as the patient and relevant family members before proceeding with the surgery.

Table 5.2 ASA physical status classes

Class 1. A healthy patient (no physiologic, physical, or psychological abnormalities)
Class 2. A patient with a mild systemic disease without limitation of daily activities
Class 3. A patient with severe systemic disease that limits activity but is not incapacitating
Class 4. A patient with incapacitating systemic disease that is a constant threat to life
Class 5. A moribund patient not expected to survive 24 h with or without the operation
Class 6. A brain-dead patient whose organs are being removed for donor purposes

Add "E" to denote emergency surgery

The ASA physical status (ASA PS) classification is universally used to stratify patients preoperatively. The classification takes into consideration the preoperative systemic comorbid illnesses and their impact on daily function (Table 5.2). However the ASA PS has some significant limitations. It does not take into consideration the age of the patient or the underlying functional and physiological reserves and it does not include the inherent risk associated with the surgical procedure in the estimation of a risk profile. The ASA classification system does provide a useful way for healthcare providers from multiple disciplines to communicate about the severity of illness of an individual or group of patients.

POSSUM Scale

POSSUM stands for Physiological and Operative Severity Score for the enUmeration of Mortality and Morbidity. It is a risk assessment scale which is popular in the United Kingdom and takes into consideration the physiological impact of the surgical procedure. For example the scoring takes into account if the procedure is emergent vs. elective, the amount of anticipated blood loss and the projected length of the procedure. Age is included as an independent risk factor. Although the POSSUM scale has been reported to overestimate the risk of morbidity in a healthier cohort of patients, it appears to be an accurate and comprehensive risk assessment tool that can be valuable in sicker elderly patients. It is most commonly used as a comparative tool to assess outcomes—for individual surgeons or groups of providers. It is not commonly used by anesthesiologists preoperatively.

Organ-Specific Risk Assessment

Cardiovascular System

Cardiovascular complications represent the primary source of perioperative complications in elderly patients. Preexisting cardiac conditions such as coronary artery disease, hypertension, and abnormal left ventricular function put the patient

Table 5.3 Cardiac risk for noncardiac surgery

High risk >5%
• Emergency
• Aortic and major vascular
• Peripheral vascular
• Lengthy procedures with major blood loss or fluid shifts
Intermediate risk <5%
• Carotid endarterectomy
• Head and neck
• Intraperitoneal and intrathoracic
• Orthopedic
• Prostate
Low risk <1%
• Endoscopic surgeries
• Superficial procedures
• Cataract surgery
• Breast procedures

at risk for a postoperative cardiac event. Adverse outcomes may be minimized by identifying patients at risk and the implementation of risk reduction strategies.

The incidence of cardiovascular complications in the elderly is also higher in the elderly population by virtue of increased prevalence of coronary artery disease, hypertension and diabetes in this population. This risk is compounded by the various age-related changes that occur in the cardiovascular system which limit the patient's ability to compensate for the stress of illness and surgery.

The decision to send a patient for further cardiac evaluation is complex and includes consideration of patient comorbidities as well as the level of risk of the planned procedure. The American College of Cardiology and the American Heart Association have published guidelines for preoperative evaluation and risk assessment of patients undergoing noncardiac surgery. These guidelines formulate a composite risk of perioperative cardiac events based on the preoperative history of cardiovascular events and risk factors. Recommendations have been formulated based on the acuity of surgical procedure and severity of the disease process. The surgical procedures have been classified into major, intermediate and minor risk procedures based on the likelihood for postoperative morbidity and mortality associated with them (Table 5.3).

Major Risk Factors

Active cardiac conditions can increase the risk of major complications following noncardiac surgery. These include acute myocardial infarction, unstable angina, decompensated heart failure, significant arrhythmias, and severe valvular disease (Table 5.4). These risk factors may warrant cancelation of nonemergent or non-life saving surgery

Table 5.4 Active cardiac conditions as defined by ACC/AHA 2007 guidelines

Unstable coronary syndromes
Unstable or severe angina
May include stable angina in unusually sedentary patients
Recent MI (within 30 days)
Decompensated heart failure; worsening or new-onset heart failure
Significant arrhythmias
Mobitz II atrioventricular block
Third-degree atrioventricular block
Symptomatic ventricular arrhythmias
Supraventricular arrhythmias with uncontrolled ventricular rate
Symptomatic bradycardia
Severe valvular disease
Severe aortic stenosis (mean pressure gradient more than 40 mm Hg, aortic valve area less than 1.0 cm^2, or symptomatic)
Symptomatic mitral stenosis

due to the significant risk of a perioperative adverse cardiac event or even death. Further medical or surgical management of these conditions should occur before proceeding with surgery. However if the surgery is truly emergent, the risk benefit should be carefully weighed and discussed with the surgeon, patient and family.

Cardiac Risk Factors

The Revised Cardiac Risk Indices have replaced the intermediate risk factors of prior guidelines. These are ischemic heart disease, CHF, cerebrovascular disease, insulin-dependent diabetes mellitus, and a serum creatinine >2 mg/dl. The incidence of postoperative cardiac complications increase from 0.4 to 11% depending on the number of predictors (1, 2, or more than 3).

Minor Risk Factors

Minor predictors are recognized markers for cardiovascular disease that have not been proven to increase perioperative risk independently, for example, advanced age (>70 years), abnormal ECG (LV hypertrophy, left bundle-branch block, ST-T abnormalities), rhythm other than sinus, and uncontrolled systemic hypertension. The presence of multiple minor predictors might lead to a higher suspicion of CAD but is not incorporated into the recommendations for treatment.

The stepwise algorithm for preoperative assessment of a patient for noncardiac surgery is summarized in the flow chart.

Exercise Tolerance

Functional status has been shown to be reliable predictor for perioperative and long-term cardiac complications. For a patient without active or major cardiac conditions an assessment of the patient's functional status is a critical step in the testing algorithm. Functional capacity can be expressed as metabolic equivalents (METs). A MET describes the resting or basal oxygen consumption (VO_2); 1 MET is the equivalent of an expenditure of 3.5 mL/kg/min. The MET of common activities and exercise is shown in Table 5.5. According to these guidelines, if the patient's functional status is good (>4 METS), even higher-risk procedures may be undertaken without further cardiac noninvasive testing.

When it is not possible to establish the functional capacity of a patient with significant clinical risk factors for coronary artery disease and those who are undergoing high-risk surgery, noninvasive cardiac testing may be required. The rationale for further evaluation should also be determined by the impact of the test results on plan of care for that particular surgery. For example what if anything would be done differently based on the test results.

Physiological capacity (PC) is an assessment tool that may provide an accurate assessment of the functional reserve. PC defines an individual's metabolic response, measured by gas exchange, during cardiopulmonary exercise testing (CPET). Gas exchange measurements reflect the efficiency of oxygen utilization and the integrated efficiency of the oxygen transport system. A CPET is an individual, noninvasive, evaluator-independent, controlled metabolic stress test. The results obtained

Table 5.5 Functional assessment scale

1 MET	Can you take care of yourself?
↓	Eat, dress, use the toilet?
	Walk indoors around the house?
	Walk 1–2 blocks on level ground at 2–3 mph?
	Do light housework?
4 METS	Climb a flight of stairs? Carry groceries?
↓	Walk on level ground at 4 mph?
	Run a short distance
	Do heavy housework?
	Do moderate sports—golf, dance, doubles tennis?
10 METS	Play competitive sports? Singles tennis? Ski?

from CPET may define the degree of physiological reserve that determines an individual's ability to adjust to perioperative stress. However this is not routinely performed in the preoperative setting.

Pulmonary System

Pulmonary reserve decreases with age, and it can often be difficult to separate age-related changes from those secondary to disease and environmental factors. The influences of prior smoking and environmental exposures are particularly difficult to distinguish from senescence.

The major changes that occur with aging can be broadly attributed to the following factors: blunting of the central nervous system reflexes, a decrease in the compliance of the thoracic wall, a decrease in alveolar gas exchange surface, and a generalized deconditioning of chest wall musculature. Functionally this translates into increased work of breathing and an increased predisposition to hypoxemia. Overall there is a decrease in the maximal breathing capacity.

A history of COPD and smoking and limited functional capacity secondary to dyspnea predict postoperative pulmonary complications. A detailed history of the patient's functional capacity and 6-min walk test may be helpful to establish a baseline pulmonary function. Smokers should be counseled on cessation of smoking at least 6 weeks prior to surgery, and preoperative breathing exercises should be recommended.

A chest X-ray, lung function tests, and/or arterial blood gases may be recommended in patients who have a significant history of COPD and active symptoms of respiratory disease.

Airway history should be attained during the preoperative evaluation. A prior intubation or course in the intensive care unit may result in residual damage such as tracheal stenosis. A history of a difficult intubation should prompt an attempt to obtain prior medical records.

Nervous System

Neurological conditions such as Parkinson's disease, cerebrovascular disease, and early and advanced dementia may all impact anesthetic administration and are more common in the elderly population. The preoperative evaluation is an opportunity to carefully assess and document the diagnosis, medications currently prescribed, and status of current symptomatology. Dementia is becoming increasingly common in the elderly population; in these patients, it is vital to involve the family or caretakers early for consent and appropriate perioperative planning. A mini mental state examination may help to delineate baseline cognitive disabilities which would predict postoperative complications. Postoperative delirium and confusion are more common in patients with preexisting neurological conditions.

Renal Function

As many as 30% of elderly patients have renal impairment prior to surgery, predisposing them to acute tubular necrosis after major surgery and trauma. Acute renal failure accounts for a fifth of postoperative deaths in the elderly. Chronic renal failure is a complex systemic disease that may result from many conditions common in the aging population; diabetes mellitus, hypertension, and glomerulonephritis are among the most common causes. Volume status and electrolyte balance are important issues in dialysis patients. The preoperative assessment should include a description of the frequency, the mode of administration of dialysis, and the timing of dialysis perioperatively. Generally dialysis should be performed the day before a surgery, and a potassium level may be required on the day of surgery. Volume control is a critical issue in dialysis patients, and in the elderly patient with potential autonomic dysfunction blood pressure, liability is a frequent problem. Older patients without overt renal failure may need a preoperative assessment of renal function before major surgery. Blood urea nitrogen and creatinine can establish baseline renal function, although the serum creatinine can be misleading in the elderly patient and underestimate renal insufficiency. More recently many laboratories will report out a calculated GFR based on the patient's age and laboratories; this can enhance detection of chronic renal insufficiency.

Anesthetic History

As electronic anesthetic records become increasingly popular, it is easier to locate and compare previous anesthetic charts. The anesthetic history is a key element of the preoperative assessment. For an elderly patient, a few features should be emphasized, such as the cardiovascular response to the anesthetic induction and maintenance, the need for pressors during a case, the volume tolerated, and the overall ability of the blood pressure. It is also important to obtain information from the patient and their family—for example, was the patient excessively groggy or sleepy afterwards, or were they confused or less independent? This type of assessment can lead to positive recommendations regarding blood pressure expectations, pain control, and medication dosing.

Medications

Polypharmacy is a major issue in the elderly population. All patients should be instructed to provide a detailed list of medications—including both prescription and over-the-counter medication. In general, most medications should be continued until the night before surgery; in the morning of surgery, patients may be advised to hold diuretic medication and nonessential medications and supplements. Angiotensin-converting enzyme inhibitors can result in significant post-induction vasodilatation and hypotension, and holding these medications the day of surgery is recommended.

Laboratory Evaluation

Although older patients frequently have multiple comorbid illnesses, preoperative laboratory testing should be directed by the type of surgery planned and the patient's current medical status. Routine screening can lead to excessive cost as well as potential morbidity for further investigation of false positive results.

Hemoglobin or Hematocrit. A hemoglobin or hematocrit is commonly indicated in older patients with multiple comorbidities and poor nutrition undergoing surgery associated with significant blood loss. Even in patients undergoing moderate-risk surgery, a baseline hemoglobin may be valuable in a patient with a complex systemic disease and ongoing anemia. Elevated hemoglobin in a very old patient is unusual and may indicate hemoconcentration from dehydration or an underlying hematological disorder.

Coagulation Studies. Patients on anticoagulants such as warfarin should have coagulation studies drawn and/or generally repeated in the morning of the surgery if warfarin has been discontinued, so that normal coagulation parameters can be documented. Other indications include significant liver disease or known coagulopathic conditions.

Electrolytes and Blood Chemistry. Elderly ambulatory patients with mild to moderate systemic disease such as hypertension do not need routine electrolytes. Patients with chronic renal failure should have electrolytes, BUN, and creatinine drawn prior to any significant surgery. Renal dialysis patients should have potassium drawn immediately prior to surgery. Renal insufficiency is common in older patients, and baseline electrolytes are indicated if a surgery with fluid requirements or blood loss is planned. Albumin has been shown to be a predictor of poor outcome in older patients, but even if low, it is unlikely to lead to a change in perioperative management.

Electrocardiograms. An ECG should be done in patients with cardiac risk factors and a history of cardiac disease undergoing intermediate or major surgery. Occult cardiac disease is extremely common in older patients; however, many institutions are moving away from using age-based criteria for EKG screening in healthy elderly undergoing surgery. A prior ECG within 3–6 months of the surgery in the absence of ongoing symptoms or changes in cardiac status is generally acceptable.

Chest Radiographs. These should only be ordered preoperatively if the medical history or examination suggests an underlying disorder such as pneumonia or pleural effusions. Several studies have demonstrated that widespread routine chest X-rays can often lead to significant morbidity but rarely discover unexpected findings resulting in a change in management.

Type and Screen. These should be drawn prior to surgeries with the potential for significant blood loss. The presence of antibodies may make it difficult and time consuming to find compatible products.

As with all preoperative testing, requests for laboratory studies or further investigations should be directed by the history and a physical examination that includes a functional assessment. Further testing beyond the history and physical will be determined by the risk associated with the surgical procedure and the baseline comorbidities of the patient. For instance, a patient with significant cardiac morbidity coming in for a low-risk cataract surgery may not need further cardiac evaluation, whereas a patient with lesser cardiac risk factors coming in for high-risk surgery will need a comprehensive cardiac evaluation.

Special Considerations in the Elderly

The preoperative evaluation in patients with complicated medical histories can be very difficult in patients with baseline dementia and memory loss, and every effort should be made to obtain prior medical records and contact the primary care physician taking care of the patient. Preoperative depression and alcohol abuse are relatively common and not always admitted by the patient or family, but will increase the risk of delirium in the postoperative period.

In addition to a high incidence of comorbidities, the overall health status of the aged patient may also significantly influence the choice of anesthetic technique. For instance, chronic pain, agitation, and dementia may prohibit the patient from lying still during the procedure, making a plan for deep sedation unfeasible even though the procedure may be minor, for example, a cataract extraction.

The preoperative visit helps to identify medical or socioeconomic conditions which could cause a delay or cancelation of the procedure on the day of surgery. The early identification of patients requiring further investigations or those with social issues may help with advance planning and room scheduling. For instance, a patient with minimal social and family support would be admitted postoperatively after a minor procedure.

During the course of the preoperative evaluation, it may become obvious that patient may not be able to provide informed consent for the procedure due to a variety of reasons. In that case a health care proxy who is determined by the patient may have to be contacted.

Outside Facilities

The preoperative assessment of institutionalized patients can be especially challenging. It may be difficult or impractical to require these patients to come to a hospital or facility for a preoperative visit. In these instances a remote preoperative screen can be conducted. If possible the facility physician should provide a brief history and physical assessment and the results of any laboratory testing done recently. These can be reviewed by the anesthesiology team who may decide if more testing is indicated. The preoperative examination can be completed the day of the surgery. Arrangements for consent from a legal guardian or family member should be made in advance to prevent delays on the day of surgery.

Conclusion

The geriatric population is a group of people above the age of 65 years with a wide range of physical capabilities and organ reserves. The effect of age-related illness on organ systems can be difficult to distinguish from the disease process itself which poses a challenge in the perioperative setting. The preoperative visit is crucial in this population to establish the baseline health status of the individual, determine the level of optimization of the comorbidities, provide a realistic risk assessment for the procedure, and, with this information, formulate a plan of care that would provide optimum and efficient care to the elderly and minimize the risk of morbidity and mortality.

Key Points

- Individuals over the age of 65 years have on average three or four medical diseases, often limiting function and increasing morbidity.
- Polypharmacy is a major issue in this population; patients should be instructed to bring in an accurate list of medications preoperatively.
- Risk assessment should be performed and must take into account patient factors and procedure risk.
- Functional capacity is an important factor in the preoperative assessment.
- A disproportionate increase in perioperative risk may occur without adequate preoperative optimization, and adverse events are more frequent when cases are done on an emergent basis.
- Preoperative laboratory testing should be performed only when indicated by the patient's history, physical examination, and the procedure planned.

References

American Society of Anesthesiologists Task Force on Preanesthesia Evaluation. Practice advisory for preanesthesia evaluation: a report by the American Society of Anesthesiologists Task Force on Preanesthesia Evaluation. Anesthesiology. 2002; 96:485.

American College of Cardiology/American Heart Association Task Force on Practice Guidelines (Writing Committee to Revise the 2002 Guidelines on Perioperative Cardiovascular Evaluation for Noncardiac Surgery); Executive summary of the ACC/AHA task force report: Guidelines for Perioperative Cardiovascular Evaluation for noncardiac surgery. Anesth Analg. 1996; 82:854–860.

Fischer SP. Development and effectiveness of an anesthesia preoperative evaluation clinic in a teaching hospital. Anesthesiology. 1996; 85:196–206.

Fleisher LA, et al. ACC/AHA 2007 Guidelines on Perioperative Cardiovascular Evaluation and Care for Noncardiac Surgery: Executive Summary: A Report of the American College of Cardiology/American Heart Association Task Force on Practice Guidelines. Circulation. 2007; 116(17):1971–1996.

Hightower CE, et al. A pilot study evaluating predictors of postoperative outcomes after major abdominal surgery: physiological capacity compared with the ASA physical status classification system. Br J Anaesth. 2010 April; 104(4): 465–471.

Joehl RJ. Preoperative evaluation: pulmonary, cardiac, renal dysfunction and comorbidities. Surg Clin North Am. 2005; 85(6):1061–1073.

Lawrence VA, Cornell JE, Smetana GW. Strategies to reduce postoperative pulmonary complications after noncardiothoracic surgery: systematic review for the American College of Physicians. Ann Intern Med. 2006; 144(8):596–608.

Liu LL, et al. Predicting adverse post operative outcomes in patients aged 80 years or older. J of Am Geriatric Soc. 2000; 48:405–1.

Liu LL, Dzankic S, Leung JM. Preoperative electrocardiogram abnormalities do not predict postoperative cardiac complications in geriatric surgical patients. J Am Geriatr Soc. 2002; 50:1186.

Narr BJ. Outcomes of patients with no laboratory assessment before anesthesia and a surgical procedure. Mayo Clin Proc. 1997; 72:505–509.

Noordzij PG, Boersma E, et al. Prognostic value of routine preoperative electrocardiography in patients undergoing noncardiac surgery. Am J Cardiol. 2006; 97(7):1103–1106.

Poldermans D, et al. The effect of bisoprolol on perioperative mortality and myocardial infarction in high risk patients undergoing vascular surgery. N Engl J Med. 1999; 341:1789–1794.

Polanczyk CA, Marcantonio E, Goldman E, et al. Impact of age on perioperative complications and length of stay in patients undergoing noncardiac surgery. Ann Intern Med. 2001; 134:637–643.

Schein Oliver D, et al The value of routine preoperative medical testing before cataract surgery. N Engl J Med. 2000; 342:168–175.

Silverstein JH, Central nervous system dysfunction after noncardiac surgery and anesthesia in the elderly. Anesthesiology. 2007; 106:622–628.

Thompson JS, Baxter BT, Allison JG, Johnson FE, Lee KK, Park WY. Temporal Patterns of Postoperative Complications Arch Surg. 2003; 138:596–603.

Chapter 6
Analgesics and Sedatives

Julia I. Metzner and G. Alec Rooke

Introduction

Of primary importance for the clinical anesthesiologist is the realization that the older adult is often not an ordinary, straightforward patient. Aging affects the pharmacokinetics and pharmacodynamics of the most commonly used anesthetic drugs, and opioids and benzodiazepines do not represent an exception to this rule. This chapter will portray the unique features and pharmacological differences of sedative/analgesic drugs in the elderly along with evidence-based practical strategies to reduce side effects and improve patient safety.

Opioid Analgesics

Acute pain, one of the most frustrating symptoms experienced by surgical patients, has historically been poorly evaluated and frequently undertreated. In the twenty-first century the concept of anesthesia is inextricably intertwined with those of pain control or analgesia. Analgesics, by themselves or combined with sedative/anxiolytics, provide a more comfortable patient experience, reduce induction and intraoperative anesthetic requirements, and generally improve patient satisfaction.

Managing pain in older patients requires consideration of a multiplicity of age-related factors that affect the safety and efficacy of treatment.

J.I. Metzner, MD (✉) • G.A. Rooke, MD, PhD
Department of Anesthesiology and Pain Medicine, University of Washington Medical Center, 1959 NE Pacific Street, P.O. Box 356540, Seattle, WA 98195-6540, USA
e-mail: metznj@uw.edu; rooke@uw.edu

S.R. Barnett (ed.), *Manual of Geriatric Anesthesia*, DOI 10.1007/978-1-4614-3888-5_6,

General Considerations

Snyder and colleagues in the United States and Terenius and colleagues in Sweden simultaneously established the existence of specific opioid receptors in 1973. Afterward, specific opioid receptors were identified and classified in three major classes: μ, δ, and κ. Sophisticated pharmacologic and recently genetic studies on knockout mice confirmed that activation of all these receptors will result in analgesia. However, in the clinical practice, morphine-like drugs gained use, which are mostly selective for μ-receptors.

μ-receptors are further divided into μ_1, μ_2, and μ_3 subtypes. The μ_1-receptors found in the periaqueductal gray matter, the nucleus raphe magnus, and the locus caeruleus are postulated to have supraspinal analgesic properties. The μ_1-receptors are responsible for almost all opioid analgesic properties and, to some extent, their side effects. The μ_2-receptors, characterized by a lower affinity for opioids than μ_1, are responsible for the untoward side effects of opioids, including respiratory depression, delayed GI motility (nausea, vomiting, and constipation), urinary retention, bradycardia, miosis, euphoria, and physical dependence. The μ_3-receptor, located in the vascular endothelium, releases nitric oxide and might be partially implicated in the vasodilatatory effect of opioids.

At the cellular level, the interaction between opioid and receptor is extremely complex and only partially understood. All opioid receptors are G-protein coupled, which coordinates the function of second messengers, including adenylate cyclase, phospholipase C, and various ion channels. Activation of opioid receptors decreases Ca^{2+} ion entry into the cell and inhibits presynaptic neurotransmitter release, including substance P and calcitonin gene-related peptide in the dorsal horn of the spinal cord. Enhancement of K^+ efflux resulting in the hyperpolarization of postsynaptic neurons and inhibition of [gamma]-aminobutyric acid (GABA)-ergic transmission in the brain stem also contribute to the activation of a descending circuit with an inhibitory function on pain transmission.

Data from pain threshold studies showed a decreased tolerance to long-standing and intense pain, opposite to an increased pain threshold to mild and short-duration stimulus. Similar studies demonstrated both peripheral and central sensitization, mechanisms that may contribute considerably to increased pain responses and hyperalgesia following tissue damage.

However, it is not clear if the observed changes are caused by the aging itself or are correlated with the higher prevalence of comorbid diseases seen in this age group. Advancing age is associated with a progressive decrease in the density of myelinated and unmyelinated fibers and a slowing in peripheral nerve conduction velocity. These changes may contribute to age-related differences in the perception of pain. There is also a reduction in the content and turnover of neurotransmitter systems, particularly affecting the glutamate, serotonin, and GABA receptors, known to be important mediators of nociception.

In addition, functional neuroimaging (fMRI) studies have shown that with aging, there is a progressive decrease in the volume of brain regions responsible for pain processing. This finding mirrors the decreased number of opioid receptors found in the brains of aged rats.

Therefore, the experimental data appears to suggest that although aging is associated with important changes in nociception and pain perception, aging does not appear to be associated with a substantive functional change over the pain stimulus–response curve. In short, the elderly feel and react to pain and are particularly vulnerable to the negative impact of untreated pain.

Pharmacokinetic Properties and Pharmacodynamic Effects of Specific Opioids

The older patient often displays exaggerated clinical responses to drugs affecting the CNS. For opioids, the most important clinical change is an approximate doubling of the sensitivity of the brain to a given tissue level of the opioid. There are also significant pharmacokinetic differences between young and old adults that are variable among the opioids.

Traditionally, morphine has been considered the prototype of μ-receptor agonist to which all other related agonists are compared. As with all opioids commonly used during anesthesia, after a bolus intravenous injection, morphine is rapidly distributed throughout the body. However, compared to fentanyl, its onset and offset is slower and duration of action longer due to the lower lipophilicity of morphine, which causes a slower movement in and out of the brain. The concentrations of morphine in the brain and CSF are far behind the concentration in plasma. In adults, the average elimination halftime of morphine is 3 h, but approaches 4 h in patients older than 65 years.

Morphine is metabolized (>90%) mainly in the liver, with most of the conversion to morphine-3-glucuronide (M3G) but also smaller amounts of morphine-6-glucuronide (M6G) and normorphine. All three metabolites are active. M6G is thought to contribute to morphine's analgesic effect, while M3G has neurostimulating properties.

The glucuronides are eliminated via renal excretion; thus, unimpaired renal function is critical to avoid the accumulation of these metabolites. Respiratory depression and excessive sedation have been reported and attributed to M6G toxicity not only in patients suffering from renal dysfunction, but in healthy volunteers and in patients on chronic morphine therapy as well.

For accurate dosing in patients with renal insufficiency, creatinine clearance rather than creatinine should be measured. Dose should be reduced to 75% for a glomerular filtration rate (GFR) between 20 and 50 mL/min, to 50% for GFR between 10 and 20 mL/min, and to 25% for GFR <10 mL/min. In the elderly, M6G may accumulate because of an age-related reduction in renal clearance and exacerbate the clinical effects of the drug.

Common sense and clinical studies indicate that slow titration to effect and dose adjustments can avoid undesirable side effects. When used for postsurgical pain management, the elderly required less morphine (boluses of 2 mg every 5 min versus 3 mg in younger patients) to achieve comparable levels of analgesia. Interestingly, the number of boluses to achieve adequate pain relief was similar in both groups, suggesting that although older patients might be susceptible to the CNS effects of morphine, their pain experience is identical to those younger.

Hydromorphone is a semisynthetic opioid that modulates the nociceptive process by binding to μ-opioid receptors. In comparison to morphine, hydromorphone has a more rapid onset and shorter duration of action. Given orally, hydromorphone is approximately five times as potent as morphine, whereas with intravenous administration, hydromorphone is 7–8 times more potent.

Unlike morphine, hydromorphone does not have an analgesically active 6-glucuronide metabolite that can accumulate in renal failure. The safety of hydromorphone has been recently described in patients on chronic hemodialysis: no signs of opioid toxicity have been observed. Theoretically the findings of this and other similar reports could be extrapolated to the elderly; however, given the lack of age-specific studies, dosage reduction and careful titration are advised for acute pain management in the elderly.

The pharmacologic properties of fentanyl and alfentanil in the elderly have been intensively studied. The first studies date back to the 1980s, when Bentley et al. reported that fentanyl had decreased clearance and consequently a prolonged effect in aged patients. Scott and Stansky were the first to shed light on the pharmacokinetics and pharmacodynamics of fentanyl and alfentanil. They used power spectral analysis of EEG changes to evaluate the brain effect of a continuous infusion in older patients and observed that the dose requirements for both fentanyl and alfentanil decreased by 50% over the age range from 20 to 89 years. Curiously, the pharmacokinetic parameters were not affected by age. Other investigations have confirmed these findings. These results suggest that with age, the brain becomes more sensitive to the opioids and indicate the necessity of an ~50% reduction in the dosage given to elderly patients. However, because only the pharmacodynamics and not the pharmacokinetics of fentanyl and alfentanil are dependent of age, it would be logical to consider that the effect of a given dose will dissipate no less rapidly in the elderly in comparison to younger patients.

The pharmacokinetic parameters obtained by Scott and Stansky were validated during target-controlled infusion for delivery of alfentanil to two study groups consisting of young women and aged men. The target serum concentrations of alfentanil were accurately achieved by the model, thereby confirming that the pharmacokinetic of alfentanil is independent of age.

Sufentanil is about ten times more potent than fentanyl and is more rapidly eliminated. Its context-sensitive half-life (i.e., the time required to obtain a 50% reduction in the plasma drug concentration after the end of the infusion) is sevenfold smaller than fentanyl, making it less likely to have a prolonged recovery time if a long-term infusion is required. The data on the pharmacologic profile of sufentanil in the elderly is limited. When pooling together the available research data, apparently the pharmacokinetics of sufentanil is minimally affected by age. One recent study that assessed the linearity of the pharmacokinetics of sufentanil concluded that the distribution and clearance of sufentanil is unaffected by dose and that age did not affect the pharmacokinetics of sufentanil. However, Matteo et al. observed a prolonged effect of sufentanil in elderly neurosurgical patients. Six of seven elderly patients required administration of naloxone at the termination of surgery to reverse the respiratory depressant effect of sufentanil while only one younger patient required antagonism of ventilatory depression. They speculated that geriatric patients exhibit sensitivity to a given concentration of sufentanil, similar to what has been observed with fentanyl and alfentanil.

Introduced in clinical practice in 1996, remifentanil is the first ultrashort acting mu-receptor agonist. Although its pharmacodynamic properties are comparable to those of other opioids, what makes remifentanil distinctive is its chemical structure and unique pharmacokinetic profile. Due to its methyl-ester side chain, remifentanil is quickly hydrolyzed by nonspecific plasma and tissue esterases to essentially inactive compounds, which are excreted by the kidneys. As a direct consequence, remifentanil does not accumulate in the peripheral compartment, allowing rapid clearance of 9–10 min and fast recovery. Moreover compared to its congeners, the context-sensitive halftime of remifentanil is constant (~3 min) and independent from the duration of the infusion, in contrast to fentanyl and alfentanil where 180 and, respectively, 47 min will be needed to halve the plasma concentration following a 3-h infusion.

Despite its extreme pharmacologic versatility, advanced age is associated with important effects on the pharmacokinetics and pharmacodynamics of remifentanil. As demonstrated by Minto et al., the central volume of distribution decreases about 25%, and the clearance decreases by about 33% from age 20 to 85 (Fig. 6.1).

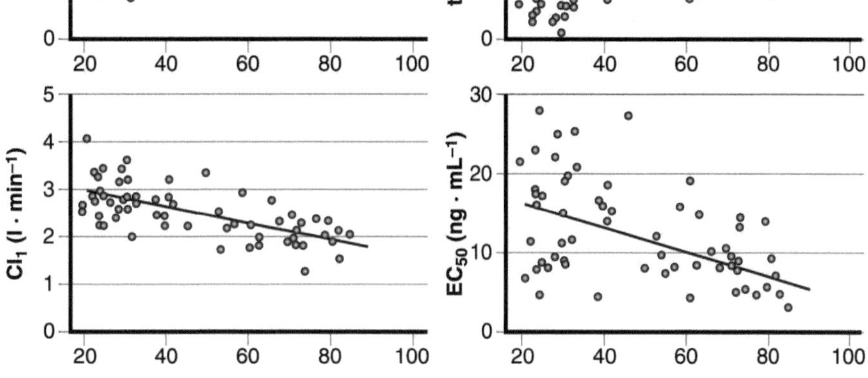

Fig. 6.1 Relationship between pharmacokinetic and pharmacodynamic parameters and age for remifentanil

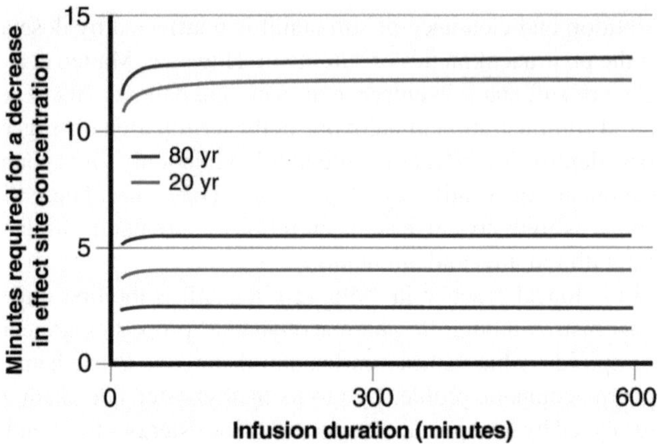

Fig. 6.2 The time required for decreases in effect-site concentration of 20%, 50%, and 80% as a function of remifentanil duration

In addition, age influences the pharmacodynamic response to remifentanil. Using EEG depression as a surrogate measure for opioid potency, the effect-site concentration (EC50) is reduced by 50% in the elderly, suggesting that the CNS sensitivity to remifentanil is twice that of younger patients. Additionally, the onset of the clinical effect is delayed by almost twofold, probably due to a slower equilibration between the blood and the brain. The evidence for this is a longer $t_{1/2}k_{eo}$, the plasma effect-site equilibration rate constant in minutes. In light of these changes, one should reduce a bolus dose of remifentanil by 50% and expect a slightly longer time to achieve clinical effect. Because of the reduced clearance, the infusion rate should only be ~34% of the rate for a young adult. On discontinuation of the infusion, it may take slightly longer for the plasma concentration to decline, but given the rapidity of remifentanil metabolism, that change is not very significant clinically (Fig. 6.2).

A simulation has been performed illustrating the time necessary to achieve 20%, 50%, and 80% decrease in effect-site drug concentration after infusions of variable length in 20- and 80-year olds with lean body mass of 55 kg. For each desired decrease, it requires one to two more minutes for the older patient (Fig. 6.2). The simulation model also revealed the effects of boluses of remifentanil on effect-site concentrations. After a single bolus of remifentanil, the peak effect-site concentration is minimally affected by age; however, peak effect will be reached ~1 min later in the 80-year-old individual.

Meperidine is perhaps the one opioid not suitable for use in elderly patients for analgesia. Meperidine is a phenylpiperidine derivative and 8–10 times less potent than morphine. It has a redistribution half-life of 4–15 min and an elimination halftime of 3–5 h. Similar is metabolized in the liver to form active compounds, which are then excreted via the kidneys. Normeperidine, the major metabolite, has a markedly longer half-life (14–24 h) than meperidine, accumulates with high and repeated doses, and may cause neuroexcitation (delirium, restlessness) and seizures. Patients who are particularly vulnerable to this side effect include the elderly, patients who are dehydrated, and those with renal impairment. As the metabolite toxicity is dose dependent, meperidine in low doses (12.5–25 mg) for the treatment of postoperative shivering should be acceptable use in the elderly.

Methadone has several unique features that distinguish it from other opioids. It lacks active metabolites, and its clearance is unaffected by renal or hepatic dysfunction. It is a strong mu-agonist, but in addition has *N*-methyl-D-aspartate (NMDA)-blocking properties, which apparently plays a role in reducing opioid tolerance and the attenuation of postoperative hyperalgesia. Following a single intravenous dose of 10–20 mg, the onset and duration of action mimic those of morphine. However, with repeated doses, the plasma concentration tends to rise, and the analgesic effect extends over 20 h. Furthermore, methadone has a long and unpredictable elimination half-life ranging from 8 to 87 h and the potential for unexpected toxicity from accumulation with repetitive doses. Although clinical studies of methadone in the elderly are lacking, an understanding of these unique properties plus experience in how to titrate the drug and closely monitor the patient should provide safe perioperative use in the elderly in selected circumstances.

The effect of age on the pharmacokinetics and pharmacodynamics of opioids is summarized in Table 6.1.

Nonopioid Analgesics

In the modern multimodal approach of perioperative pain control, nonsteroidal anti-inflammatory drugs (NSAIDs) represent a distinctive category. Their mechanism of action is characterized by the inhibition of cyclooxygenase (COX) enzyme activity, which in turn will decrease the synthesis of prostaglandin (PG). Because prostaglandins enhance nociception and modulate pain sensations in the periphery, spinal cord, and CNS, their inhibition will result in analgesia.

The benefits of NSAIDs are particularly notable when they are used in combination with an opioid for the management of acute pain. By reducing the amount of opioid use, opioid-related side effects are lessened, including sedation, respiratory depression, nausea, and vomiting. However, NSAIDs may cause important adverse effects and must be used carefully in the elderly, particularly in those suffering from renal dysfunction, bleeding diathesis, peptic ulcer disease, or chronic antiplatelet therapy.

COX-2-selective inhibitors are superior over COX-1 inhibitors in the perioperative setting because they do not cause renal compromise or increase the risk of bleeding. However, in the light of scrutiny related to increased cardiac morbidity and mortality, rofecoxib and valdecoxib have been withdrawn for the US market, leaving only celecoxib available. In a randomized trial of adjunctive celecoxib therapy versus placebo, initial 24-h PCA morphine usage was reduced (15.1 versus 19.7 mg with placebo). In addition, the visual analogue pain scores at rest were lower in the celecoxib group than with placebo, and the use of celecoxib improved

Table 6.1 The influence of age on the pharmacology of intravenous opioids

Drug	Pharmacokinetic changes with age	Pharmacodynamic changes with age	Comments and recommendations for dosing in elderly
Fentanyl, sufentanil	Minimal change	Twofold ↑ in brain sensitivity	Reduce dose by 50%
Alfentanil	Modest ↓ in terminal half-life	↑ Potency attributed to ↑ brain sensitivity	Reduce dose by 50%
Remifentanil	Slower onset and offset	Twofold ↑ in brain sensitivity	Reduce bolus doses by 50%
	Moderate↓ in clearance (~60–70%) from age 20 to 80		Decrease infusion rates by 60–70%
Morphine	Slow onset	↑ Brain sensitivity	Reduce bolus dose by 50%
	Delayed peak effect (90 min after a bolus)		Avoid in patients with renal impairment
	Up to 35% reduction in plasma clearance		Accumulation of active metabolites
Hydromorphone	No studies in elderly	Probable ↑ brain sensitivity	
	Compared with morphine faster onset and no active metabolites		
Methadone	Lack of studies in elderly	Probable ↑ brain sensitivity	Prudent to reduce doses by about 50%
	Very long half-life		
Meperidine	↑ Clearance	Probable ↑ brain sensitivity	Not recommended
	Potential accumulation of toxic metabolites	Negative inotropic and positive chronotropic effect	Use only for postoperative shivering

knee range of motion over the first three postoperative days. Another study of abdominal laparoscopic procedures demonstrated improved gastrointestinal function, resumption of physical activities, and patient satisfaction with the use of celecoxib 400 mg/day on the day of surgery and for the first three postoperative days after laparoscopy.

Ketorolac is available for intravenous administration, and it is considered to be one of the strongest NSAIDs, capable to relieve acute pain that traditionally would require an opioid. Ketorolac should be avoided in patients with a history of gastropathy, platelet dysfunction, and thrombocytopenia or patients with renal impairment or hypovolemia. It should be used with caution in elderly patients. A loading dose of 15 mg IV, followed by 15 mg IV every 6 h for a short course, can provide effective analgesia for mild to moderate pain or can be a useful adjunct for moderate to severe pain when combined with opioids or other analgesic techniques.

Benzodiazepines

In the perioperative setting, the four most commonly used benzodiazepines are the agonists midazolam (Versed), lorazepam (Ativan), diazepam (Valium), and the antagonist flumazenil. The spectrum of their clinical effects is wide and includes sedation, amnesia, anxiolysis, hypnosis, centrally mediated muscle relaxation, and antiseizure activity.

The benzodiazepines are low molecular weight crystalline compounds and, except for midazolam, insoluble in water. Prepared for commercial use in an acidic media ($pH < 4$), midazolam becomes water soluble causing minimal pain and venous irritation on injection compared with diazepam that is formulated in propylene glycol. At physiologic pH, midazolam becomes highly lipophilic and so achieves a rapid and predictable onset of action (Table 6.2).

The effects of benzodiazepines appear to be mediated via stimulation of $GABA_A$ receptors within the CNS, thereby potentiating the GABA effects on the chloride channel at the $GABA_A$ receptor. The increase in chloride ion flux hyperpolarizes the cell and diminishes the ability of the nerve cell to initiate an action potential. Because receptor occupancy is dose dependent, lower doses produce anxiolysis and sedation, whereas higher doses achieve hypnosis.

Table 6.2 Physicochemical properties of commonly used benzodiazepines

	Midazolam	Diazepam	Lorazepam
pK_a	6.2	3.2	11.5
Water solubility	Good at $pH < 4$	Insoluble	Insoluble
Lipid solubility	Good at $pH > 4$	Good	Moderate
Venous irritation and pain on injection	No	Yes	Yes

Table 6.3 Pharmacokinetic data of intravenous BDZ's in adults

Drug	VSD (L/kg)	T1/2 α (min)	T1/2 β (h)	Clearance (mL/kg/min)	Protein binding (%)
Midazolam	1.1–1.7	7–15	2–3	6–11	96
Diazepam	0.7–1.7	10–15	20–50	0.2–0.5	98
Lorazepam	0.8–1.3	3–10	11–22	0.8–1.8	90

VSD volume of distribution at steady state, *T1/2 α* distribution half-life, *T1/2 β* elimination half-life

Benzodiazepines are metabolized in the liver. Biotransformation involves two principal pathways: hepatic microsomal oxidation and/or glucuronide conjugation. Lorazepam is dependent on glucuronide conjugation whereas midazolam and diazepam are metabolized through oxidation via the cytochrome P450 (CYP) enzyme system. The oxidative process may be altered by factors such as old age, coexistent diseases (e.g., liver cirrhosis, congestive heart failure), as well as administration of drugs that modulate the CYP system, e.g., calcium-channel blockers, antiarrhythmics, cimetidine.

Both midazolam and diazepam yield to form pharmacologically active metabolites. In normal conditions these metabolites are rapidly cleaved to inactive compounds and eliminated via renal excretion. However, they may accumulate during continuous infusion in the critically ill causing prolonged sedation as seen in the elderly and in patients with renal or hepatic dysfunction and decreased albumin levels.

The pharmacokinetic profiles of the benzodiazepines differ significantly, including lipid solubility, distribution, metabolism, and clearance (Table 6.3). Midazolam is highly lipophilic and following intravenous administration quickly reaches the central compartment, producing an onset of action in <1 min. The duration of action after a single bolus dose depends mainly on the speed of redistribution from the CNS compartment to the peripheral tissue (muscle, fat).

Compared to young adults, the elimination halftime of midazolam is increased in elderly (5.6 versus 2.1 h) because of decreased liver clearance. The volume of distribution of midazolam is minimally affected by age, but will be increased in obesity and chronic liver disease resulting in delayed elimination.

As with midazolam, the lipid solubility of diazepam is high, and after a single bolus dose (IV 5–10 mg), the onset of effect occurs within 1 min with duration of effect from 1 to 6 h. Although liver clearance appears to remain preserved in the elderly, the elimination halftime of diazepam is greatly prolonged, attributed mostly to an increase in volume of distribution.

The CNS effects of benzodiazepines are dose dependent, with increasing dose providing initially anxiolysis and antiseizure activity followed by sedation, decrease in muscular tone, and finally hypnosis. It is important to remember that the amnestic effects are superior and longer lasting than the sedative effects. Intense amnesia may be present for hours, although the patient appears fully conscious.

Benzodiazepines decrease cerebral metabolic rate and cerebral blood flow (CBF), although to a lesser extent than barbiturates or propofol. A ceiling effect on these

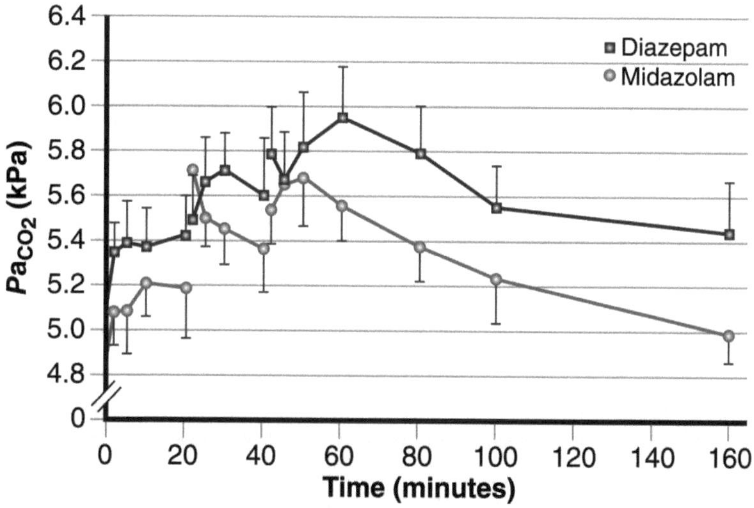

Fig. 6.3 Time course of respiratory depression after a bolus of diazepam or midazolam

parameters has been observed, which may represent saturation of receptor-specific binding sites. Unlike in animal studies, there is no clear evidence that benzodiazepines have neuroprotective properties in humans.

Several studies demonstrate that enhancement in clinical manifestations, such as prolonged sedation and cognitive and psychomotor impairment, is primarily the result of age-related increased sensitivity (pharmacodynamics) and not due to pharmacokinetic changes. Proposed changes responsible for the increased sensitivity include an increase in benzodiazepine receptor binding, higher benzodiazepine concentrations in the CNS due to alterations in blood–brain membrane permeability, and decline of general organ function.

Benzodiazepines produce dose-related central respiratory depression. The mechanism involves a decrease in hypoxic drive, which is enhanced in patients with chronic obstructive pulmonary disease and obstructive sleep apnea. The ventilatory response curve to CO_2 is flattened but not shifted to the right as seen with opioid administration (Fig. 6.3). The peak onset of respiratory depression after a midazolam bolus of 0.15–0.2 mg/kg occurs in 3 min and lasts 60–120 min. The decrease in tidal volume and minute volume that occurs is amplified by coadministration of opioids or other sedatives. In addition, analogous to propofol, benzodiazepines decrease upper respiratory muscle tone activity, which may contribute to airway obstruction during sedation and anesthesia induction.

Intravenous administration of benzodiazepines causes mild systemic vasodilation and moderate reduction in blood pressure and cardiac output. However, these hemodynamic changes may be exaggerated in hypovolemic patients or in those with little cardiac reserve, particularly when large doses are administered or if combined with an opioid.

Benzodiazepines are commonly used preoperatively for premedication, intraoperatively for sedation during local or regional anesthesia, outside of the operating room for procedural sedation, postoperatively for sedation in ICU, and to a lesser extent for the induction and maintenance of general anesthesia. When used for sedation, it is important to consider the significant variability of effect among individual patients. Careful monitoring and slow titration to the desired effect is recommended to prevent oversedation and avoid respiratory compromise.

Midazolam

The initial intravenous (IV) dose for sedation with midazolam in adult patients is usually 1–2 mg over 30 s, followed by doses of 0.5–1 mg at intervals of about 2 min as required. The onset of effect after bolus administration occurs within 30–60 s, peak effect after 3–5 min, and an offset of sedation ranging from 15 to 80 min. The time of onset is affected by the dose administered, concurrent administration of other sedatives/analgesics, age, and concurrent diseases.

Clinical studies and daily experience convincingly demonstrate that sedation with midazolam is safe and well tolerated in the elderly. However, as pointed out by several investigators, the sensitivity of the geriatric patients to the sedative/hypnotic effects of midazolam is significantly increased. For instance, Jacobs et al. used a logistic regression model to demonstrate that the steady-state plasma concentration, Cp50 of midazolam (a value comparable to the concept of MAC during inhalational anesthesia) capable to obliterate response to verbal command at 80 years old, was <25% of the value at 40 years. Bell et al. found a strong correlation between age and the dose of midazolam required for sedation during upper gastrointestinal endoscopy. In this study 90% of the patients older than 70 years required <5 mg of midazolam to tolerate the procedure. Another study investigated the safety of low-dose midazolam (30 mcg/kg) in octogenarians. They found that postendoscopy desaturation ($SPO2<92\%$) occurred frequently and concluded that careful monitoring is necessary to outweigh the risk of sedation in older people (Fig. 6.4).

Induction of general anesthesia with midazolam in the elderly is possible; however, based on pharmacokinetic studies, significant reduction in dose is required in order to preserve hemodynamic stability and prevent prolonged cognitive dysfunction. A 20–25% reduction in induction dose is recommended in patients older than 55 years and ASA physical status equal or greater than III (Table 6.4).

In a recent article, Shafer reviewed and summarized the results of previous studies and concluded that in the light of pharmacodynamic data, the induction dose of midazolam should be lowered by 75% in elderly patients. Based on this, the induction dose of midazolam would be 0.1–0.15 mg/kg in the elderly, with further reduction in the dose to <0.1 mg/kg if synergistic drugs, such as opioids, are used.

In young, healthy volunteers, emergence following induction with midazolam is about 2–2.5 times longer compared to induction with thiopental; however, recovery times do not differ significantly. With a lack of data in elderly patients, we may

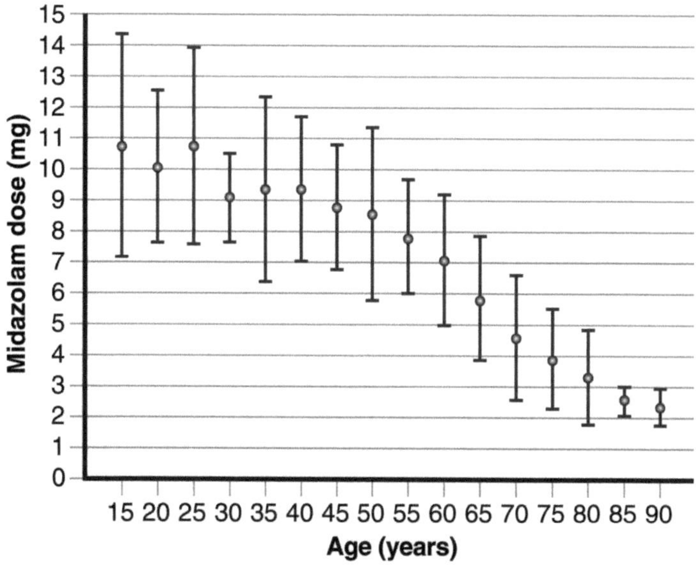

Fig. 6.4 Relationship between age of patient and the mean dose of intravenous midazolam required to produce adequate sedation prior to upper gastrointestinal endoscopy

assume there is a prolonged effect and longer emergence and recovery times due to increased central nervous system sensitivity to benzodiazepines and the prolonged metabolic half-life. Furthermore, when midazolam is used for the maintenance of GA, the context-sensitive halftime (the time required for a 50% decrease in plasma concentration as a function of infusion duration) of midazolam will be almost doubled in an 80-year-old patient, compared to 20-year old. Additionally, the longer the drug is administered, the greater the difference in recovery time between younger and older subjects.

Diazepam

For many years diazepam had been considered the gold standard for preoperative premedication and anxiolysis. Currently, it is used for sedation during nonpainful minor procedures. For this purpose, an intravenous dose of 0.1–0.2 mg/kg is recommended. With a single dose the onset of sedation occurs within 1 min, with duration of sedation between 1 and 6 h (Table 6.4).

Although diazepam is 2–3 times less potent than midazolam, its CNS depressant effect is significant in the elderly. Dose reduction and slow titration to the desired effect are advisable to avoid oversedation and delayed emergence, particularly when older age is associated with other comorbidities (e.g., cirrhosis) or other sedatives are coadministered. Because of the prolonged context-sensitive halftime, diazepam is not well suited for the induction and maintenance of anesthesia or sedation.

Table 6.4 Dosing guidelines for intravenous BDZ's

	Midazolam		Diazepam		Lorazepam	
Indications	Healthy adult	Elderly	Healthy adult	Elderly	Healthy adult	Elderly
[a]Sedation	1–2 mg	0.5–1 mg	2–5 mg	1–2.5 mg	0.5–1 mg	0.25 mg
GA induction	0.2–0.3 mg/kg	0.05–0.15 mg/kg	0.3–0.5 mg/kg	[b]Not recommended	0.1 mg/kg	[b]Not recommended
Maintenance infusion	0.5–1 μ/kg/min	N/A	0.03–0.1 mg/kg at 6 h interval	N/A	0.01–0.02 mg/kg	N/A

N/A data not available; perhaps doses should be reduced by 25–50% and carefully titrated to the desired effect
[a]Always titrate slowly to the desired level of sedation
[b]Prolonged effect

Lorazepam

Lorazepam is by far more potent than midazolam or diazepam. However, unlike midazolam, its onset of sedation is delayed with a peak effect occurring some 20–30 min after IV administration. The duration of action is also prolonged and can last more than 8–10 h (Table 6.4). Because of this, lorazepam is a poor choice for the induction or maintenance of anesthesia or for titration to achieve moderate sedation. For preoperative anxiolysis, the usual dose is between 2 and 4 mg administered orally and at least 2 h before surgery. Alternatively, a dose of 0.5–2 mg IV may be injected ~30 min before the procedure. However, one should realize that even small doses might significantly slow the emergence and prolong amnesia postoperatively. This is particularly important in the geriatric population where there is a tendency for enhanced drug effect. Based on pharmacologic studies conducted in elderly patients who were sedated, intubated, and mechanically ventilated in the ICU, for every 10 years of patient age over 60 years, lorazepam potency increases by about 18%; thus, the sedation dose should be lessened accordingly (Fig. 6.5).

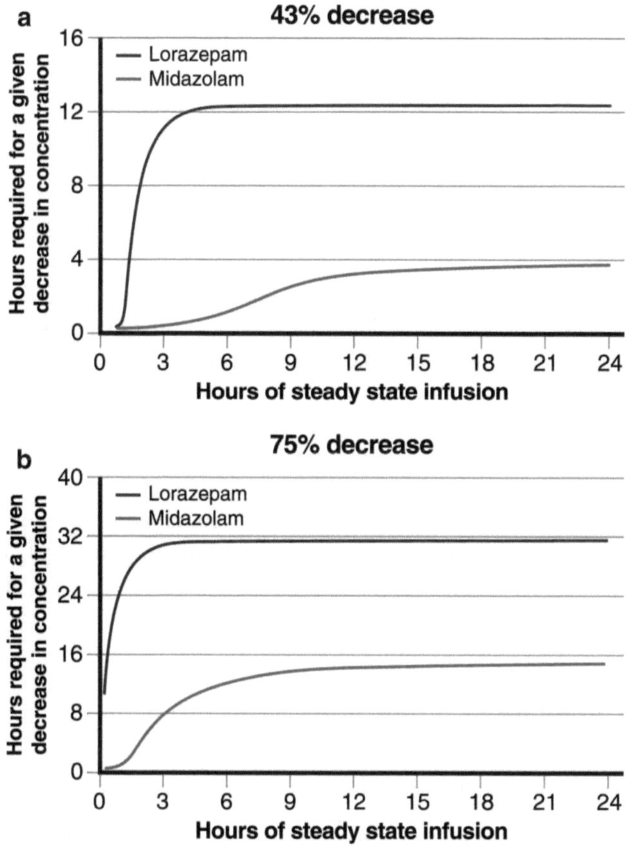

Fig. 6.5 Time necessary for 43% and 75% decreases, respectively, in blood lorazepam and midazolam concentrations

Flumazenil

Flumazenil is a competitive and highly specific benzodiazepine receptor antagonist used to reverse the unwanted effects of benzodiazepine overdose. In the CNS, flumazenil competes with the benzodiazepine binding sites and replaces the agonist drug in a dose-dependent manner. However, because the binding is competitive and the duration of action is short compared to benzodiazepines, the receptor site may become reoccupied by the agonist with resulting resedation of the patient.

The initial dose for reversal is typically given in incremental boluses of 0.2–0.3 mg IV every minute, up to a total dose of 3 mg. The onset of effect is very rapid (1–2 min) with a maximum effect after 2–10 min and duration of action between 45 and 90 min.

Flumazenil promptly reverses the CNS and cardiorespiratory manifestations associated with benzodiazepine oversedation. It has also been shown to be effective in reversing paradoxical agitation related to benzodiazepine administration in geriatric patients.

Flumazenil is contraindicated in tricyclic antidepressant overdose and in patients treated with benzodiazepines to control seizures. Flumazenil is best to be avoided in patients with benzodiazepine dependence because of the potential of acute withdrawal symptom.

Key Points

- Older patients are much more sensitive to opioids and benzodiazepines than young adults.
- This increase in sensitivity is principally due to pharmacodynamic rather than pharmacokinetic changes: the elderly brain is more sensitive to these drugs.
- In general, opioid doses should be decreased by 50% in the elderly and side effects carefully monitored.
- Midazolam doses should be decreased by 25–50% in elderly patients (even more so in the very old) and carefully titrated particularly in patients receiving opioids or other sedatives.
- Nonsteroidal medications are an important component of the multimodal approach to pain management of the geriatric patient. However, these drugs should be used cautiously in the elderly with a history of renal insufficiency, peptic ulcer disease, or associated anticoagulant therapy.

Suggested Reading

Albrecht S, Ihmsen H. The effect of age on the pharmacokinetics and pharmacodynamics of midazolam. Clin Pharmacol Ther. 1999;65(6):630–39.

Barr J, Zomorodi K, Bertaccini EJ,et al. A double-blind, randomized comparison of i.v. lorazepam versus midazolam for sedation of ICU patients via a pharmacologic model. Anesthesiology. 2001;95(2):286–98.

Buvanendran A, Kroin JS, Tuman KJ, et al. Effects of perioperative administration of a selective cyclooxygenase-2 inhibitor on pain management and recovery of function after knee replacement. A randomized controlled trial. JAMA. 2003;290:2411–18.
Christe C, Janssens JP. Midazolam sedation for upper gastrointestinal endoscopy in older persons: a randomized, double-blind, placebo-controlled study. J Am Geriatr Soc. 2000 Nov; 48(11):1398–403.
Coloma M, White PF, Huber PJ, et al. Effect of ketorolac on recovery after anorectal surgery: Intravenous vs local administration. Anesth Analg. 2000;90:1107.
Davis M, Glare P, Hardy J, ed. Opioids in Cancer Pain, Oxford, UK: Oxford University Press; 2005:247–65.
Eilers H, Niemann CU. Clinically Important Drug Interactions with Intravenous Anaesthetics in Older Patients. Drugs Aging. 2003;20(13):969–80.
Evers AS, Maze M. Anesthetic Pharmacology. Churchill Livingstone, 2004.
Geppetti P, Benemei S. Pain treatment with opioids achieving the minimal effective and the minimal interacting dose. Clin Drug Investig. 2009;29 Suppl 1:3–16.
Gibson SJ, Farrell M. A review of age differences in the neurophysiology of nociception and the perceptual experience of pain. Clin. J. Pain. 2004;20:227–239.
Jacobs JR, Reves JG. Aging increases pharmacodynamic sensitivity to the hypnotic effects of midazolam. Anesth Analg. 1995;80(1):143–8.
Keïta H, Tubach F. Age-adapted morphine titration produces equivalent analgesia and adverse effects in younger and older patients. Eur J Anaesthesiol. 2008;25(5):352–356.
Klotz U. Pharmacokinetics and drug metabolism in the elderly. Drug Metabolism Reviews. 2009; 41(2):67–76.
Kurella M, Bennett WM, Chertow GM. Analgesia in patients with ESRD: a review of available evidence. Am J Kidney Dis. 2003;42:217–228.
Latta KS, Ginsberg B, Barkin RL. Meperidine: a critical review. Am J Ther. 2002;9:53–68.
Lötsch J. Opioid metabolites. J Pain Symptom Manage. 2005;29(5 Suppl):S10–24.
Minto CF, Schnider TW, Shafer SL. The influence of age and gender on the pharmacokinetics and pharmacodynamics of remifentanil : I. Model development. Anesthesiology. 1997;86:10–23.
Norton JR, Ward DS. Differences between midazolam and propofol sedation on upper airway collapsibility using dynamic negative airway pressure. Anesthesiology. 2006;104(6):1155–64.
Olkkola KT, Ahonen J. Midazolam and other Benzodiazepines. Handb Exp Pharmacol. 2008;(182):335–60.
Pasternak GW. The pharmacology of mu analgesics: from patients to genes. Neuroscientist. 2001; 7(3):220–31.
Shafer SL. The pharmacology of anaesthetic drugs in elderly patients. Anesthesiol Clin North Am. 2000;18(1):1–29.
Shafer SL. The pharmacology of anesthetic drugs in elderly patients. Anesthesiol Clin North America. 2000;18(1):1–29.
Silverstein JH, Rooke GA. Geriatric Anesthesiology, Springer 2008, pg.217.
Walhovd KB, Fjell AM, Reinvang I, et al. Effects of age on volumes of cortex, white matter and subcortical structures. Neurobiol Aging. 2005;26(9):1261-1–70.
Weinbroum AA, Szold O.The midazolam-induced paradox phenomenon is reversible by flumazenil. Epidemiology, patient characteristics and review of the literature. Eur J Anaesthesiol. 2001; 18(12):789–97.
White PF, Sacan O, Tufanogullari B, et al. Effect of short-term postoperative celecoxib administration on patient outcome after outpatient laparoscopic surgery. Can J Anaesth. 2007;54:342–48.

Chapter 7
General Anesthesia: Intravenous Induction Agents, Inhalational Agents, and Neuromuscular Blockers

Yulia Ivashkov, Alexander A. Vitin, and G. Alec Rooke

Intravenous Induction Agents

Intravenous medication has been the most common method of induction of general anesthesia for many decades, primarily due to the speed of onset, lack of patient discomfort as unconsciousness develops, and the ability to select a drug (or drugs) and dosages tailored to the patient's medical status. As there is no single ideal induction agent, the relative advantages and disadvantages of each agent must be understood in order to make a rational choice, especially for the older patient whose organ systems demonstrate diminished reserve with greater sensitivity and more adverse effects than their younger counterparts.

There is perhaps no greater effect of aging than what happens to drug pharmacokinetics and pharmacodynamics. Pharmacokinetic changes with aging alter initial drug concentrations in the blood, drug redistribution into tissue, and drug metabolism and excretion. Pharmacodynamic changes involve the change in sensitivity of the brain to the drug. An understanding of the common physiologic age-related changes is helpful to anticipate age-related differences in the older patient's response to medications.

Y. Ivashkov, MD (✉)
Department of Anesthesiology and Pain Medicine, Harborview Medical Center, University of Washington, 325 Ninth Avenue, Box 359724, Seattle, WA 98104, USA
e-mail: ivashy@u.washington.edu

A.A. Vitin, MD, PhD. • G.A. Rooke, MD, PhD
Department of Anesthesiology and Pain Medicine, University of Washington Medical Center, 1959 NE Pacific Street, P.O. Box 356540, Seattle, WA 98195-6540, USA
e-mail: vitin@u.washington.edu; rooke@u.washington.edu

S.R. Barnett (ed.), *Manual of Geriatric Anesthesia*, DOI 10.1007/978-1-4614-3888-5_7,

Pharmacokinetics

Changes in Distribution

Around the third decade the human body starts to undergo a decrease in total body water, a decrease in muscle mass, and an increase in body fat. These changes occur at about 1% per year, and by the age of 65, 25–30% of muscle may be lost and replaced by fat tissue. Total body water at this age also decreases to a similar degree. These changes in body composition may influence the volume of distribution for certain drugs.

A decrease in water content leads to reduction in initial volume of distribution of water-soluble drugs. As a result, blood levels for a given drug dose are higher in the elderly, causing a greater brain concentration and resulting in a greater effect.

Increases in total body fat may prolong the elimination half-life for lipid-soluble drugs. With an increase in adipose tissue, drugs accumulate more extensively in fat, thereby increasing the volume of distribution. A larger volume of distribution (V_d) increases the metabolic half-life by making less drug available in the blood ($t_{1/2} \sim V_d/$Clearance, where Clearance is the volume of blood from which drug is eliminated on a per-time unit basis). This phenomenon is especially applicable to lipophilic drugs such as the benzodiazepines and many of the opioids such as the fentanyl family (except remifentanil). Figure 7.1 shows the relationship between lipid

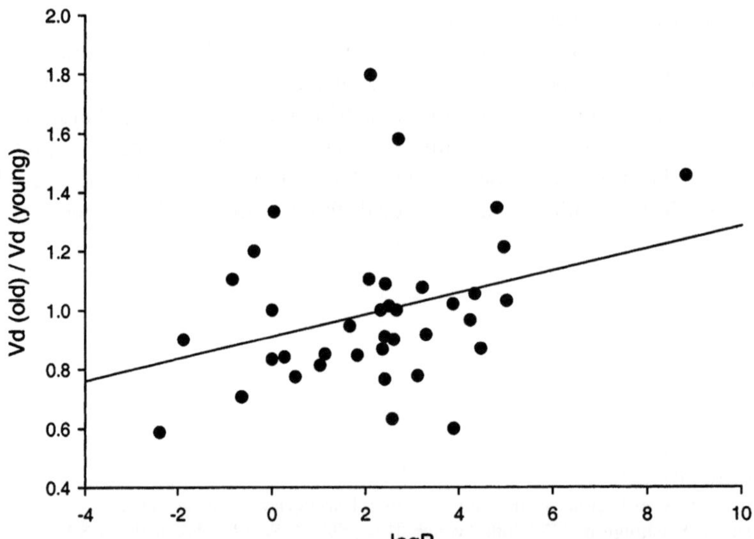

Fig. 7.1 The relationship between the log of the octanol–water partition coefficient [logP], determined from Interactive LogKow and the ratio between the volume of distribution of the drug in older people compared with younger people. If one outlier (amikacin) is excluded, the relationship is borderline significant ($P=0.053$) (Reprint with permission from ASPET Copyright Department; McLean AJ, Le Couteur DG. Pharmacological Reviews. 2004;56:163–184)

solubility of drugs and changes in their volume of distribution with aging. Curiously, with extreme age and frailty, total body fat typically declines and therefore the volume of distribution for lipophilic drugs may decrease. In theory, metabolic half-life would therefore decrease (faster elimination), but only if clearance did not change with age.

Changes in Metabolism

As might be expected, drug elimination typically does decrease with age. Both drug metabolism by the liver and drug excretion by the kidneys decrease, even in healthy elderly. The liver mass in a patient of advanced age can decrease by 20–40% and is accompanied by a 35% decrease in hepatic blood flow. The rate of glomerular filtration also decreases ~10% per decade after age 50 and is accompanied with a loss of renal parenchyma. It is important to remember that decline in renal function may not be reflected by creatinine levels due to a reduction in muscle mass and a corresponding decrease in creatinine production. Thus, the decrease in clearance and the increase in the volume of distribution conspire to slow drug metabolism in the elderly patient. The magnitude of the decrease in metabolism can be dramatic. For example, diazepam has a half-life in hours that is approximately equal to the patient's age, meaning that a 72-year-old patient has a metabolic half-life for diazepam of ~3 days.

Changes in Protein Binding

Age-related changes in plasma proteins have not been investigated to a full extent, and clinical significance of these changes is not completely clear. Healthy elderly may experience decrease in albumin levels up to 10%, but it may decrease more in frail and malnourished individuals. But not all the proteins decrease with advanced age; α1-acid glycoprotein may increase, possibly due to an underlying inflammatory processes. However, in general, protein binding decreases in the elderly. Since only protein-unbound drugs produce tissue effects, a decrease in protein binding increases the amount of active drug, reducing the necessary drug dose. This is particularly true regarding the drugs that undergo liver metabolism, are highly protein bound, and are administered intravenously, for example, lidocaine, fentanyl, and midazolam.

Pharmacodynamics

Pharmacodynamics studies the effect of medications on a body and describes a change in sensitivity of the target organ to the drug. Due to complex methodology, pharmacodynamics is far less explored and hence less understood than pharmacokinetics.

The target organ for intravenous anesthetics is the central nervous system. Age-related alteration of CNS includes anatomical and functional loss of neurons, reduction in receptor number and affinity, and alterations in signal transduction, and homeostatic regulation.

Loss of Neurons

Even though that age-related decline in neuron number through apoptosis and neuron death is not very prominent in normal aging, significant neuronal loss in elderly is often associated with neurodegenerative diseases such as Alzheimer's disease, Parkinson's disease, or stroke. The healthy elderly may also experience age-related cognitive decline such as memory impairment, which may be explained not only by absolute decrease in neurons, but rather by anatomical and functional changes at the synaptic level. These changes may be represented as a decrease in the number of active synapses, or loss of function of some existing synapses.

Receptor Changes

Multiple changes in receptor activity and expression occur in an aging nervous system. These changes are very complex and vary in different areas of brain. The resulting imbalance in neurotransmission may affect the reaction of elderly to anesthetics.

Age is associated with a decrease in the number of μ- and κ-opioid receptors. This change may be related to memory impairment in healthy elderly. Number of dopaminergic neurons and dopamine D_2 receptors also declines. GABA(A) receptors not only decrease in number, but also undergo changes in composition with loss of presynaptic GABA release. That may explain the increase in sensitivity to benzodiazepines with advanced age. Other CNS receptors that decrease in number and/or in binding with age include cholinergic (nicotinic and muscarinic) and *N*-methyl-D-aspartate (NMDA) receptors. Receptor changes outside the CNS also include down-regulation of β-adrenoceptors and diminished responsiveness of adenosine A-1 receptors that carry out cardioprotective effect. Though the clinical significance of the receptor-related alterations is not completely clear, they may explain why elderly require less anesthetic agents to produce the desired end-organ effect.

Signal Transduction and Homeostatic Mechanisms

Decrease in cell proliferation with age may be related to changes in signal transduction mechanisms. One of the critical components of signal transduction is CREB (cyclic AMP response element binding protein). CREB is an important element for neuroplasticity, and inadequate expression of CREB leads to short-term memory impairment. Brains of humans with Alzheimer's disease have decreased level of phosphorylated CREB, though it is still unclear whether loss of pCREB regulation contributes to cognitive dysfunction in normal aging.

A progressive decline in homeostatic mechanisms is a hallmark of aging. When cognitive reserve is exhausted, aging patients will be more sensitive to the drugs and require more time to return to baseline after drug administration.

There are other aging phenomena that may be deleterious. CNS homeostatic changes include an increase in duration of cytoplasmic Ca^{2+} signals. Increased intracellular Ca^{2+} is cytotoxic and may affect adversely neurons and synapses. Insulin resistance also develops with aging, and it is associated with endothelial dysfunction, inflammation, and progression of atherosclerosis.

Other Implications of Aging

Anesthesia personnel should also be aware of expected changes in hemodynamic response to intravenous sedatives and hypnotics. Loss of elasticity of connective tissue stiffens blood vessels and the myocardium. By the age of 80 blood vessels lose 90% of distensibility compared to the age of 20. The autonomous nervous system also undergoes functional decline. Older people have lower basal vagal tone and higher sympathetic tone. The baroreceptor reflex-mediated heart rate response to hypotension decreases as well. The cardiovascular system becomes noncompliant, and much like an outdated plumbing system, it cannot effectively buffer sudden changes in pressure or volume.

In addition, the elderly are more likely to have hypertension, coronary artery disease, and valvular abnormalities. Comorbidities reduce tolerance to cardiovascular instability and increase the probability of adverse events such as exacerbation of congestive heart failure or myocardial ischemia.

Patients with comorbidities may receive either no routine medical treatment at all or may present with a long list of regular medications. Both situations need careful attention. Untreated disease such as hypertension predisposes patient to a marked hemodynamic lability in situations when surgical care is emergent and does not allow time for medical optimization.

Conversely, routine medications may have undesired interactions with anesthetic agents. ACE inhibitors may cause refractory hypotension with general anesthesia, diuretics may lead to hypokalemic arrhythmias, and β-blockers may contribute to profound bradycardia and mask preexisting hypovolemia.

From the preceding, one can conclude that pharmacokinetic changes associated with age most likely increase the elderly patient's sensitivity to both the desired drug effects and to the side effects. As such, the elderly require smaller induction doses than younger adults. In addition, the onset of action may be slower (mechanism not entirely understood), and the emergence may be prolonged.

Unfortunately, no single predictive factor gives the anesthesiologist a definitive measure of the pharmacokinetic age-related changes, and drug dosage must be tailored to each patient to achieve the desired effect.

Intravenous Agents

Propofol

Propofol [2,6-disopropylphenol] is an alkyl phenol. It acts mainly by activation of $GABA_A$ receptors, though it also inhibits the NMDA receptor. Propofol also has been shown to produce relaxation of preconstricted airway smooth muscle by the inhibition of calcium mobilization through slow calcium ion channels in smooth muscle cells. Propofol has rapidly become the most popular induction drug due to its rapid onset and termination of action, predictable dose-related hypnotic effect, and antiemetic properties. It also has some amnestic effects, and although the effect may be weak and not always reliable, it still could be useful during sedation in the elderly when benzodiazepines are deliberately avoided to reduce the risk of cognitive impairment in the postoperative period. Although propofol has no direct analgesic properties, it may lower analgesic requirements.

The cardiovascular side effects of propofol, along with pain on injection, are the features that hold it back from being an almost ideal induction medication. Propofol inhibits sympathetic vasoconstriction and causes dramatic decreases in systemic vascular resistance. It also suppresses reflex tachycardia which is already diminished in the elderly. These processes may lead to profound hypotension from both a decrease in vascular resistance as well as a decrease in cardiac output, especially in volume depleted individuals.

Propofol is a potent lipophilic drug, and it is also highly protein bound. Since the volume of distribution and protein binding undergo significant alteration with age, as described earlier, propofol pharmacokinetics change remarkably in elderly, and there may be a modest pharmacodynamic increase in brain sensitivity as well. To avoid undesirable effects, the induction dose of propofol should be reduced by at least 20% in older people, with the decrease of bolus dose to 1.5–1.8 mg/kg. The dose of a maintenance infusion decreases by at least 30% (Fig. 7.2). Failure to adjust the dose of propofol may result in frank hypotension upon induction and delayed emergence after prolonged infusion.

Thiopental

Thiopental causes hypnosis by activation of $GABA_A$ receptors. Thiopental decreases myocardial contractility and lowers systemic vascular resistance, thereby typically

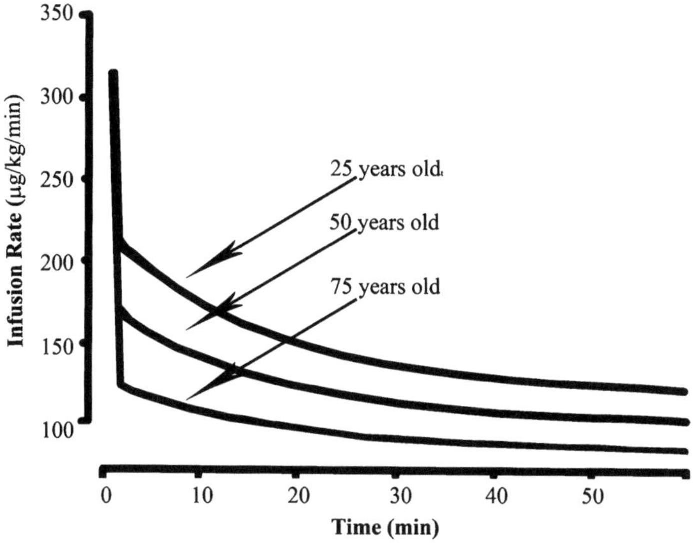

Fig. 7.2 Age-adjusted infusion regimens to maintain adequate anesthesia with propofol. An elderly patient requires a reduction in propofol infusion rate of 30–50%, compared to a younger patient, to maintain the same anesthetic effect (Reprint with permission from Wolters Kluwer Health; Schnider TW, Minto CF. Anesthesiology. 1998;88:1170–1182)

causing a decrease in blood pressure when given as a large bolus at induction. It causes less suppression of the baroreflex compared to propofol, and therefore is more likely to cause tachycardia than propofol. The combination of decreased blood pressure and increased heart rate may prove unfavorable to the elderly patient with coronary artery disease, which is not uncommon in elderly.

The hyperalgesic properties of thiopental were widely discussed through the last decade of the twentieth century, but have not been revisited since then. Thiopental creates less favorable conditions to laryngoscopy compared to propofol, and it does lower pain threshold in rodents, but the question whether it produces clinically significant hyperalgesia in humans remains open.

Thiopental and other barbiturates can provoke an attack of acute liver porphyria. It does not cause discomfort with intravenous injection, but with extravasation or intraarterial administration, severe arterial constriction and tissue necrosis may occur.

The pharmacodynamics of thiopental does not change with age in that the elderly brain is not more sensitive to thiopental; however, the pharmacokinetics of thiopental do change with age, mostly due to a change in the initial volume of distribution. The octogenarian requires a 15–20% reduction of the induction dose suitable to a 20 year old. As long as the dose is appropriately adjusted for age, the recovery time from either bolus or infusion will be similar for all age groups.

Methohexital

Methohexital is commonly used for short procedures such as electroconvulsive therapy. Unlike thiopental, methohexital may cause discomfort with intravenous injection. The clearance of methohexital is higher than thiopental and is more dependent on hepatic blood flow, resulting in shorter elimination half-life (3–6 versus 12 h for thiopental). However, hepatic blood flow declines with age, making emergence from methohexital slower than in younger individuals.

Experience with methohexital in anesthesia for ambulatory dental patients in prepropofol era was described by Benjamin S. Recant, D.D.S in 1960: "Particularly gratifying was the older patient's rapid emergence from the anesthetic state, inevitably a problem with thiobarbiturates when given in intermittent administration. These patient's rapid return to awareness and their obvious early alert reactivity were remarkable." Doses of methohexital in elderly when used without addition of opioids range from 0.9 to 1.2 mg/kg.

Etomidate

Etomidate preserves cardiovascular stability on induction: a desirable feature in volume-depleted patients and in patients with an unstable cardiovascular system as is present in many elderly patients. It does not depress myocardial contractility unless used in large doses (0.45 mg/kg). Heart rate, systolic pressure, ejection time, and the velocity of myocardial contraction are the main determinants of the metabolic demand of the heart. Since etomidate does not significantly alter these parameters, it provides better myocardial oxygen supply to demand ratio in comparison to propofol.

Unfortunately, its inhibition of corticosteroid production warrants caution. Etomidate inhibits conversion of cholesterol to cortisol. Some decrease of cortisol levels starts within an hour after single induction dose and lasts up to 15 h. This side effect is more clinically relevant to infusions rather than to a single bolus but nevertheless it is considered by many as a serious drawback. Etomidate has no anticonvulsant properties and it has been used successfully for electroconvulsive therapy in elderly seizure-resistant patients.

The pharmacodynamics of etomidate does not change with age, but the pharmacokinetics do. An 80-year-old patient requires less than half the dose of etomidate to reach the same stage EEG end point as a 22-year-old patient.

Midazolam

Although midazolam is a useful, short-acting benzodiazepine, it may be associated with postoperative cognitive impairment and/or delirium in elderly patients and therefore should be used judiciously and not as a matter of routine. CNS dysfunction caused by midazolam in elderly is probably related to some age-related changes in pharmacodynamics that are not yet fully understood. Midazolam is highly lipid soluble, and it is metabolized by the liver. Since total body fat increases with age, the volume of distribution of midazolam slightly increases, whereas hepatic perfusion decreases and both these effects decrease clearance. The net result is a reduction of induction dose by 20% after age of 55 and even more with advanced age.

Ketamine

Ketamine is a water-soluble compound that is structurally related to phencyclidine. Ketamine antagonizes the excitatory neurotransmitter glutamate by blocking NMDA receptor sites. It produces a so-called dissociative anesthesia by interference with interpretation of pain signals. Ketamine acts as sympathomimetic, hence it stimulates the cardiovascular system and causes bronchodilation. Due to its undesirable effects on the central nervous system ketamine currently has a limited place as a general anesthetic and in the elderly in particular. However, it could be used in small doses (10 mg increments) as an adjunct to sedation as long as all the possible undesirable side effects have been considered.

Dexmedetomidine

The α_2-adrenergic receptor agonist dexmedetomidine is gaining popularity as a sedative. It is used in intensive care units and in the operating rooms. It produces genuine conscious sedation, anxiolysis, and analgesia without respiratory depression. Presynaptic activation of the α_2 adrenoreceptor inhibits the release of norepinephrine, preventing the propagation of pain signals, and postsynaptic action in the central nervous system inhibits sympathetic tone. Side effects include mild to moderate cardiovascular depression with slight decrease in heart rate and blood pressure. Dexmedetomidine has dose-dependent α_2 adrenoreceptor selectivity; it is eight times more selective for α_2 adrenoreceptors than clonidine. The initial bolus of dexmedetomidine may result in a transient increase of blood pressure due to peripheral α_{2B} adrenoreceptor stimulation in vascular smooth muscle. This response can be attenuated by a slow bolus administration. It is a promising drug, especially for use with fast developing surgical techniques of endovascular repair of intraabdominal aneurysms, though its pharmacokinetics and pharmacodynamics in elderly has not been studied fully yet.

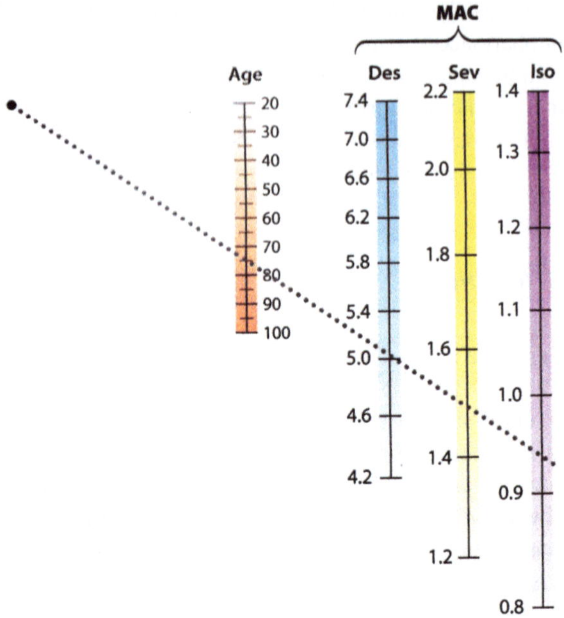

Fig. 7.3 Nomogram for Minimum Alveolar Concentration (MAC) as a function of age for isoflurane, sevoflurane, and desflurane (Reprint with permission from Wolters Kluwer Health; Rivera R, Antognini JF. Anesthesiology. 2009;110:1176–81)

Inhalational Anesthesia and the Aging Patient

Use of the inhalational anesthetic agents remains the popular and simplest mode of anesthetic maintenance and, in selective cases, induction of general anesthesia, despite the emerging trend in favor of total intravenous anesthesia for elderly patients. Over the last decade the marketplace has demonstrated a clear preference for sevoflurane, desflurane, isoflurane, and nitrous oxide, over other agents such as halothane or enflurane. In consequence, these latter agents will not be discussed in this chapter.

Advanced age causes significant anatomical and physiological changes in every organ system, thus affecting the pharmacokinetics and pharmacodynamics of all drugs, including inhalational agents. However, no credible evidence is found to date that age-related decrease of alveolar gas exchange surface and mismatching of perfusion and ventilation significantly influences the processes of volatile anesthetic uptake. Factors that affect volatile anesthetic pharmacokinetics include the age-related 50–70% increase in body fat percentage, the decrease in muscle mass, and the concomitant decrease in the total body water. These changes result in greater body accumulation of highly lipid soluble inhalational agents, thereby increasing body stores of volatile anesthetics and delaying emergence from anesthesia. The relatively low lipid solubility of desflurane and sevoflurane allows significantly faster emergence in the elderly patients than that with halothane and isoflurane.

MAC, minimal alveolar concentration, serves as a definition of volatile anesthetic potency and provides a guideline for its dosage. In healthy, young adults, MAC is 1.15% for isoflurane and 1.85% for sevoflurane. The MAC for desflurane is 6.0%, defined in subjects aged 31–65. Presumably on the basis of decreased CNS reserve, MAC decreases with age at an approximate rate of 6% per decade. The relationship is nonlinear; however, as the decline accelerates after 40–50 years of age. Nomograms for estimation of the age-related changes in MAC are available (Fig. 7.3).

For practical purposes, the dosage of volatile anesthetics can potentially be guided by the hemodynamic response and the BIS value rather than strictly by end-tidal gas concentration. However, when combined with opioids and/or nitrous oxide, total anesthetic dosage may exceed one MAC, and therefore represent an overdose. Specifically, in patients older than 65, MAC for desflurane has been defined as 5.17% with oxygen and 1.67% with 60% nitrous oxide. End-expired concentration of only 0.25% isoflurane with 67% of nitrous oxide has been reported to be required for 95-year-old patient.

Other medical conditions and pharmacological interactions also influence MAC in patients, including the elderly. Of those factors that increase MAC, chronic ethanol abuse, amphetamine, and cocaine use, and also drugs like levodopa, MAO inhibitors, and ephedrine are the best known. Factors that decrease MAC are much more numerous. Opioids, clonidine, lithium, barbiturates, benzodiazepines, chlorpromazine, verapamil, and also hypoxia, hypotension, and metabolic acidosis may effectively decrease MAC.

Inhalational anesthetics may affect the aged cardiovascular system in many ways. Direct myocardial depression, however in different degrees, has been demonstrated for all inhalational agents. One of the most important desirable characteristics of an inhalational agent is to ensure the hemodynamic stability, and the great advantage of the modern volatile agents over halothane and enflurane is that they exert significantly less effects on myocardial function, specifically contractility and diastolic relaxation, and are therefore better tolerated by elderly patients. Moreover, desflurane and sevoflurane, and to a lesser extent isoflurane, have been demonstrated to possess ischemic cardioprotective effects, and had shown no significant depressant effects on myocardial performance in comparison with propofol as part as TIVA for elderly cardiac patients. Use of these agents has also been associated with significant reduction in postoperative cardiac morbidity and mortality.

Desflurane has been shown to preserve and protect myocardial function in conditions of either hypotension or significant hypertension. At low fresh gas flow rates (around 1 L/min), anesthesia with desflurane provides more stable conditions than that with isoflurane. It also causes transient sinus tachycardia and hypertension with an abrupt increase in concentration to 1.5 MAC, which, in comparison with sevoflurane, may be attributed to maintenance of the initial level of catecholamines for at least 5 min after induction with desflurane and also possibly to the irritant effects of desflurane on upper airway. Desflurane, in concentrations of 2 MAC, unlike sevoflurane, also prolongs the QT interval. In patients with medical conditions, predisposing to rhythm disturbances, sevoflurane also causes significantly less postoperative atrial fibrillation and supraventricular arrhythmias than does desflurane.

In contrast to halothane and enflurane, sevoflurane, desflurane, and isoflurane decrease blood pressure more by decreasing peripheral vascular resistance than by decreasing cardiac output (via myocardial depression). Sevoflurane decreases systemic vascular resistance almost immediately after induction, while desflurane causes even more significant drop of SVR only after ~7 min. Aged patients may be especially sensitive to swings in blood pressure and the associated fluctuations in coronary and cerebral blood flow.

Although isoflurane decreases systemic vascular resistance (major mechanism for hypotension) while causing relatively little depression of contractility and cardiac output in concentrations up to ~1 MAC, these observations have only been verified in patients up to approximately age 60. Of all other volatile anesthetics, isoflurane does depress the early phase of the left ventricle relaxation to the greatest degree, which considerably affects diastolic function and actually decreases end-diastolic volume. Isoflurane typically increases the heart rate in younger patients, but may actually cause bradycardia in the elderly, thus worsening the older patient's ability to combat hypotension.

Even with prolonged exposure, sevoflurane and isoflurane do not appear to cause significant nephrotoxicity, despite the increase in fluoride concentration. Only sporadic cases of significant hepatotoxicity of sevoflurane, desflurane, and isoflurane have been reported. Compound A (fluoromethyl-2,2-difluoro-1-[trifluoromethyl] vinyl ether) is a breakdown product of sevoflurane produced by its interaction with carbon dioxide absorbents in the anesthesia machine. It has been shown to cause transient nephrotoxicity in laboratory animals, but its nephrotoxicity in humans has not been proved to date.

Nitrous oxide has enjoyed an exceptional longevity in anesthesia and is still in common use. Its MAC appears to be additive to the MAC of the more potent inhalational agents. Sixty percent nitrous oxide, given in combination with volatile agents, has demonstrated sympathomimetic as well as direct cardiodepressive effects and has been shown to decrease cardiac index by 10–15%, as well as left and right ventricular stroke work index. When used in combination with isoflurane, initiation of nitrous oxide is associated with tachycardia and preserved blood pressure, followed by sinus bradycardia and arterial hypotension. In a relatively high risk (vascular surgery) cohort of elderly patients, the use of nitrous oxide was associated with an increased incidence of postoperative myocardial ischemia. Consideration should therefore be given to avoiding the use of nitrous oxide altogether in the aged population.

The various agents are different with respect to speed of emergence and postanesthesia recovery. Compared to sevoflurane, desflurane, isoflurane, or an infusion of propofol, isoflurane is associated with the most delayed emergence, as demonstrated by the longest times for spontaneous eye opening, extubation, response to verbal stimuli, and full orientation. Recovery from desflurane is significantly faster than sevoflurane. Specifically, time to extubation, eye opening, following commands, and orientation in time and place were all ~2–4 min shorter with desflurane, and recovery room stay was reduced by 10–25 min. With respect to postoperative cognitive decline, even when the Mini-Mental State is examined as soon as 1 h after extubation, no significant differences have been observed between desflurane and sevoflurane. More sophisticated cognitive testing as early as 6 h after extubation have also shown no differences between the two agents.

Use of Neuromuscular Blockers and Reversal Agents in Aged Patient

Although initiation of neuromuscular blockade may well be necessary for tracheal intubation, maintenance of the blockade during surgery largely depends on the surgical need for relaxation. If neuromuscular blockade is used during the maintenance of anesthesia, and immediate extubation is planned, then the risks associated with inadvertent residual neuromuscular blockade become an issue. In many cases, adequate surgical relaxation can be attained with inhalational anesthetics and opioids.

A variety of factors related to aging may affect the action of neuromuscular blocking agents. These include anatomical and physiological changes, from the structure of the neuromuscular junction to cortical coordination of voluntary movements, changes in body composition, cardiovascular performance, drug clearance, and also numerous diseases.

With aging, the neuromuscular junction undergoes mostly degenerative change. The distance between the preterminal axon and the motor end plate (synaptic cleft) widens, thus increasing the diffusion time for acetylcholine molecules to traverse the cleft and bind to the postjunctional receptors (Fig. 7.4). The number of acethylcholine receptors does not appear to change significantly after age of 60, however, their organization is different. NM receptors tend to be organized in groups. With age, there may be more groups, but the number of receptors per group decreases. There is also a flattening of the folds and lengthening of the end plate. Also, an increase in the number of preterminal axons occurs, with more of them connected to a single end plate. Despite these changes, there is no evidence that the speed or completeness of neuromuscular transmission suffers any functional impairment in advanced age.

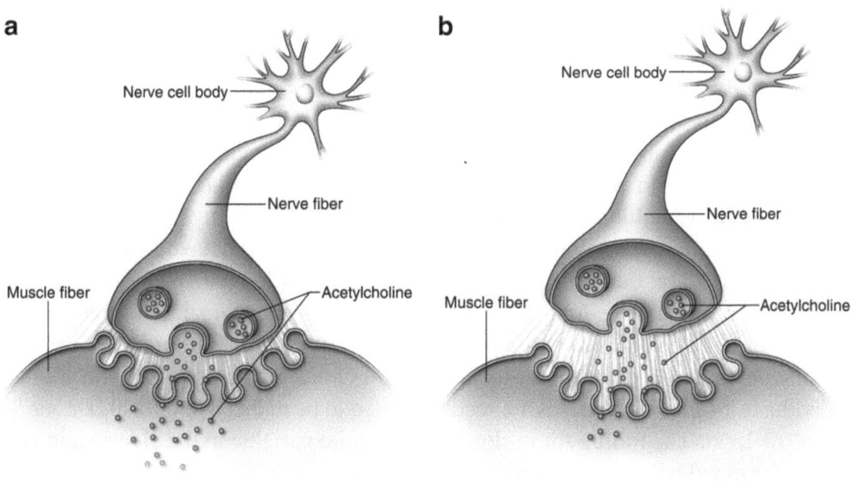

Fig. 7.4 Normal neuromuscular junction of younger person (**a**) versus that of elderly individual (**b**): Synaptic cleft is widened, end plate folds are flattened, smaller conglomerates of acetylcholine receptors (Used with permission from Muscular Dystrophy Association)

Aged muscles demonstrate a modest degree of denervation and proliferation of extrajunctional acetylcholine receptors, such as observed in disuse atrophy. There is also a reduction in the number of motor neurons in the spinal cord and ventral root fibers. These changes, however, have not been shown to cause either increased resistance or sensitivity to muscle relaxants, particularly to succinylcholine, in elderly patients.

Succinylcholine dosing for 95% neuromuscular block does not appear to change with age, despite the decrease in water content and lean body mass, and the increase in fat, and the decrease in the initial volume of distribution. Prolonged duration of action/prolonged recovery times have been observed in the elderly as well. Although it is commonly thought that succinylcholine-induced fasciculations are less severe in the elderly, such a difference has not been documented.

For most intermediate and long-acting nondepolarizing muscle relaxants, the time to block onset lengthens with age (Table 7.1). For *rocuronium* and *cisatracurium*, for example, onset delays of 36–60 s and 45–60 s, respectively, have been demonstrated. Failure to take these delays into account may prompt the caregiver to incorrectly assume that the administered dose was too small, and therefore give additional agent, thereby ending up with a duration of blockade much longer than desired.

Duration of action and recovery are affected by age, but in different ways and to different degrees for the commonly used nondepolarizing neuromuscular blocking agents. Mivacurium, although rarely used, is the only nondepolarizer with a short duration of action due to its metabolism by plasma cholinesterase. Metabolism, and therefore recovery time, is prolonged by ~30% in elderly patients. Consequently, it is recommended that the intubation dose be decreased to 100 mcg/kg, recognizing that the time to achieve an intubation-quality block will be 3–7 min (1.5 min later than for a younger population receiving a larger dose). Decrease in plasma cholinesterase activity, common in advanced age, prolongs the duration of action of mivacurium by 15–20% (normally 14–28 min). 25–75% recovery time is on average 5 min longer than in a nongeriatric population. Maintenance dosage is recommended to be about 25–35 mcg/kg, and re-dose timing should be guided by train-of-four testing.

Vecuronium is eliminated primarily by direct excretion into the bile, with only 25–30% excreted in the urine. Vecuronium provides remarkably stable hemodynamic conditions in patients with significant cardiovascular disease, including congestive heart failure. The intubation dose of 0.08–0.1 mg/kg is supposed to produce intubation conditions in 2.5–3 min, which may be delayed by ~1.5 min in older patients. The duration of action is similarly prolonged, with some elderly subjects exhibiting very long recovery times. Recovery from just initial dose of 0.1 mg/kg has been shown to be prolonged to ~50 versus 35 min in nongeriatric population. In one study, recovery took three times longer in comparison with younger individuals. Maintenance doses are recommended to be reduced to 0.01–0.008 mg/kg (30–40% less). The timing for re-dose may be quite variable in the elderly and so is best determined by clinical criteria and use of the twitch monitor.

Rocuronium is another intermediate-acting agent with increasing popularity. Metabolism is primarily hepatic, but clearance of rocuronium is also decreased and duration time is prolonged in patients with renal failure. As with vecuronium, onset

Table 7.1 Estimated intubation and maintenance dosages and onset and duration times for elderly patients in comparison to young adults

	Young patient (18–65 years old)				Elderly (65–90 years old)			
Neuromuscular blockers	Intub. dose (mg/kg)	Onset time (min)	Duration (min)	Maint. dose (mg/kg)	Intub. dose (mg/kg)	Onset time (min)	Duration (min)	Maint. dose (mg/kg)
Succinylcholine	0.5–1	0.3–1.1	4–6	0.01–0.07	0.5–1	1–1.5	4–6	0.01–0.07
Rocuronium	0.1–06	1–2 (0.4–6)	31 (15–85)	0.1–02	0.05–0.4	3 (1.3–11)	35–46	0.08–0.1
Vecuronium	0.02–0.06	2.5–3	25–40	0.01–0.015	0.01–0.04	4–5.5	35–137	0.01–0.008
Pancuronium	0.02–0.1	2–3	60–180	0.01–0.02	0.01–0.05	4–5	180–220	0.005–0.008
Cis-atracurium	0.05–0.2	2–3	40–60	0.03–0.04	0.05–0.2	2.5–3.5	45–55	0.03–0.04
Atracurium	0.2–0.5	2.5–3	20–45	0.08–0.1	0.2–0.5	2.5–3.5	40–50	0.08–0.1
Doxacurium	0.01–0.03	5–6	100–160	0.005–0.01	0.005–0.03	6–8	120–180	0.005–0.1
Mivacurium	0.15	2.5–4.5	14–25	0.04–0.05	0.1	3–7	17–37	0.025–0.035

Duration time is defined as spontaneous return of T1 twitch height to 25% of control (Data used with permission from Wolters Kluwer Health; Rivera R, Antognini JF. Anesthesiology. 2009;110:1176-81, with changes)

time is longer by ~35–60 s. Clearance decreases with age by ~27%; consequently, duration of action and recovery times are prolonged by ~3–4 min. There is no difference, however, in the potency of rocuronium in the elderly and young patients. With an initial dose of 0.6 mg/kg, intubation conditions in elderly may require anywhere from 1.3 to 11 min (versus 60–75 s in young patients), and the average duration of action is about 46 min (versus 22–35 min in the young).

Atracurium, as well as its isomer cis-atracurium, depends to a large extent on temperature-dependent, spontaneous Hoffman degradation for its elimination. As such, its metabolism is largely unaffected by age, with only a 15% increase in the elimination half-life. Except for some delay in onset time (45–60 s for cis-atracurium), duration of action and recovery time are almost identical to nongeriatric subjects. No differences in dosage requirements in elderly patients have been found to date. The recommended initial doses of 0.15 mg/kg for cis-atracurium and 0.4–0.5 mg/kg for atracurium provide good intubation conditions in 120–180 s. Maintenance doses of 0.03 and 0.08–0.1 mg/kg, respectively, have an approximate duration of action of 45–55 min. Both drugs possess excellent hemodynamic stability, even elderly patients with poor cardiac function.

Elimination of all long-acting neuromuscular blocking agents is primarily dependent on the kidney: 85% for pancuronium bromide and 90–98% for pipecuronium, doxacurium, and metocurine. With the age-related decline in renal function, the pharmacodynamics of these long-acting agents is significantly affected (Table 7.1). For all these compounds, onset is delayed, the duration of action is increased (by 40–50%, which comprises up to 180–220 min, for pancuronium), and recovery times are significantly prolonged (by 60% for pancuronium). The use of long-acting agents is associated with an increased need for prolonged postoperative ventilation, an increased incidence of pulmonary complications, and higher tracheostomy rates. If at all possible, long-acting muscle relaxants should be avoided in elderly patients.

Age-related changes in the pharmacology of anticholinesterases are similar to that of nondepolarizing muscle relaxants. However, the dose of the anticholinesterase required to antagonize neuromuscular blockade may be greater than the dose in younger patients. For example, the dose of neostigmine required to reverse vecuronium-induced blockade was found to be 39% greater in young adults (~60–70 versus 40–50 mcg/kg in older patients). Neostigmine duration of action and elimination half-life are prolonged with age, which is potentially advantageous in elderly patients because of the likelihood that the duration of the neuromuscular blocking agent will also be prolonged. Sugammadex, the novel selective relaxant-binding agent, in bolus doses 2 mg/kg have been demonstrated to be safe and effective in rapid reversal of rocuronium, and recovery was only slightly faster in patients younger than 65 years of age.

Key Points

- Doses of most intravenous induction agents are reduced in elderly due to changes in pharmacokinetics and/or pharmacodynamics.

- Elderly are susceptible to wide hemodynamic swings during the induction of anesthesia. Slow and careful titration along with dose adjustment is helpful in prevention of hemodynamic instability.
- Midazolam may cause cognitive impairment in elderly, and it should be used with caution.
- Ketamine use is not recommended in the elderly, except in small doses as a sedative–analgesic.
- Minimal Alveolar Concentration of isoflurane, sevoflurane, and desflurane decreases with age, with considerable acceleration after approximately age 50. MAC may be estimated from published nomograms.
- Elderly patients are much more likely to suffer hemodynamic instability with any anesthetic, including inhalational anesthetics.
- Isoflurane provides generally less favorable hemodynamic conditions than sevoflurance or desflurane and produces the longest recovery times.
- Sevoflurane and desflurane are similar in terms of hemodynamic stability. However, desflurane may cause tachycardia and transient hypertension if its concentration is rapidly increased.
- Desflurane provides the shortest recovery times but does not appear to improve cognitive function in comparison to sevoflurane.
- Isoflurane, sevoflurane, and desflurane demonstrate no measurable nephrotoxicity.
- Use of nitrous oxide may be associated with substantial myocardial depression and increased incidence of perioperative cardiac morbidity and mortality. Consideration should therefore be given to avoidance of nitrous oxide in elderly patients.
- Pharmacology of succinylcholine is apparently unaffected by age-related physiological changes. No dose adjustment is required.
- Intermediate-acting agents vecuronium and rocuronium have delayed onset, prolonged duration of action and recovery times in elderly. Doses of both compounds should be decreased, and titration to effect is mandatory.
- Duration of action and recovery times of atracurium and cis-atracurium are practically identical to a young population. No significant dose adjustment is necessary beyond individual variability.
- Long-acting neuromuscular blockers are best avoided in elderly patients.
- The dose of neostigmine may need to be increased for at least vecuronium-produced neuromuscular blockade.

Suggested Reading

Arain SR, Kern S, Ficke DJ, Ebert TJ. Variability of duration of action of neuromuscular blocking drugs in elderly patients. Acta Anesthesiol Scand. 2005 Mar;49(3):312–5.

Chen X, et al. The recovery of cognitive function after general anesthesia in elderly patients: a comparison of desflurane and sevoflurane. Anesth Analg. 2001;93:1489–94.

Cope TM, Hunter JM. Selecting neuromuscular-blocking drugs for elderly patients. Drugs Aging. 2003;20(2):125–40.

Eger EI. Age, minimum alveolar anesthetic concentration, and minimum alveolar anesthetic concentration-awake. Anesth Analg. 2001;93:947–53.

Haynes GR. Inhalational anesthetics. In: Silverstein JH, Rooke GA, Reves JG, Macleskey CH. Geriatric anesthesiology, 2008, Springer, pp246–65.

Hogg RMG, Mirahur RK. Reversal of neuromuscular blockade: current concepts and Future developments. J Anaesth Clin Pharmacol. 2009;25(4):403–12.

Hutchison LC, O'Brien CE. Changes in Pharmacokinetics and Pharmacodynamics in the Elderly Patient. Journal of Pharmacy Practice. 2007;20(1):4–12.

Lien CA, Suzuki T. Relaxants and their reversal agents. In: Silverstein JH, Rooke GA, Reves JG, Macleskey CH. Geriatric anesthesiology. New York: Springer; 2008:266–77.

Macario A, Dexter F, Lubarsky D. Meta-analysis of trials comparing postoperative recoveryafter anesthesia with sevoflurane and desflurane. Am J Health-Syst Pharm. Jan 1, 2005;62:63–7.

Myles PS, Leslie K, Peyton P, et al. Nitrous oxide and perioperative cardiac morbidity (ENIGMA-II) Trial: rationale and design. Am Heart J. 2009 Mar;157:488-94.e1.

Nickalls RWD, Mapleson WW. Age-related iso-MAC charts for isoflurane, sevoflurane and desflurane in man. British J Anesth. 2003;91(2):170–4.

Ornstein E, et al. Pharmacodynamics and pharmacokinetics of Cisatracurium in geriatric surgical patients. Anesth. 1996 March;84(3):520–25.

Priebe HJ. The aged cardiovascular risk patient. British journal of anesthesia. 2000;85(5):763–78.

Rivera R, Antognini JF. Perioperative drug therapy in elderly patients. Anesthesiology. 2009;110:1176–81.

Sadean MR, Glass PS. Best Pract Res ClinAnaesthesiol. 2003;17(2):191–205.

Shafer SL. The pharmacology of anesthetic drugs in elderly patients. Anesthesiology Clinics of North America. 2000;18(1):1–29.

Turnheim K. When drug therapy gets old:pharmacokinetics and pharmacodynamics in the elderly. Experimental gerontology. 2003;38(8):843–53.

Vuyk J. Pharmacodynamics in the elderly. Best Practice & Research Clinical Anaesthesiology. 2003;17(2):207–18.

Chapter 8
Regional Anesthesia and Joint Replacement Surgery

Jacques E. Chelly, Anna Uskova, Qing Liu, Richa Wardhan, and Uchenna O. Umeh

Introduction

As the population ages there is an increase in demand for anesthetic regimens that provide a safe and positive outcome for the very elderly patient. Regional anesthesia offers many advantages to older patients especially with respect to postoperative pain relief and the immediate recovery from surgery. This chapter will address some of the important issues regarding the use of regional anesthesia in very elderly patients.

J.E. Chelly, MD, PhD, MBA (✉)
University of Pittsburgh Medical Center Shadyside-Presbyterian Hospitals, Posner Pain Center, Aiken Medical Building, 532 South Aiken Avenue, Suite 407, Pittsburgh, PA 15232, USA
e-mail: chelje@anes.upmc.edu

A. Uskova, MD
Department of Anesthesiology, Shadyside Presbyterian University of Pittsburgh Medical center, 5230 Center Avenue, Suite#205, Pittsburgh, PA 15206, USA

Q. Liu, MD, PhD
Department of Anesthesiology, UPMC Presbyterian-Montefior Hospital, 3550 Terrace Street, A1305 Scaife Hall, Pittsburgh, PA 15261, USA

R. Wardhan, MD
Department of Anesthesiology, Yale New Haven Hospital, 333 Cedar Street, New Haven, CT 06511, USA

U.O. Umeh, MD
Department of Anesthesiology, New York University Hospital for Joint Diseases, 301 East 17th Street, New York, NY 10003, USA

S.R. Barnett (ed.), *Manual of Geriatric Anesthesia*, DOI 10.1007/978-1-4614-3888-5_8,

Age-Related Physiologic Changes and the Impact of Regional Anesthesia

It is well established that aging is associated with many physiologic changes that may play an important role in the patient's outcome (Table 8.1). These changes may also impact upon the administration and utilization of regional anesthesia techniques. Although the mechanisms controlling the rate of aging are still poorly understood, it is recognized that basic organ function declines around 1% per year after the age of 30. With this decline there is also a concomitant decline in the body's responsiveness to stress.

Cardiovascular changes are probably one of the most important when considering the use of a regional technique in an older patient. A regional technique may alter the cardiovascular response to stress, and this may have negative effects in an elderly patient with reduced physiologic reserve. For example, a spinal or epidural anesthetic may be associated with hypotension that in a young patient may be insignificant but in an older patient with underlying cardiac ischemia or valvular disease can lead to an adverse event.

In brief, aging is associated with a decrease in the vessel and heart compliance leading to eventual systolic hypertension with or without diastolic hypertension, decreased myocardial function and cardiac output, and a decrease in the baroreceptor function. The parasympathetic nervous system dominates, and autonomic nervous system dysfunction occurs. Consequently, elderly patients have a decreased maximum heart rate and a blunted ability to increase cardiac output during times of stress. They become more preload dependent and also exhibit less of a chronotropic response to catecholamines, making them less likely to compensate by an increase in heart rate in the case of hypotension. When hypotensive, the older person may thus be less likely to maintain autoregulation of tissue perfusion at the level of the brain, the heart, and the kidney. These deleterious consequences associated with aging are confounded by the fact that elderly patients may present for anesthesia and surgery hypovolemic and anemic. These factors make the maintenance of hemodynamic stability even more challenging for anesthesiologists. Hypotension is not uncommon after performing regional anesthesia techniques such as neuraxial and lumbar plexus blocks. For the reasons described above, the older patient may not be able to compensate rapidly, and this can lead to a significant drop in cardiac output, heart failure, and myocardial ischemia or even infarction as well as low perfusion of other vital organs such as the brain, the kidney, and the intestine. The use of regional techniques for anesthesia can provide benefits such as reduced blood loss and a reduction in the occurrence of thromboemboli. Regional anesthesia may reduce the need for opioids in the postoperative period and thus avoid their related complications. However it must be emphasized that the benefit of regional anesthesia is only realized when hemodynamic stability is strictly maintained.

Table 8.1 Physiologic changes associated with aging and the consequences of regional anesthesia

Physiologic changes	Effect of regional anesthetic	Implications
Cardiovascular		
Parasympathetic dominance	Sympathectomy resulting in hypotension secondary to decreased SVR, inability to compensate with tachycardia	Lower dose of local anesthetic in both spinal and epidural techniques
Stiff myocardium and vasculature	Rhythm disturbances with accidental intravascular injections of local anesthetic	Cautious rehydration
Preload dependence		Consideration for use of paravertebral nerve block in place of epidural where possible
Chronotropic response decreased		Normal precautions, use of ultrasound, frequent aspiration during dosing
Higher prevalence of dysrhythmias		
Respiratory		
Decreased vital capacity, increased residual volume, increased FRC (loss in elasticity)	High spinal causing respiratory compromise and possible GA	Lower dose for spinal anesthesia
Closing capacity exceeds FRC	Unilateral diaphragmatic palsy secondary to phrenic nerve block	Avoid interscalene nerve block in high-risk patients, use ultrasound to decrease volume of local anesthetic and decrease risk of phrenic nerve palsy
		Paravertebral blocks and epidurals to help prevent postoperative respiratory failure from inadequate analgesia or opioid consumption
Neurologic—CNS		
Increased incidence of all-cause dementia	Hypotension and decreased cardiac reserve secondary to epidural/spinal anesthesia	Lower dose in neuraxial techniques
Increased required cerebral perfusion pressure (CPP)	Decreased CPP	Consider vasopressors where necessary to preserve CPP
Decreased MAC, increased sensitivity to sedation	Increased risk of respiratory failure and confusion from over sedation	Decrease sedation during preoperative nerve block and intraoperative sedation
Increased incidence of spinal stenosis and decreased epidural fat		

(continued)

Table 8.1 (continued)

Physiologic changes	Effect of regional anesthetic	Implications
Neurologic—PNS		
Increased incidence of neuropathy	Faster onset of peripheral nerve blocks	Lower dose of local anesthetic
Decreased myelinated nerve fibers, decreased conduction velocity	Prolonged blockade and increased sensitivity to local anesthetics Increased risk for weakness and risk for falls	Frequent neurologic exams, good communication with physical therapy team to decrease risk of falls secondary to motor blockade
Kidney		
Decreased GFR	Decreased clearance of drugs	Decrease sedation
Liver		
Decreased liver mass	Rarely affects metabolism in elderly without liver disease	Consider lower doses in drugs with hepatic metabolism in patients with liver disease and malnutrition
Decreased plasma cholinesterase levels	Decreased drug binding/ increased free drug levels	
Decreased albumin levels in elderly with poor nutrition		

Regional Anesthesia and Surgical Stress

Other factors that could significantly affect the outcome of the elderly patient during the perioperative period are the consequence and magnitude of associated pain and surgical stress. In this respect, regional anesthesia and especially epidural techniques have been shown to prevent the development of the stress response associated with pain. Similar beneficial effects have not been observed by the use of opioids alone. Epidural anesthesia has also been shown to blunt the hormonal stress-related response. This may lead to better control of perioperative glycemia and a blunted steroid and catecholamine release from the adrenal gland.

Pharmacodynamic and Pharmacokinetic Consequences of Aging

The pharmacokinetic and pharmacodynamics of many drugs including local anesthetics are significantly affected by aging. Clinically a longer duration of sensory and motor block following a brachial plexus block has been observed in those older than 70 versus those of a younger age group. The same observation is true in the case of neuraxial techniques. Although the mechanism is not established, it is clear that there are several factors that contribute to the observed prolongation of a block in the elderly:

1. A decrease in peripheral circulation and blood flow associated with aging leading to delayed systemic reabsorption of the local anesthetic resulting in an increase in the amount of local anesthetics available at the receptor sites.
2. The degeneration of the neuronal function, for example, in patients with peripheral neuropathy. This leads to a decrease in the number of receptors at the effector site able to bind the local anesthetics. This also indirectly increases the relative concentration of the drug at the receptor site.
3. In the case of neuraxial techniques, the degeneration of the connective tissues, reduced epidural fat, and a reduction in the volume of distribution of the local anesthetic mixture injected intrathecally. Spinal stenosis in the elderly occurs commonly and also contributes to the prolongation of the block. Overall the age-related changes lead to a shorter onset, a higher level of block achieved, and a longer duration of epidural anesthesia.
4. Aging is associated with a decrease in the number of nerve fibers, and the conduction velocity in motor and sensory fibers is lower. There is also an age-related decrease in the number of myelinated nerve fibers, leading to an increase in the speed in which local anesthetics penetrate the nerve sheaths.

Local Anesthetic Metabolism

Local anesthetics are metabolized by the liver, and their elimination is dependent on a high clearance mechanism. Although aging is associated with a reduction of the size of the liver, it is unlikely that a decrease in the local anesthetic metabolism plays a role in the prolongation of the duration of a block observed in the elderly. However poor nutrition, common in older patients, may be associated with a decrease in albumin level, thus affecting the drug binding of medications administered.

Practical Implications of Regional Anesthesia

The choice of the regional technique will depend on the type of surgery. Acceptable regional techniques include epidural or paravertebral nerve blocks for abdominal, pelvic, and thoracic procedures and the use of peripheral nerve blocks (PNBs) for upper and lower extremity surgery. These techniques not only allow for the preservation of respiratory function by avoiding the need for management of the airway and the use of mechanical ventilation but also have been demonstrated to provide excellent perioperative analgesia, decreasing the need for opioids and the related side effects. In addition, in certain instances, greater hemodynamic stability has been observed especially in the case of peripheral nerve and paravertebral blocks.

Paravertebral nerve blocks have a wide range of indications and a low incidence of complications when properly placed. Epidural blocks provide excellent analgesia; however, their use is frequently associated with hypotension that may compromise the perioperative outcome in the elderly. In the recovery period hypotensive episodes frequently lead to premature discontinuation of an epidural infusion. This can create a vicious cycle of recurring inadequate analgesia, an increased need for parental opioids, and a renewed stress response. In addition the use of epidural catheters creates a special challenge when it is time to discontinue the infusion as any anticoagulants must be briefly discontinued. There appears to be a higher risk of developing an epidural hematoma in patients receiving thromboprophylaxis.

Benefits of Regional Anesthesia in the Elderly

Epidural anesthesia has been inconsistently shown to block the stress response as measured through cortisol and other biomarkers of stress intraoperatively. However postoperative epidural analgesia has been more consistently observed to produce positive benefits for patients. Patients undergoing thoracotomy and upper abdominal surgery appear to benefit the most from postoperative epidural analgesia. This is most likely due to the improved respiratory mechanic and function postoperatively. Other reported advantages for regional anesthesia during the postoperative period include reduced opioid use, earlier mobilization, and quicker time to discharge. Early patient mobilization has been shown to be a determinant factor of a patient's immediate outcome. Decreased mobilization leads to an increased risk of deep venous thrombosis (DVT), pressure ulcers, and infection. In an older patient with a potentially compromised immune system, pneumonia, delirium, confusion, and cognitive dysfunction may result. For vulnerable elderly patients, earlier ambulation and increased interaction with staff and other patients, particularly in physical therapy, can lead to significant improvements and an earlier recuperation.

Indication of Regional Anesthesia in the Elderly

Regional anesthesia/analgesia in the elderly population may be indicated either for anesthesia or perioperative analgesia. Regional anesthesia can benefit the elderly following multiple surgeries including general, thoracic, gynecologic, urologic, vascular, orthopedics, and surgeries related to trauma. These surgeries reflect the growing burden of elderly-related medical problems such as heart disease, cancer, arthritis, and osteoporosis. Heart disease is the leading cause of mortality, while arthritis is the leading cause of disability and morbidity.

Orthopedic Surgery and Lower Extremity Joint Replacement

Orthopedic surgery and joint replacements in particular are some of the most commonly performed surgeries in the elderly population. Eighty percent of the geriatric population have musculoskeletal complaints requiring a physician encounter and some form of treatment. It is estimated that ~68% of total hip arthroplasty (THA) and 74% of total knee replacement (TKR) are performed on people over the age of 65 years. With the current growth of the elderly population, it is estimated that the number of joint replacements will increase from 500,000 to around 3.5 million in 2030. Although age alone is not a barrier to hip and knee arthroplasty surgery, the postoperative outcome is correlated with preoperative comorbidities. Regional anesthesia can be beneficial in this population.

Preoperative Evaluation

The preoperative assessment for older patients scheduled to undergo THA or TKR is an important part of the anesthesia management plan. The preoperative evaluation establishes the comorbidities and risk assessment profile. A complete history, physical examination, laboratory examinations, and an assessment of the surgical risks should be included. The next section highlights important issues surrounding the preoperative assessment in the older orthopedic patient.

Cardiovascular Issues

A practice guideline for perioperative cardiovascular evaluation for noncardiac surgery has been established by the American College of Cardiology and American Heart Association Task Force. Using this guideline, patients are assessed through a stepwise approach according to clinical predictors, the risk of the proposed operation, and the patient's functional capacity.

Thromboembolic Issues

It has been reported that 60% of the hospitalized patients who have undergone joint arthroplasty develop venographically detectable DVT. It is widely accepted that pharmacologic thromboprophylaxis should be used for joint replacement procedures in the elderly; however, the choice of prophylaxis remains a subject of continued controversy. The current American College of Chest Physicians (ACCP) Consensus Conference on Antithrombotic Therapy recommends the following for older surgical patients:

- Total hip replacement: postoperative low molecular weight heparins (LMWH) should be given every 12 h, low-intensity warfarin therapy (to keep international normalized ratio of 2–3) should be initiated preoperatively or immediately postoperatively.
- TKR: postoperative LMWH should be given every 12 h. Intermittent pneumatic compression (IPC) is the most effective nonpharmacologic regimen and is comparable to LMWH. Low-intensity warfarin can also be used.
- Hip fracture repair: fixed-dose fondaparinux should be started preoperatively.

There is an increased risk of bleeding complications in patients treated with anticoagulants, especially in patients with concomitant conditions such as diabetes, renal impairment, and cardiovascular disease. The patient's creatinine clearance and age should be taken into account when dosing older patients as both of these affect the drug elimination and pharmacokinetics of anticoagulants, such as fondaparinux and LMWH.

Pain and Functional Status

It is not uncommon to find elderly joint replacement patients to be chronically exposed to narcotics prior to surgery. Since long-term narcotic exposure decreases the patient's overall pain threshold, the demand for the use of narcotics to manage postoperative pain is significantly higher in this patient population. This can make pain control challenging in the perioperative period. Preoperative functional status is one of the most important predictors of outcome in the elderly patient. The ability of the patient to mobilize postoperatively will in part depend on muscle strength prior to surgery.

Infection

Deep periprosthetic infection is one of the leading causes of reoperation after joint arthroplasty. Management of the infection relies heavily on prevention. Prophylactic antibiotics given within 1 h of skin incision and continued for 24 h after surgery have greatly reduced the incidence of infection in primary joint replacements to 1–4%.

Intraoperative Anesthesia Management

Joint arthroplasty procedures can be performed either under general anesthesia (GA) or regional anesthesia (RA). Regional anesthesia techniques include neuraxial block and PNB. Many studies have been conducted to compare the postoperative outcomes associated with the two anesthetic techniques for hip or knee replacement surgeries. A recent meta-analysis of ten independent trials, which compared neuraxial block with general anesthesia for total hip replacement, reported that total hip replacement under neuraxial block has a lower incidence of blood transfusion, DVT, and thromboembolic events than those under general anesthesia. Neuraxial block can also reduce the operative time by 7 min/case and intraoperative blood loss by 275 mL/case. Other suggested benefits of neuraxial block compared to GA include a decreased alteration in a patient's cardiopulmonary condition and less cognitive impairment. However this is controversial, and furthermore most of this data was derived from studies on total hip replacement. Further studies need to be done to truly delineate the benefits of RA versus GA in joint replacement surgery.

Prior to administering a neuraxial block for joint replacement procedures, it is important to review potential contraindications. These include patient refusal, infection at the site of injection, coagulopathy (acquired, induced, genetic), severe hypovolemia, increased intracranial pressure (i.e., brain tumor or recent head injury), severe valvular diseases (i.e., aortic stenosis, mitral stenosis), severe uncorrected anemia, and an allergy to local anesthetics.

When using a regional technique, consideration should be given to the level of sedation required. The choice of the anesthesia technique may also be dependent upon the preference of the surgeon and, more importantly, surgical time. Although short surgical times (20–45 min) present an opportunity to maximize the benefits of regional anesthesia, in some cases, 4–6 h are still required when performing a joint replacement. In these cases the use of regional anesthesia may be difficult to implement, making the combination of general anesthesia and an epidural a potential alternative. In this situation the use of regional anesthesia is associated with a reduction of perioperative blood loss and therefore the need for perioperative transfusion.

Postoperative Pain Management and Care

Pain management following THA or TKA is a major challenge. 50% of THA patients and 60% of TKA patients experience severe pain. If not appropriately managed, such pain can delay the start of physical therapy and be a factor limiting the success of rehabilitation. Traditionally, patient-controlled analgesia (PCA) and epidural analgesia used with local anesthetics and opioids have been used to provide postoperative pain relief. Unfortunately, the use of opioids in the elderly has been associated with significant side effects. More recently, PNBs, when used as part of a multimodal approach, have been advocated. Single-injection and continuous PNBs are efficacious adjuncts optimizing patient outcome, satisfaction, and rehabilitation while minimizing complications and reducing costs and length of hospital stay. Plus, they can be safely used in elderly patients with significant comorbidities, specifically those with cardiopulmonary disease and obesity.

PNBs for lower extremity surgeries include lumbar plexus (LP) blocks, femoral nerve blocks, and sciatic nerve blocks. Continuous LP blocks, together with a single injection of sciatic nerve block, may provide adequate postoperative analgesia for THA, while continuous femoral and sciatic nerve blocks are indicated for TKA.

The true benefits of the PNB emerge when these procedures are compared with traditional spinal or epidural analgesia and PCA methods. PNB techniques reduce postoperative nausea and vomiting and are not associated with urinary retention that often manifest in those patients who receive neuraxial blocks and other standard analgesic techniques. Lower extremity nerve blocks can be safely used in patients who receive anticoagulation therapy, which is known to increase the risk of hematoma formation in patients undergoing spinal anesthesia. This is particularly beneficial for geriatric patients, who are frequently anticoagulated pre- and postoperatively. Moreover, PNBs reduce opioid requirements and blood loss after THA and TKA.

Besides the intrinsic risk of local anesthetic toxicity and nerve injury associated with the performance of PNB, LP blocks carry a risk of retroperitoneal hematoma. This is a rare complication, but it is important to recognize that hip and knee replacement and the use of anticoagulants can lead to retroperitoneal hematoma. In patients undergoing total hip and knee replacement, sciatic nerve injuries represent an important complication. The cause of the injury is sometimes difficult to determine, especially when a sciatic nerve block is performed. Sciatic nerve block and/or surgery also causes self-limiting dysesthesias usually responsive to gabapentin or pregabalin. The risks associated with the performance of a femoral nerve block are considered to be of less consequence. However, femoral nerve injury can occur not only because of the performance of a femoral block but also because of a tourniquet.

The benefits of PNBs have been proven to be complemented by the use of cyclooxygenase 2 (COX-2) inhibitors and nonsteroidal anti-inflammatory drugs (NSAIDS). In the elderly patient, special consideration should be given to the bleeding, cardiac, and renal consequences of their administrations. This approach has been proven to reduce the need for postoperative opioids by over 70%. During surgery, the use of a small dose of ketamine (0.1 mg/kg IV) has also been used to reduce postoperative pain and opioid consumption.

Early functional recovery is an important determinant of the long-term functional recovery of patients undergoing total joint replacement. Unfortunately, as patients become more mobile, there is an increased risk for falls. Some reports claim that the use of nerve blocks increases the risk of fall following joint replacement; however, it is important to recognize that falls following joint replacement occur independently of the performance of a block. The etiology of a fall is usually multifactorial. Important contributors include advanced age, the administration of sedatives, cardiac arrhythmia, etc. The prevention of falls, especially in the elderly, is complex and requires considerable education and resources.

Patients who have THA and TKA attain improved mobility and significant improvements in quality of life, with postoperative quality of life often equal to or exceeding the population norm. This translates into retained independence and self-care and decreased health care costs. THA and TKA surgeries are among the most successful interventions available to the geriatric population, as measured by the Medical Outcomes Study 36-Item Short-Form Health Survey (SF-36) in terms of improvement in quality-of-life years gained. Appropriate perioperative anesthetic management of these patients should minimize the risk of developing devastating complications associated with surgical procedures, reassuring excellent outcomes in patients exposed to joint arthroplasty.

Orthopedic Trauma

Hip, wrist, and multiple rib fractures represent some of the most important indications for the use of regional technique following trauma. Evidence supports the concept that the morbidity and mortality associated with trauma can be decreased by early mobilization, maintenance of cognitive function, and maintenance of hemodynamic stability. This can be achieved with the use of regional anesthesia for anesthesia and aggressive perioperative management of pain. The use of neuraxial blocks have long been advocated in the case of hip fractures whereas the use of PNB can be valuable for the repair of wrist fractures. However in the past few years, perioperative thromboprophylaxis such as with LMWH has become more common, limiting the use of spinal and epidural techniques. Consequently peripheral and paravertebral blocks are becoming increasingly popular for perioperative pain management. Rib fracture pain can lead to significant respiratory consequences and various regional techniques have been used to manage pain in patients with rib fractures. These include intercostal nerve block, epidural analgesia, and intrapleural and paravertebral nerve blocks. Regional techniques like these should be considered as a first-line treatment for the management of pain in patients with severe blunt thoracic trauma. In patients older than 65 years with greater than four rib fractures, these techniques have been shown to reduce mortality. In addition, the use of regional decreases the need for parental opioids and their associated side effects.

Conclusion

As more elderly and very elderly patients are present for surgery, the use of regional techniques is becoming increasingly recognized as an important alternative to traditional general anesthesia.

Key Points

- Age alone should not be considered as a contraindication to a regional anesthesia technique for surgery or post operative pain.
- The use of Regional anesthesia may lead to a reduction in stress response associated with surgery.

- Hemodynamic stability can be challenging to maintain with certain regional techniques in older patients.
- Regional anesthesia can be very beneficial in patient undergoing joint replacement.
- The use of regional anesthesia can be associated with earlier mobilization and better postoperative outcomes in older patients.
- The use of regional techniques for postoperative pain management can lead to a reduction in perioperative opioid consumption.
- Age-related changes in physiology and anatomy lead to a reduction in local anesthesia requirement in the aged patient.

Suggested Reading

Ben-Ari A, Moreno M, Chelly JE, Bigeleisen PE. Ultrasound-guided paravertebral block using an intercostal approach. Anesth Analg. 2009 Nov; 109(5):1691–4.

Ben-David B, Frankel R, Arzumonov T, Marchevsky Y, Volpin G. Minidose bupivacaine-fentanyl spinal anesthesia for surgical repair of hip fracture in the aged. Anesthesiology. 2000 Jan; 92(1):6–10.

Burns DA, Ben-David B, Chelly JE, Greensmith JE. Intercostally placed paravertebral catheterization: an alternative approach to continuous paravertebral blockade. Anesth Analg. 2008 Jul; 107(1):339–41.

Buvanendran A, Tuman KJ, McCoy DD, Matusic B, Chelly JE. Anesthetic techniques for minimally invasive total knee arthroplasty. J Knee Surg. 2006 Apr; 19(2):133–6.

Chelly JE, Greger J, Gebhard R, Coupe K, Clyburn TA, Buckle R, Criswell A. Continuous femoral blocks improve recovery and outcome of patients undergoing total knee arthroplasty. J Arthroplasty. 2001 Jun; 16(4):436–45.

Macfarlane AJ, Prasad GA, Chan VW, Brull R. Does regional anaesthesia improve outcome after total hip arthroplasty? A systematic review.Br J Anaesth. 2009 Sep; 103(3):335–45.

Marino J, Russo J, Herenstein R, Kenny M, Chelly JE. Continuous psoas compartment block vs. continuous femoral block or PCA for total hip arthroplasty. J Bone Joint Surg Am. 2009; 91: 29–37.

Matot I, Oppenheim-Eden A, Ratrot R, Baranova J, Davidson E, Eylon S, Peyser A, Liebergall M. Preoperative cardiac events in elderly patients with hip fracture randomized to epidural or conventional analgesia. Anesthesiology. 2003 Jan; 98(1):156–63.

Mears DC, Mears SC, Chelly JE, Dai F, Vulakovich KL. THA with a minimally invasive technique, multi-modal anesthesia, and home rehabilitation: Factors associated with early discharge? Clin Orthop Relat Res, 2009; 467:1412–7.

Motamed S, Klubien K, Edwardes M, Mazza L, Carli F. Metabolic changes during recovery in normothermic versus hypothermic patients undergoing surgery and receiving general anesthesia and epidural local anesthetic agents. Anesthesiology. 1998 May; 88(5):1211–8.

Newman S, Stygall J, Hirani S, Shaefi S, Maze M. Postoperative cognitive dysfunction after noncardiac surgery: a systematic review. Anesthesiology. 2007 Mar; 106(3):572–90.

O'Hara DA, Duff A, Berlin JA, Poses RM, Lawrence VA, Huber EC, Noveck H, Strom BL, Carson JL. The effect of anesthetic technique on postoperative outcomes in hip fracture repair. Anesthesiology. 2000 Apr; 92(4):947–57.

Paqueron X, Boccara G, Bendahou M, Coriat P, Riou B Brachial plexus nerve block exhibits prolonged duration in the elderly. Anesthesiology. 2002 Nov; 97(5):1245–9.

Silverstein JH, Timberger M, Reich DL, Uysal S. Central nervous system dysfunction after noncardiac surgery and anesthesia in the elderly. Anesthesiology. 2007 Mar; 106(3):622–8.
Stevens RD, Van Gessel E, Flory N, Fournier R, Gamulin Z.Lumbar plexus block reduces pain and blood loss associated with total hip arthroplasty. Anesthesiology. 2000 Jul; 93(1):115–21.
Urwin SC, Parker MJ, Griffiths R. General versus regional anaesthesia for hip fracture surgery: a meta-analysis of randomized trials. Br J Anaesth. 2000 Apr; 84(4):450–5.

Chapter 9
Fluid Management and Blood Transfusion

Gerardo Rodriguez and Keith P. Lewis

Introduction

"Fluid or no fluid?" This is a recurring question confronting anesthesiologists caring for patients in the perioperative settings. Some of the triggers for this query include preoperative fasting state, intraoperative hypotension, and postoperative oliguria. Controversy continues regarding how clinicians should assess volume status and determine end points of fluid therapy. Blood transfusion is often equally controversial, with few exceptions. Issues surrounding fluid and blood products are especially complex in the aged patient. In this chapter, fluid management and blood transfusion therapy in the context of care of the geriatric patient will be addressed.

The Aged Kidney

With increasing age, the kidney undergoes progressive deterioration in both function and structure. Medical comorbidities, in addition to genetic predisposition, may alter the acceleration of age-related renal changes. How these changes impact fluid management in the aged patient are in part predictable; however, much remains to be answered.

G. Rodriguez, MD (✉) • K.P. Lewis, RPh, MD
Department of Anesthesiology, Boston Medical Center, Boston University School of Medicine, Room 2817, 88 East Newton Street, Boston, MA 02118, USA
e-mail: Gerardo.Rodriguez@bmc.org

S.R. Barnett (ed.), *Manual of Geriatric Anesthesia*, DOI 10.1007/978-1-4614-3888-5_9,

Renal Structure

The human kidney undergoes progressive atrophy beginning the fourth decade of life. Specific renal deterioration includes a number of changes. The cortex—the renal corpuscles and renal tubules—degenerates more so than renal medulla consisting of the loops of Henle and cortical collecting ducts. The glomerular basement membrane, the major site of renal filtration, thickens with hyaline membrane deposition, leading to its eventual destruction. Renal tubule atrophy, and their reduction, is accompanied by arteriole sclerosis and mesangial-cell-mediated fibrosis with eventual nephron losses.

Renal Function

Age-related declines in renal filtration reduce overall renal reserve from acute and chronic insults, such as hemorrhagic shock and hypertension, respectively.

Renal Blood Flow

An aged kidney's ability to handle large fluid shifts is partially explained by reduction in renal blood flow (RBF). Normal RBF is ~25% of cardiac output or 1.5 L/min in a 70-kg male. RBF decreases progressively each decade of adult life. By the ninth decade of life, RBF, adjusted for body surface area (BSA), is reduced by about 50% from ~600 ml per minute per 1.73-m^2 BSA to 300 ml per minute per 1.73-m^2 BSA. Thus it is not surprising that administration of large volumes of fluid may not be handled efficiently in the aged kidney, resulting in hypervolemia, and subsequent cardiopulmonary complications.

Glomerular Filtration Rate

A broad range of changes in glomerular filtration rate (GFR) are found in the aging kidney. However for the majority of healthy geriatric patients, without significant comorbidities, one can expect a decline of ~10% from baseline GFR. Renal creatinine clearance (CrCl) is a key determinant of GFR. Associated age-related losses in muscle mass result in lower creatinine and serum creatinine that are relatively constant despite reduced GFR. In older patients it is important to be prepared to calculate the creatinine clearance, rather than rely on a single serum creatinine value which is likely to underestimate true renal function and reserve.

A number of formulas exist for CrCl calculation. An acceptable formula, despite limited applicability to extremely aged persons, to calculate CrCl in an adult is the Cockcroft–Gault equation:

$$\text{CrCl(ml / min)} = \frac{[(140 - \text{age (years)}] \times \text{Weight (kg)}}{72 - \text{serum creatinine (mg / dL)}} \times (0.85 \text{ if female}).$$

Using this formula, a Cr_{serum} of 1 mg/dl in an 80-year-old male may correlate to only 50% of creatinine clearance of a 40-year-old adult. Thus in the elderly patient, increases in Cr_{serum} likely represent significant impairment in CrCl. Renally cleared medications should be adjusted for CrCl to minimize renal impairment. GFR reduction may be hastened in the presence of comorbidities such as cardiovascular disease or diabetes.

Renal Tubular Function

The aged renal tubules have both a limited urinary concentrating ability and a greater susceptibility to acute injury. The former is demonstrated by a limited urinary acidification when the kidney is faced with an acid load. The latter is theorized to be a function of renal vascular and autocrine changes, ultimately resulting in less resistance to renal ischemia and nephrotoxicity. Eventually, as nephrons are lost with age, tubules succumb to interstitial fibrosis.

Intravascular Volume Assessment

The need for fluid therapy can be predicated on the following question: "is the tank full or empty?" That is, does the patient have adequate circulating blood volume or not? How this is determined if often complex. Fluid compartments change with age. Physical exam and lab findings may be altered or less reliable in the elderly, making the assessment of volume status more challenging. Newer hemodynamic monitors provide clinicians sophisticated approaches to determining the intravascular volume status.

Fluid Compartments and Body Composition

Total body water (TBW) is optimal at young adulthood. In the young adult male, 60% of body weight is TBW, which is divided into two-thirds intracellular fluid (ICF) and one-third extracellular fluid (ECF). The ECF is further divided into one-quarter plasma and three-quarter interstitial fluid. Potassium is the major cation of ICF, whereas, sodium is the major cation of ECF.

With advancing age TBW decreases. A geriatric patient may contain 10% less TBW per kilogram body weight compared to a young adult. Therefore, the geriatric patient starts at a lower TBW content, and thus, identical TBW losses in a geriatric patient represent a greater loss per weight when compared to a young adult.

As TBW declines, aging leads to a shift towards increased adipose tissue and decreased lean muscle mass. Aging-related muscle loss represents both a significant source of TBW loss and circulating creatinine, a marker of muscle metabolism.

Physical Exam

In general the physical exam is a limited tool for assessing volume status of the geriatric patient. Extremes in volume status may be identified relatively easily, for example, significant jugular venous distention (JVD) with orthopnea and dependent peripheral edema are consistent with congested heart failure or hypervolemia. But in other instances in patients with multiple comorbid conditions, volume status may not be easy to estimate based on exam alone in an elderly patient.

The classical physical assessment of volume status in the geriatric patient can be confounded by normal physical changes, debilitation, comorbidities, and medications. For example, skin turgor is normally lost with aging due to changes in elastin and collagen within the skin itself, rendering skin turgor unreliable marker of hydration. Mucus membranes may be dried from common psychiatric medications, such as donepezil for Alzheimer's dementia. Dysrhythmias are common in the aged, making pulse quality and rate extrapolation invalid. Inexperienced JVD measurement, morbid obesity, and right-sided heart lesions, such as tricuspid regurgitation, may make JVD assessment an impractical tool in the perioperative setting. Peripheral edema might be due to non-cardiogenic sources such as lymphedema or malnutrition.

The traditional utilization of urine output as a surrogate marker for intravascular volume status can be difficult and misleading in the geriatric patient. Preoperatively assessing urinary output based on history of voiding and diuretic-use is practically impossible, and difficult at best. Intraoperatively, patient position, anesthetic choice, or surgery type may all affect reliability of urinary output to volume status. Postoperatively, determination of adequate urine output is confounded by urinary retention due to residual anesthetics, anticholinergics, or benign prostatic hypertrophy. Furthermore, oliguria may occur due to postsurgical syndrome-of-inappropriate-antidiuretic hormone secretion or increased activation of the renin–angiotensin–aldosterone system in hypertension, both well-described occurrences.

Laboratory and Radiographic Assessment

Signs of hypovolemia and hypervolemia may be extrapolated from laboratory and radiographic markers (Table 9.1). In general laboratory markers can be used to evaluate for signs of hypoperfusion secondary to hypovolemia. Unfortunately in the

Table 9.1 Surrogate markers of intravascular volume status

Laboratory	Signs of hypovolemia
Hematocrit	Increasing from baseline
Metabolic acidosis, HCO_3^-	<21 mmol/L
Lactate	>2.0 mmol/L
Urine specific gravity	>1.010
BUN: creatinine	>20
Fractional sodium excretion (FeNa)	<1%
Urine sodium	<10 mEq/L
Urine osmolality	>450 mOsm/kg
Radiography	*Signs of hypervolemia*
Chest X-ray	Pulmonary edema, perihilar fullness

elderly patients, there are many challenges associated with the interpretation of these common laboratory markers. For example, approximately, 25–45% of elderly patients, 65 years or older, are prescribed diuretics. Ingestion of diuretics may lead to predictable laboratory abnormalities. For example hypokalemia is commonly observed in patients taking thiazide diuretics, and indeed hypovolemic patients on low-salt diets (the classic geriatric hypertensive patient) frequently develop a metabolic alkalosis as well while on thiazide diuretics. Another extremely common diuretic, furosemide is known to alter the reliability of fractional excretion of sodium (FENa) and urine sodium excretion, rendering this test invalid. Markers of hypoperfusion, such as lactate, reflect the end result of prolonged hypovolemia and, are not as useful when a more routine assessment of volume status is indicated.

Radiographic signs of hypervolemia, such as perihilar fullness or bilateral venous congestion, are well described. Unfortunately, chest x-ray findings are often delayed, insensitive to early signs of hypervolemia, and nonpredictive of acute decompensated heart failure risk. Its practical application is limited to the preoperative and postoperative setting.

Hemodynamic Monitoring

Invasive Hemodynamic Monitoring

Various hemodynamic devices exist for guiding fluid management that can aid clinicians in predicting a patient's location on the Frank–Starling curve. Location on the steep part of the curve suggests fluid responsiveness or state of potential cardiac output augmentation via intravenous fluid delivery. Location on the flat part of the curve may suggest a lack of fluid responsive state. Significant cardiopulmonary comorbidities in the geriatric population, and the greater risk of serious adverse effects due to hypervolemia and hypovolemia, often lower clinician's threshold to utilize these monitors.

Static Hemodynamic Parameters

Measurement of static cardiopulmonary pressures via an intravascular central venous catheter has traditionally been used to guide fluid management in the perioperative and critical care setting. Recently, however, this practice has been questioned due to its limited predictive value and utility in assessing preload or volumetric status.

Central Venous Pressures

Right ventricular preload, or end-diastolic volume, has historically been extrapolated from right atrial pressure or central venous pressure (CVP). A CVP of 5–10-cm H_2O in a normal patient is traditionally believed to indicate an adequate preload status, and, therefore, would imply that intravenous fluid loading would not result in augmented stroke volume. Recently, however, the clinical reliability of this age-old physiologic concept has been challenged based on numerous clinical studies demonstrating a poor correlation between CVP, a static parameter, and fluid responsiveness, a dynamic parameter. Furthermore, a number of confounding factors, such as mechanical ventilation or tricuspid valve disease, will alter the interpretability of CVP, further complicating any possible correlation to volume status.

Pulmonary Artery Catheter

A pulmonary artery catheter (PAC) may be used to obtain static parameters, such as pulmonary artery occlusion pressure (PAOP) or wedge pressure. Traditionally preload assessment and fluid management have been targeted to physiologic parameters often based on cardiac filling pressures by PAC, in an attempt to determine or adjust where the patient might exist on the Frank–Starling curve. A wedged PAC, theoretically, establishes continuity from the pulmonary circulation to the left ventricle, such that the following pressure-to-volume relationship is postulated: PAOP = left atrial pressure (LAP) = left ventricular end-diastolic pressure (LVEDP) = left ventricular end-diastolic volume (LVEDV). Hence, PAOP by PAC is interpreted as a surrogate for LVEDV. This presumed cardiac pressure-to-volume relationship has also been questioned based on recent findings demonstrating that cardiac filling pressures by PAC provide poor predictive value of fluid responsiveness. PAC-guided goal-directed therapy compared to CVP-guided care in elderly, high-risk, non-cardiac surgery patients has not been shown to reduce mortality. A similar negative finding in adult patients with shock and ARDS has further disputed the role of PAC in fluid management. Complications related to pulmonary artery catheterization include pulmonary embolism, arrhythmias, and line infection.

Dynamic Hemodynamic Parameters

A distinctive feature of dynamic hemodynamic monitors is their reported ability to provide clinicians the ability to guide fluid management based on measured preload variation indices that discriminate fluid responders from non-fluid responders. Wide cyclic changes in preload during positive pressure ventilation, as occurs during hypovolemia and increase venous capacitance, predict fluid responsiveness. Conditions that induce such a dynamic preload state are dehydration, significant hemorrhage, and general anesthesia. Despite this understanding, clinicians must still discern if a fluid-responsive patient requires fluid therapy.

Invasive Hemodynamic Monitors

Fluid management is a complex task affected by factors related to fluid responsiveness, intracardiac volume status, cardiac output, and consequences of excessive fluid delivery. Dynamic invasive hemodynamic monitors provide real-time hemodynamic data that may assist the clinicians in managing these interdependent categories.

Vigileo Monitor

Stroke volume variation (SVV) is the key dynamic index available from this monitor. SVV is a physiologic phenomenon produced by the cyclic changes in intrathoracic pressure during positive pressure ventilation, which produce concurrent changes in stroke volume. Continuous arterial beat-to-beat wave analysis or pulse contour analysis generates SVV measurements and extrapolations of stroke volume and cardiac output. Cyclic variation is marked in hypovolemic patients. SVV values above threshold suggest fluid responsiveness. When attached to a functioning arterial line, the Vigileo monitor and its FloTrac sensor (Edwards Lifesciences LLC) provide continuous SVV and cardiac output measures. Monitoring reliability is dependent on several factors, such as arterial waveform quality, controlled mechanical ventilation, greater than 8cc-per-kg tidal volumes, and avoidance of arrhythmias. Small intraoperative trials with substantial geriatric participants have demonstrated some reliability of SVV to predict fluid responsiveness during controlled mechanical ventilation.

PiCCO Monitor

Unique to the PiCCO monitor are intracardiac volumetric and lung water indices that provide dynamic measures of hemodynamics, fluid responsiveness, and pulmonary edema.

Fluid responsiveness, similar to other devices, is measured by both arterial pulse pressure variation (PPV) and SVV. PPV, similar to SVV, is derived from the phenomenon of cyclic SVV during positive pressure ventilation in which pulse pressure (PP) varies between maximum width (PPmax) and minimum width (PPmin). The following formula for PPV describes this relationship: $(\mathrm{PPmax}-\mathrm{PPmin})/[(\mathrm{PPmax}-\mathrm{PPmin})/2)]\times 100$.

Cardiac output measurement is determined by both arterial pulse contour analysis and transpulmonary thermodilution. Based on thermal indicator injectate detection over time, cardiopulmonary blood volumes may be measured, thereby allowing for extrapolation of volumetric preload, or global end-diastolic volume (GEDV), and extravascular lung water (EVLW).

Pulmonary edema, or excessive EVLW, has been demonstrated to correlate with increased mortality in critically ill patients. Improvements in oxygenation and lung mechanics have been associated with conservative fluid strategies that aim to reduce EVLW. Clinical exam, laboratory testing, and radiographic assessment are unreliable and insensitive to early EVLW changes.

Noninvasive Hemodynamic Monitoring

Echocardiography

Echocardiography provides point-of-care, rapid assessment of cardiovascular physiology and fluid responsiveness. Transthoracic, transesophageal, and esophageal Doppler are echocardiography devices available for hemodynamic monitoring. Heart–lung interaction during ventilation results in volume and afterload shifts between the right and left ventricles that are appreciable by two-dimensional and Doppler ultrasound. During a positive pressure breath, right ventricular afterload increases and preload decreases, while in the left ventricle, afterload decreases and preload increases. During exhalation, the reverse occurs. Cyclic respiratory variation in peak systolic blood pressure and stroke volume during mechanical ventilation is pronounced in hypovolemic patients. Doppler ultrasound can quantify these variations by continuous blood velocity measurements during left ventricular ejection. Similarly, degree of superior and inferior vena cava compression during mechanical ventilation can predict fluid responsiveness by esophageal echocardiography. Esophageal Doppler-guided, perioperative fluid expansion in elderly patients undergoing cardiac and noncardiac surgery has been shown to reduce postoperative morbidity and hospital length of stay.

Fluid Therapy

Optimal perioperative fluid strategies continue to be debated. Choice of fluid—crystalloid versus colloid, “conservative” versus “liberal” fluid strategies—and magnitude of presumed fluid shifts are areas of ongoing controversy.

Fluid Physiology

Starling fluid flux postulates that as fluid moves through a capillary, filtration across the wall of a capillary is determined by the hydrostatic pressure gradient, oncotic pressure gradient, and a capillary filtration and permeability correction coefficients. This relationship is calculated by Starling's formula:

$$\text{Net Fluid Flux} = K[(\text{Pc} - \text{Pi}) - r(\prod \text{c} - \prod \text{i})],$$

where K = filtration coefficient, Pc = capillary hydrostatic pressure, Pi = interstitial hydrostatic pressure, r = reflection coefficient, $\prod$c = capillary oncotic pressure, and $\prod$i = interstitial oncotic pressure.

Fluid Shifts

Capillary fluid homeostasis is susceptible to disruption. Malnutrition, a common condition in fragile, aged patients, may decrease systemic oncotic pressure, thereby making capillaries leaky. Inflammation and tissue trauma, as occurs during surgery, are known to increase capillary permeability. Inordinate attempts to compensate for fluid extravasation may produce a hypervolemic state, which may lead to capillary pressure increases, oncotic load dilution, and lymphatic reabsorption overload. Tissue edema due to hypervolemia may compromise wound healing and increase risk of infections. Significant perioperative fluid weight gain has been correlated with decreased survival.

Fluid Types

Crystalloids

Perioperatively, crystalloids are the preferred intravenous, low-cost, fluid choice for resuscitation. Crystalloids are glucose-free, isotonic salt solutions (Table 9.2). Their volume expansion efficiency is limited by intravascular oncotic force dilution. Therefore, a significant proportion of crystalloid volume expansion extravasates immediately post-infusion. The "3:1 rule" implies that 1/3 of infused crystalloids remain intravascular. Recent animal studies, however, suggest a readjustment of this ratio to "5:1" during normovolemia.

Table 9.2 Common crystalloid solutions administered perioperatively for fluid resuscitation

Isotonic crystalloid solutions	pH	Na^+ (mEq/L)	Cl^+ (mEq/L)	K^+ (mEq/L)	$Lactate^+$ (mEq/L)
Normal saline (0.9%)	6.0	154	154	–	
Lactate Ringer's	6.5	130	109	4	28
Plasmalyte[a]	7.4	140	98	5	

[a]Contains (mEq/L) Mg^+, acetate, and gluconate

Table 9.3 Common colloid solutions administered perioperatively for fluid resuscitation in the USA

Colloid solutions	Characteristics	Risks
Albumin	Human-plasma derived, sterile, filtered	Allergic reaction (low incidence)
Sodium hetastarch (Hespan)	Polysaccharides modified with hydroxyethyl-group substitutions, resistant to degradation Volume expanders, rheology effects, coagulation effects	Allergic reaction (low incidence)
Dextran	Bacteria-generated colloid molecules of various size, shape, and interaction strength Volume expander (dextran-70), significant rheologic effect (dextran-40)	Acquired von Willebrand's syndrome Factor VIII activity reduction Anaphylaxis

Colloids

Colloids solutions are fluid suspensions composed of large molecules with oncotic pressure potential (Table 9.3). Theoretically, these solutions are designed to stay intravascularly longer, thereby minimizing significant fluid extravasation into the interstitium. Colloids are a costly fluid resuscitation option with potential allergic and coagulation risks. Cost per milliliter is significantly greater for albumin than hetastarch solutions.

Crystalloid Versus Colloid

Preferential colloid administration, over crystalloid, in the perioperative setting is often justified based on their potential to maintain volume expansion while reducing extravascular redistribution into vulnerable organ sites, such as lungs and gut. On the other hand, crystalloids may be chosen for being inexpensive, readily available, and the traditional choice for fluid resuscitation. To date randomized controlled trials refute the theory that fluid resuscitation with colloids compared to crystalloids, are superior. Fluid resuscitation with colloids, compared to crystalloids, does not improve survival in critically ill patients.

"Restrictive" Versus "Liberal"

Controversy remains regarding "restrictive" and "liberal" fluid resuscitation. "Restrictive" strategies aim to limit fluid excess, primarily extravascular redistribution. Excess perioperative weight gain has been correlated with greater pressor dependence, greater number of ventilator days, and increased mortality in patients with similar disease severity. During major abdominal surgery, a mix of 'restrictive' fluid strategies has been shown to reduce hospital length of stay, improved return of bowel function, and reduced complications, such as wound infection, wound dehiscence, pulmonary edema, pneumonia, and cardiac dysrhythmias. Given crystalloid fluids' high propensity for extravascular redistribution, elderly patients with limited renal function and chronic cardiopulmonary disease are at risk of developing complications when excess fluid is administered.

Fluid strategies compared to "restrictive" strategies, consequently, are labeled "liberal." This label is usually applied to the standard of care at any given institution. Clinicians applying "liberal" strategies are likely attempting to provide "optimal" fluid delivery, in order to maintain adequate organ perfusion, stable hemodynamics, and prevent postoperative nausea and vomiting in minor elective surgeries.

Evaluation and implementation of "restrictive" and "liberal" strategies from various studies is hindered by their heterogeneous perioperative methodology. Currently, no evidence-based recommendations can be made on choice of fluid, whether colloid or crystalloid, or optimal fluid amounts. Nonetheless, suggested strategies to limit crystalloid use include (1) strict adherence to a theoretical "optimal" fluid range, (2) judicious use of vasopressors intraoperatively, in order to counter vasodilatory effects of general anesthesia, (3) balanced administration of colloid and crystalloid and (4) consideration of significant comorbidities, such as end-stage renal disease and congestive heart failure. Ultimately, fluid optimization by either "liberal" or "conservative" fluid strategies must be patient centered and based on clinical judgment.

Perioperative Packed Red Blood Cell Transfusion

A large quantity of allogeneic blood is transfused in the perioperative setting. Transfusion targets are often made by estimation of blood loss, comorbidities, surgeon request, hematocrit levels, coagulation status, hemodynamics, improved myocardial oxygen delivery, or transfusion guidelines. Clinicians' ability to gauge short-term effectiveness and long-term complication rates of blood component transfusion is difficult given the labile nature of perioperative care.

Recent, community survey data reveals that anemia is common in 11% of men and 10% of women over 65 years of age. Precipitating factors include nutritional deficiency, iron deficiency, chronic disease, or myelodysplastic syndrome. Whether correcting anemia with blood transfusion or treating underlying anemia-inducing disease improves morbidity and mortality is still unclear. Few studies have demonstrated overwhelming benefit or risk with blood transfusion.

Benefits

Transfusion benefit in acute cardiac disease in elderly patients has been demonstrated from observational data. Thirty-day mortality in elderly patients with anemia and acute myocardial infarction may be improved with correction of 33% hematocrit or lower.

Risks

Greater proinflammatory cytokine release from transfused leukocyte-containing allogeneic blood, compared to leukocyte-depleted blood, has been demonstrated. This observed immunologic phenomenon may aggravate altered capillary permeability and extravascular edema perioperatively.

The transfusion requirements in critical care (TRICC) trial remains one of the most significant trials to comprehensively evaluate "restrictive" and "liberal" blood transfusion strategies in normovolemic adults. Critical patients maintained at a "liberal" hemoglobin level of 10–12 g/dL, compared to a "restrictive" hemoglobin level of 7–9 g/dL, had a greater incidence of myocardial infarction and pulmonary edema. No difference in 30-day and 60-day mortality existed between the two groups. Blood transfusion to an arbitrary hematocrit goal of 30% in all adults should, therefore, be questioned. Current evidence is leaning towards resetting this threshold to a hemoglobin of less than 10 g/dL in both geriatric and non-geriatric patients.

Transfusion Guidelines

Transfusion guidelines do not exist specifically for elderly patients. Nevertheless, ASA Practice Guidelines for perioperative red blood cell transfusion recommend the following:

1. Visual assessment of blood loss quantity.
2. Organ perfusion and oxygenation monitoring by noninvasive and invasive means.
3. Transfusion trigger of 6–10 g/dl should be based on ongoing blood loss, cardiopulmonary risk, signs of organ ischemia, and intravascular volume status.

Conclusion

Achieving optimal perioperative fluid management in the elderly patient is a significant challenge to clinicians. Geriatric patients may have potential fluid-handling limitations, in addition to renal-injury susceptibility, due to age-related renal degeneration. Further, cardiopulmonary comorbidities may decrease geriatric patients' resistance to complications of extravascular fluid accumulation. Assessment and management of intravascular volume status is insensitive by classic physical exam and laboratory testing and perhaps aided by noninvasive and invasive dynamic parameters. Fluid management strategies continue to be debated, though "restrictive" fluid use may be justifiable in certain surgical settings. Ultimately, the fundamental perioperative, fluid management goal sought by anesthesia care providers for every patient is the balance between organ perfusion optimization and postoperative complications reduction.

Key Points

- Renal degeneration results in limited fluid handling in the elderly.
- Both static and dynamic hemodynamic monitors may help guide fluid management; however, clinicians must ultimately decide if fluid administration is required.
- Fluid overload and cardiopulmonary comorbidities in the elderly may contribute to postoperative pulmonary edema and delay in bowel function.
- Either "liberal" or "conservative" fluid strategies may be appropriate for fluid optimization.
- Fluid resuscitation with colloids, compared to crystalloids, does not reduce mortality.
- Effectiveness of packed red blood cell (PRBC) transfusion continues to be debated though may be appropriate if hemoglobin is less than 6–10 g/dL.

Suggested Reading

Bilgin YM, van de Watering LM, Versteegh MI, van Oers MH, Brand A. Effects of allogeneic leukocytes in blood transfusions during cardiac surgery on inflammatory mediators and postoperative complications. Crit Care Med. 2010;38:546–52.

Brandstrup B, Tonnesen H, Beier-Holgersen R, et al. Effects of intravenous fluid restriction on postoperative complications: comparison of two perioperative fluid regimens: a randomized assessor-blinded multicenter trial. Ann Surg. 2003;238:641–8.

Cannesson M, Musard H, Desebbe O, et al. The ability of stroke volume variations obtained with Vigileo/FloTrac system to monitor fluid responsiveness in mechanically ventilated patients. Anesth Analg. 2009;108:513–7.

Cavallaro F, Sandroni C, Antonelli M. Functional hemodynamic monitoring and dynamic indices of fluid responsiveness. Minerva Anestesiol. 2008;74:123–35.

de Aguilar-Nascimento JE, Diniz BN, do Carmo AV, Silveira EA, Silva RM. Clinical benefits after the implementation of a protocol of restricted perioperative intravenous crystalloid fluids in major abdominal operations. World J Surg. 2009;33:925–30.

Eisenberg PR, Hansbrough JR, Anderson D, Schuster DP. A prospective study of lung water measurements during patient management in an intensive care unit. Am Rev Respir Dis. 1987;136:662–8.

Gerstle J, Shahul S, Mahmood F. Echocardiographically derived parameters of fluid responsiveness. Int Anesthesiol Clin. 2010;48:37–44.

Guralnik JM, Eisenstaedt RS, Ferrucci L, Klein HG, Woodman RC. Prevalence of anemia in persons 65 years and older in the United States: evidence for a high rate of unexplained anemia. Blood. 2004;104:2263–8.

Hebert PC, Wells G, Blajchman MA, et al. A multicenter, randomized, controlled clinical trial of transfusion requirements in critical care. Transfusion Requirements in Critical Care Investigators, Canadian Critical Care Trials Group. N Engl J Med. 1999;340:409–17.
Holte K, Kehlet H. Fluid therapy and surgical outcomes in elective surgery: a need for reassessment in fast-track surgery. J Am Coll Surg. 2006;202:971–89.
K/DOQI clinical practice guidelines for chronic kidney disease: evaluation, classification, and stratification. Am J Kidney Dis. 2002;39:S1–266.
Kelleher CL. Disorders of water and electrolyte metabolism. In: Tallis R, Fillit H, eds. Brocklehurst's textbook of geriatric medicine and gerontology. 6th ed. London: Churchill Livingstone; 2003:1109–17.
Kumar A, Anel R, Bunnell E, et al. Pulmonary artery occlusion pressure and central venous pressure fail to predict ventricular filling volume, cardiac performance, or the response to volume infusion in normal subjects. Crit Care Med. 2004;32:691–9.
Lobo DN, Bostock KA, Neal KR, Perkins AC, Rowlands BJ, Allison SP. Effect of salt and water balance on recovery of gastrointestinal function after elective colonic resection: a randomised controlled trial. Lancet. 2002;359:1812–8.
Lowell JA, Schifferdecker C, Driscoll DF, Benotti PN, Bistrian BR. Postoperative fluid overload: not a benign problem. Crit Care Med. 1990;18:728–33.
Marik PE, Baram M, Vahid B. Does central venous pressure predict fluid responsiveness? A systematic review of the literature and the tale of seven mares. Chest. 2008;134:172–8.
Michard F, Teboul JL. Using heart-lung interactions to assess fluid responsiveness during mechanical ventilation. Crit Care. 2000;4:282–9.
Nisanevich V, Felsenstein I, Almogy G, Weissman C, Einav S, Matot I. Effect of intraoperative fluid management on outcome after intraabdominal surgery. Anesthesiology. 2005;103:25–32.
Nuttall GA, Stehling LC, Beighley CM, Faust RJ. Current transfusion practices of members of the american society of anesthesiologists: a survey. Anesthesiology. 2003;99:1433–43.
Onwuanyi A, Taylor M. Acute decompensated heart failure: pathophysiology and treatment. Am J Cardiol. 2007;99:25D–30D.
Oren-Grinberg A. The PiCCO Monitor. Int Anesthesiol Clin. 2010;48:57–85.
Osman D, Ridel C, Ray P, et al. Cardiac filling pressures are not appropriate to predict hemodynamic response to volume challenge. Crit Care. Med. 2007;35:64–8.
Perel P, Roberts I. Colloids versus crystalloids for fluid resuscitation in critically ill patients. Cochrane Database Syst Rev. 2007:CD000567.
Practice Guidelines for blood component therapy: A report by the American Society of Anesthesiologists Task Force on Blood Component Therapy. Anesthesiology. 1996;84:732–47.
Practice guidelines for perioperative blood transfusion and adjuvant therapies: an updated report by the American Society of Anesthesiologists Task Force on Perioperative Blood Transfusion and Adjuvant Therapies. Anesthesiology. 2006;105:198–208.
Robin E, Costecalde M, Lebuffe G, Vallet B. Clinical relevance of data from the pulmonary artery catheter. Critical Care. 2006;10:S3.
Sandham JD, Hull RD, Brant RF, et al. A randomized, controlled trial of the use of pulmonary-artery catheters in high-risk surgical patients. N Engl J Med. 2003;348:5–14.
Spahn DR, Chassot PG. CON: Fluid restriction for cardiac patients during major noncardiac surgery should be replaced by goal-directed intravascular fluid administration. Anesth Analg. 2006;102:344–6.
Tollofsrud S, Elgjo GI, Prough DS, Williams CA, Traber DL, Kramer GC. The dynamics of vascular volume and fluid shifts of lactated Ringer's solution and hypertonic-saline-dextran solutions infused in normovolemic sheep. Anesth Analg. 2001;93:823–31.
van Kraaij DJ, Jansen RW, Gribnau FW, Hoefnagels WH. Diuretic therapy in elderly heart failure patients with and without left ventricular systolic dysfunction. Drugs Aging. 2000;16:289–300.
Wheeler AP, Bernard GR, Thompson BT, et al. Pulmonary-artery versus central venous catheter to guide treatment of acute lung injury. N Engl J Med. 2006;354:2213–24.

Wiggins J. Changes in renal function. In: Hazzard WR, Blass JP, Halter JB, Ouslander JG, Tinetti ME, eds. Principles of geriatric medicine and gerontology. 5th ed. New York: McGraw-Hill/Professional; 2003:543–9.

Wu WC, Rathore SS, Wang Y, Radford MJ, Krumholz HM. Blood transfusion in elderly patients with acute myocardial infarction. N Engl J Med. 2001;345:1230–6.

Zimmermann M, Feibicke T, Keyl C, et al. Accuracy of stroke volume variation compared with pleth variability index to predict fluid responsiveness in mechanically ventilated patients undergoing major surgery. Eur J Anaesthesiol. 2010;27(6):555–61.

Part III
Perioperative Care

Chapter 10
Acute Pain Control in the Elderly

Steve Lee and Angela Georgia Catic

As the number of elderly patients undergoing surgery rises, acute pain control in the postsurgical setting is an increasingly important concern. The consequences of poorly controlled pain in the elderly patient can be significant and lead to negative outcomes.

Chronic painful conditions are very common in the elderly preoperatively. Several studies suggest that the prevalence of pain in men and women aged >65 can be as high as 67–80%. Approximately 80% of community-dwelling older patients report taking analgesic medications at least once weekly, and 39% report daily usage. Using analgesics preoperatively can increase the difficulty in implementing optimal postoperative pain relief strategies. Suboptimal pain relief strategies in the elderly can lead to decreased mobility, decreased function, depression, agitation, restlessness, cognitive failure, and a reduction in activities of daily living. Polypharmacy exacerbations, through the addition of new medications, can occur resulting in increased confusion and falls. Overall, inadequate treatment of postoperative pain can delay recovery, increase complications, prolong hospital stays, and increase total health care costs (Table 10.1).

S. Lee, MD, MA (✉)
Department of Anesthesia, Critical Care, and Pain Medicine,
Beth Israel Deaconess Medical Center, Harvard Medical School,
330 Brookline Avenue, Boston, MA 02215, USA
e-mail: sclee@bidmc.harvard.edu

A.G. Catic, MD
Division of Gerontology, Department of Internal Medicine,
Beth Israel Deaconess Medical Center, Harvard Medical School,
110 Francis Street, Suite 1B, Boston, MA 02215, USA

S.R. Barnett (ed.), *Manual of Geriatric Anesthesia*, DOI 10.1007/978-1-4614-3888-5_10,

Table 10.1 Adverse consequences of acute pain in elderly patients

Direct suffering
Decreased physical function
Loss of independence
Decreased socialization
Depression
Delirium
Sleep disturbances
Increased health utilization costs
Increased postoperative pulmonary and cardiac morbidity
Increased length of hospitalization

Age-Related Changes in the Pain System

Multiple factors contribute to the difficulty encountered when treating and managing patients with acute postoperative pain. For a start, the aging process itself is associated with predictable changes in the physiology of pain perception. In addition common comorbidities of age such as arthritis, osteoporosis, and diabetes may exacerbate the normal age-related changes in the nociceptive primary afferent fibers, central nervous system, and endogenous pain inhibitory systems. With advanced age the density of primary afferent fibers decreases. By the age of 60, there is an ~35% decrease in the density of myelinated fibers and a 50% decrease in the density of unmyelinated fibers. The number of sensory fibers with evidence of damage or degeneration increases, and peripheral nerve conduction velocity may slow. Degenerative changes occur in the spinal dorsal horn sensory neurons with loss of myelin, axonal involution, and altered spinal neurochemistry. Significant changes in the brain occur including neuronal death, loss of dendritic arborization, appearance of neurofibrillary abnormalities, and changes in the synthesis, axonal transport, uptake, and receptor binding of neurotransmitter systems.

These changes in the nociceptive primary afferent fibers and central nervous system can lead to changes in pain perception. Similarly, alterations in the descending modulation from endogenous pain inhibitory systems may make it more difficult for elderly patients to cope with severe or persistent pain. Furthermore, aging appears to lead to an increase in the pain threshold, or point at which an individual becomes aware of pain. This threshold normally serves as a warning system that there is a risk of tissue damage. When this threshold is increased, the period between identification of pain and the onset of tissue injury is reduced, placing older patients at greater risk. Changes in pain threshold and perception may also lead to a missed or delayed diagnosis in an older patient. An example is the elderly patient who presents with an acute abdomen and peritonitis, in considerably less pain than would have been exhibited by a younger patient in the same condition.

Pain Reporting

Victor Hugo once said “Pain is as diverse as man. One suffers as one can.” This quote is especially applicable to the geriatric age group that includes a heterogeneous population with a wide spectrum of comorbidities. Various illnesses such as dementia, prior stroke, and other neurological diseases like Parkinson’s disease mean that patients may exhibit variable expressions of pain, making diagnosing and treatment challenging. The assessment of pain itself in the elderly patient can be more difficult than in younger counterparts; 23% of the elderly population have dementia and maybe nonverbal. In the postoperative period a successful pain management strategy should both provide relief from pain and ensure rapid return to presurgical function.

Pain evaluation should always start with a thorough history and physical; ideally the pain history should also be included in the preoperative assessment, so it is possible to distinguish new pain versus pain related to a chronic condition. The history should identify the quality, severity, location and nature of the pain as well as delineating exacerbating and alleviating factors contributing to the pain. In the immediate postoperative period, the source of pain is usually easy to identify and related to the recent trauma of surgery. A specific enquiry about pain is important as many older patients will not automatically report pain or complain for a variety of reasons. In general elderly patients tend to underreport pain and then only report pain they have at rest. In addition, they often assume postoperative pain is simply a consequence to be endured and thus may underplay the actual pain they are experiencing. Similarly older patients may worry about being a nuisance and do not want to complain or ask for help, or they may be fearful regarding the cause of their pain. Elderly patients may also assume that health care providers will recognize that they are experiencing pain and treat them accordingly. When examining an older patient in pain, the interview should be very directed and utilize descriptive terms about pain including discomfort, aching, and hurting (Table 10.2).

As stated the incidence of dementia is significant in the geriatric population, and a challenging part of evaluating pain in these patients is gathering a thorough history and physical from patients who are nonverbal and/or have dementia. In nonverbal patients, traditional questions are frequently inadequate, and instead observation may provide more insight into the level of pain. Pain behaviors commonly observed

Table 10.2 Acute pain assessment in geriatric patients

Proactive questions about the presence of pain
Description of pain including origin, radiation, sensory description, and severity
Question about exacerbating and relieving factors
Assessment of the functional impact of pain
Evaluation of the emotional responses to pain
Quantification of pain using a pain rating scale

include grimacing, rocking, crying, or withdrawing during the examination. Physiological expressions of pain such as increases in heart rate or respiratory rate are poor indicators of pain in the nonverbal patient.

Evaluation

An effective pain management strategy should include a reproducible assessment tool that quantifies the initial pain and can be used to reassess the impact of therapeutic interventions on pain intensity. The most common unidimensional scales used to assess pain in the general population are the verbal rating scale (VRS), numerical rating scale (NRS), and visual analogue scale (VAS) (Table 10.3). The faces pain scale is another scale that has certain advantages in the cognitively impaired or nonverbal patient.

The VRS uses a list of adjectives including no pain, mild pain, moderate pain, and severe pain to describe increasing pain intensity that characterizes different levels of pain. Patients are asked to select the level that best characterizes their pain. Although the VRS is simple to use and understand, it can be difficult to use in patients with language or comprehension barriers as the patient must understand the meaning of the words included in the rating scale.

The NRS uses a simple scale, usually 0–10, to assess pain. Patients are instructed to rate their pain along a range of pain intensities with 0 being "no pain" and 10 being "the worst pain imaginable." The NRS is easy to understand and simple to use; however, it is limited in patients with cognitive difficulties.

Table 10.3 Essentials about common unidimensional pain assessment tools

Visual analogue scale
Quick and easy to use
Requires intact visual acuity
Requires intact motor abilities
Confusing to 20% of elders
Numerical rating scale
Quick and easy to use
Typically easily understood by elders
Can be administered verbally overcoming physical and visual impairments
Verbal rating scale
Dependent on patient interpretation and understanding of descriptive terms
May lack accuracy and sensitivity of other pain scales
Preferred by some elders who can more easily describe their pain in words than numbers
Faces pain rating scale
Designed for children but has been used successfully in elders
Appropriate for patients with learning difficulties
Useful in patients with hearing impairment
Useful in patients with poor language skills

The VAS uses a horizontal line on which "no pain" is marked at the start on left to the "most intense pain imaginable" at the end on the right. The patient places a mark on the scale that corresponds to their pain intensity. The mark can then be converted into a quantifiable number for immediate assessment and follow-up pain evaluations. The VAS is slightly more complicated to use, and it is the least popular tool for pain assessment in the geriatric population.

The faces pain rating scale includes six numbered faces depicting emotions ranging from happy (no pain) to very sad (worst pain). The patient chooses the face that depicts the level of pain she or he is experiencing. While this scale was designed for children, it has been used successfully in an array of adult patients including geriatric patients, patients with learning difficulties, patients with hearing deficits, and patients with poor language skills.

An important aspect of good pain control is ongoing reevaluation and adjustment of medication regimens. The choice of pain assessment scale is less important than ensuring frequent assessments to ensure that the analgesic regimen is effective and pain is controlled.

Pain Assessment in Cognitively Impaired Elders: Pain Assessment in Advanced Dementia

One in five patients over age 80 suffers from dementia, and the number of geriatric patients with Alzheimer's disease is expected to increase to 13 million by 2050. Unfortunately, pain is traditionally poorly assessed and undertreated among patients with cognitive impairment. This is especially true when complaints are nonspecific, and vague symptoms are less likely to prompt a pain evaluation in a patient with dementia vs. a cognitively intact patient. The issue of pain control in demented patients is further impacted by inadequate treatment. Even when patients with dementia are prescribed and administered analgesics, they frequently get less analgesics than those without cognitive impairment. One reason for this is the broad misperception that these patients do not experience pain and there is little that can be accomplished by treating them with analgesics. Even though dementia can make pain assessment difficult, the patient remains the best source of information about their pain, and a thorough pain assessment is just as important for these patients as for cognitively intact postsurgical patients.

In the clinical setting cognitive impairment is a nonspecific term used to describe an array of intellectual difficulties and disease states. It can be applied to describe patients with mild cognitive impairment and very limited disability to patients with advanced dementia due to Alzheimer's disease, vascular dementia, and other etiologies. In general patients with only mild cognitive impairment will be able to use one of the pain assessment scales described. Verbal descriptors of pain (i.e., VRS) or visual scales (i.e., VAS and faces pain rating scale) are preferred and easier for patients to use. In some instances, it may be necessary to try out several scales before choosing one that the patient can comprehend and that provides an accurate

Table 10.4 The pain assessment in advanced dementia (PAINAD) scale

	0	1	2	Score
Breathing independent of vocalization	Normal	Occasional labored breathing. Short period of hyperventilation	Noisy labored breathing. Long period of hyperventilation. Cheyne–Stokes respirations	
Negative vocalization	None	Occasional moan or groan. Low level speech with a negative or disapproving quality	Repeated troubled calling out. Loud moaning or groaning. Crying	
Facial expression	Smiling, or inexpressive	Sad. Frightened. Frown	Facial grimacing	
Body language	Relaxed	Tense. Distressed pacing. Fidgeting	Rigid. Fists clenched, knees pulled up. Pulling or pushing away. Striking out	
Consolability	No need to console	Distracted or reassured by voice or touch	Unable to console, distract or reassure	

pain assessment. In nonverbal patients with advanced dementia, proxy reports and observational scales can be utilized to assess pain. It is worth noting however that healthcare provider proxy reports tend to underestimate pain. When studied, physicians appropriately identified pain in 43% of communicative patients but only in 17% of noncommunicative geriatric patients. As a pain evaluation can be subjective, it is important to avoid underestimating pain by using an observational assessment method. The pain assessment in advanced dementia (PAINAD) scale is one of the most common clinically utilized observational scales (Table 10.4). The scale is brief, easy to administer, and can be used to measure pain in nonverbal, demented individuals. The PAINAD provides an overall pain score and has the advantage of being sufficiently sensitive to detect changes in pain, thus it can also be used to evaluate the effectiveness of a pain regimen. The five domains assessed are breathing, negative vocalization, facial expression, body language, and consolability. Each domain is scored between 0 and 2 for a total possible score of 0–10. The PAINAD scale is appropriate for use in the immediate postoperative period and during the recovery period.

Joint Commission on Accreditation of Healthcare Organizations

The Joint Commission recognizes that adequate pain management is a critical element in the management of the perioperative patient. To ensure appropriate pain management, they have mandated that all healthcare providers must comply with the following requirements: (1) recognize the rights of individuals to appropriate assessment and management of pain and (2) assess the existence and, if so, the nature and intensity of pain in all patients, residents, or clients.

Key elements of acute pain assessment include an enquiry about the presence of pain; a description of the pain including origin, radiation, sensory description, and severity; discussion about exacerbating and relieving factors; and questioning regarding the functional impact of the pain. Pain rating scales are an important part of pain assessment. It is essential to understand the value, extent, and limitations of assessment tools and to recognize that a combination of tools may be need to obtain a full assessment.

Pain Management

Multiple treatment modalities including nonpharmacologic, pharmacologic, and interventional approaches should be considered when addressing pain in the postoperative elderly patient. Physicians most commonly prescribe medication and physical therapy, while it appears that some elderly patients may prefer home remedies, massage, topical agents, physical modalities (heat/cold), and informal cognitive strategies (prayer/humor). There are advantages to both treatment approaches, and it is important to customize the treatment plan for each individual patient.

Treating acute pain can be divided into two strategies, nonpharmacologic and pharmacologic, and both approaches are important. Nonpharmacologic means of treating pain may include patient education, adding therapy conducted by professionals (e.g., relaxation techniques, music therapy, art therapy, coping skills, biofeedback, and hypnosis), or intervening with appropriate nerve blocks.

World Health Organization Analgesic Ladder

The World Health Organization (WHO) analgesic ladder provides a stepwise approach to guide treatment of malignant and nonmalignant pain. The first step of the ladder utilizes nonopioid analgesics. If pain persists or worsens, the WHO ladder endorses the use of a mild opioid in conjunction with the nonopioid analgesic. Step three of the ladder provides for the use of a stronger opioid which can be titrated as needed for pain control. Obviously, in postsurgical patients, it is often necessary to use opioids immediately; however, it is still important to consider alternatives.

When considering pharmacological therapy, including implementing an analgesic regimen in elderly patients, it is important to follow the adage of "start low, go slow." Once initiated it is preferable to perform frequent pain assessments and slowly titrate opioids as indicated by persistent pain. Starting with higher initial doses can be associated with increased side effects.

The WHO three-step ladder can be used when selecting appropriate medications for the treatment of acute pain in both younger and older populations.

For step 1, mild-to-moderate pain is treated with nonopioid analgesics, such as acetaminophen. In step 2, moderate pain is treated with minor opioids, perhaps combined with adjuvants and other nonopioids. For step 3, severe pain is treated with potent opioids. Drugs with the lowest side effect profile should be utilized first, beginning with the lowest dose possible, increasing slowly. Continuous pain can be treated with long-acting or sustained-release analgesics, while episodic or breakthrough pain is better treated with short-acting, fast-onset analgesics. Adjuncts such as a COX-2 inhibitor may also help decrease pain in patients who would benefit from its anti-inflammatory action but who are at higher risk for NSAID-induced peptic ulcer disease.

For elderly patients initial doses should be reduced by 50% of the dose for a younger patient and titrated up slowly on the basis of persistent breakthrough pain.

Side Effects

In the elderly, it is important to try to avoid the development of side effects which can lead to prolonged hospitalizations, and reduced mobility and loss of independence. For example, older patients are more likely to be sensitive to side effects, such as constipation. Instituting a bowel regimen prophylactically that addresses the slowed gastrointestinal peristalsis, such as Sennakot, and adding a stool softener such as Colace can be helpful.

Respiratory depression fortunately is relatively unusual and usually occurs when long serum half-life drugs are used. These drugs require several days to achieve a steady state and render the older patient vulnerable from overdosing as doses accumulate. Another situation when respiratory depression may occur is when patients with severe pain receive escalating doses. If the underlying pain syndrome is relieved, doses that have been previously tolerated may suddenly produce hypopnea or apnea. It is also important to note that Cheyne–Stokes breathing patterns during sleep, which are not uncommon in the elderly, are different from true respiratory depression and thus should not be used as a basis for discontinuation of opioid therapy.

Nonopioid Analgesics

Acetaminophen

Scheduled acetaminophen is the first-line pain treatment and nonopioid analgesic of choice for older patients. It is surprisingly and frequently underutilized in the perioperative setting. Unless contraindicated by hepatic dysfunction, dosages of 650–1,000 mg orally or per rectum every 6 h are recommended. The intravenous formulation is now available in the USA and is a valuable alternative to parenteral routes. In the immediate postoperative setting, acetaminophen alone is often not enough for more severe pain, and opioid analgesics are usually indicated. In a systematic review, the addition of acetaminophen to a morphine patient-controlled analgesia (PCA) was associated with a morphine-sparing effect of 20%. The addition of acetaminophen was also associated with a reduction in sedation and improved pain scores.

Nonsteroidal Anti-inflammatory Drugs

In patients over age 65 years, nonsteroidal anti-inflammatory drugs (NSAIDS) are relatively contraindicated as they have a twofold increased risk of gastrointestinal bleeding and have been associated with acute renal dysfunction. However, non-acetylated drugs with a relatively simple metabolism are generally better tolerated. Indomethacin and piroxicam should be avoided since they have relatively long serum half-lives and tend to cause more gastrointestinal problems. Indomethacin is also specifically associated with delirium. A popular perioperative NSAID is ketorolac, which can be administered intravenously. However, there is a significant increased risk of gastrointestinal bleeding, ulceration, and perforation. If utilized, the dose should be reduced with a starting dose of 15 mg intravenously every 6 h not to exceed 60 mg in 24 h.

Opioid Analgesics

Opioids are the medications of choice for step two and three of the WHO analgesic ladder. The potency of opioids parallels receptor affinity and clinical efficacy. The utility of "weak" opioids (i.e., codeine, tramadol) is limited by a ceiling effect resulting in limited analgesia and dose-related adverse effects. When scheduled acetaminophen is utilized as a standard first-line pain treatment, acetaminophen toxicity must be considered with dosing of an opioid/acetaminophen combination. In general, opioid administration intervals should be extended, and dosages reduced among geriatric patients due to delayed clearance. Short-acting formulations are recommended for initial treatment until a stable dose is established. At that time, the dosage requirement can be converted to a long-acting opioid for ease of administration. Adverse effects common to all opioids include sedation, nausea, vomiting, and constipation.

Morphine Sulfate

Morphine sulfate is a popular and inexpensive postoperative analgesic. Advantages include a relatively low incidence of side effects; extensive experience; and a variety of administration routes including oral, intramuscular, intravenous, subcutaneous, and intrathecal. Postoperatively, intravenous routes are preferred as oral morphine has poor bioavailability and onset of pain relief is ~30 min compared to 5–10 min for intravenous morphine. Repeated dosing should be done cautiously as the active metabolite (morphine-6-glucuronide) can accumulate in renal dysfunction and the half-life for elimination is prolonged in geriatric patients. A reasonable starting dose of in an opioid naive, postoperative elder is 1 mg of intravenous morphine sulfate every 4 h. Studies conducted in the immediate postoperative period in the PACU have demonstrated that intravenous morphine titration can be safely administered to elderly patients using the same protocol as that used in young patients. However, these results may not apply to a frail elderly population or to patients with severe cognitive dysfunction.

Hydromorphone

Hydromorphone has similar efficacy as morphine. Oral, intravenous, intramuscular, and subcutaneous administration is available. Oral hydromorphone begins to have an analgesic effect 15–30 min following dosing with peak effect occurring at 30–60 min. The average duration of action for immediate release hydromorphone is 4–5 h, but this may be prolonged in elders due to underlying renal insufficiency. A reasonable initial dose is intravenous hydromorphone 1 mg every 6 h.

Oxycodone

Oxycodone is generally preferred when an oral analgesic is indicated, e.g., for outpatients. It is available in capsules/tablets, liquids, and concentrate form. Analgesic onset is 10–15 min following dosing with peak effect at 30–60 min. The duration of [action] is 3–6 h, but the half-life is prolonged in renal and hepatic dysfunction. In elders, a starting dose of 2.5 mg of oxycodone orally every 6 h is recommended.

Mixed Agonists–Antagonists

The mixed agonists–antagonist such as pentazocine and butorphanol tend to be more likely to produce psychomimetic effects in the elderly. Propoxyphene tends to have neurotoxic effects in the older patient. The long serum half-life drugs, such as methadone and levorphanol, require a longer time to reach steady state. Meperidine may accumulate with repeat dosing, with its active metabolite, normeperidine, causing seizures. It also has anticholinergic activity, which may cause tachycardia and agitation, and it has been associated with delirium in older patients. These opioid derivatives are not recommended in the very old patient.

Analgesic Modalities

Preemptive Premedication

Preemptive premedication with gabapentin (Neurontin) at doses ranging from 300 to 1,200 mg has been evaluated in a number of surgeries including hysterectomy, diskectomy, cholecystectomy, and mastectomy. Gabapentin works by binding the alpha-2-delta subunits of presynaptic voltage-gated calcium channels in spinal nociceptive neurons leading to inhibition of calcium influx and reduction in release of excitatory transmitters in the pain pathway. Single preoperative doses have been found to reduce pain intensity and opioid use in the first 24 h postoperatively. In addition, there was a reduced incidence of postoperative nausea and vomiting, constipation, and urinary retention. However gabapentin has been associated with an increase in sedation and a trend toward increased dizziness. Gabapentin is renally cleared, so the dose should be decreased in elders with renal dysfunction. More extensive study among elderly patients is needed to determine the optimal dosage for preemptive premedication.

Preventing postoperative pain via injection of local anesthetics via regional anesthesia has been associated with decreased length of hospital stay as well as increased patient satisfaction.

Patient-Controlled Analgesia

PCA can be a safe, effective analgesic modality in older patients. PCA may be especially effective in the treatment of acute postoperative pain in cognitively intact geriatric patients. PCA is preferred over scheduled doses of IV or IM opioids in the postoperative period, which may result in either under- or overdosages in patients where pain assessment may be challenging.

Compared to intramuscular morphine, PCA morphine in geriatric patients leads to improved pain relief, better patient satisfaction, decreased postoperative confusion, and reduced pulmonary complications; background infusions should be avoided in elderly patients as they increase respiratory depression, can lead to excessive sedation, do not reduce overall opioid requirements, and have not been shown to increase patient satisfaction.

Regional Analgesia

Both spinal and epidural anesthesia may be used effectively to provide enhanced pain control in the elderly. Intrathecal morphine has been shown to provide excellent postoperative analgesia in certain circumstances; however, in older patients, caution is advised. Intrathecal morphine is associated with dose-related adverse effects including nausea and vomiting, drowsiness, urinary retention, and delayed respiratory depression. When utilized in the older patient, the dose should be reduced, and patient should receive continuous monitoring in the immediate postoperative period. When used appropriately, intrathecal morphine may provide effective analgesia and reduce postoperative analgesic requirements while minimizing the incidence of adverse effects in the elderly.

Postoperative epidural analgesia that optimizes the synergistic effect of a local anesthetic combined with an opioid can provide excellent pain relief. In older patients the doses should be reduced to avoid side effects such as hypotension and respiratory depression. Improved postoperative outcomes compared with systemic opioids have been shown following thoracic and extensive upper abdominal surgery.

Delirium

Delirium is an acute disorder of attention and cognition which affects 25–60% of hospitalized elders including 13–61% of geriatric patients undergoing elective surgery. It is a geriatric emergency with significant associated adverse outcomes: hospital mortality rates of 22–76%, increased length of hospitalization, increased institutionalization following discharge, and increased rehospitalization within 30 days of discharge. In geriatric patients delirium is usually multifactorial in nature. Meperidine and propoxyphene are the only opioid analgesics found to specifically increase the risk of delirium. Other commonly used medications associated with delirium in elders include benzodiazepines and anticholinergic medications (i.e., diphenhydramine). Undertreated pain is also associated with delirium. In postoperative elders, low doses (<10 mg of morphine sulfate equivalents per day) or no opioid analgesics postoperatively are associated with an increased risk of delirium. Therefore, optimal pain management is vital to preventing and treating delirium in hospitalized elders.

Summary

Although pain is common among geriatric patients and results in a multitude of adverse effects, it is often poorly assessed and undertreated. Optimal pain management can be achieved by understanding the effects of aging on pain perception, accurately assigning pain in all patients, and choosing analgesic regimens on an individual basis.

Key Points

- The effects of aging on pharmacokinetics and pain perception must be considered when choosing an effective analgesic regimen. It is especially important to account for changes in excretion due to impaired renal function.
- Pain should be frequently assessed in all elders including nonverbal elders with advanced dementia. In these patients, an observational pain assessment tool such as the PAINAD is recommended.
- Pharmacologic treatment should follow the basic outline of the WHO analgesic ladder.
- Scheduled acetaminophen is first-line analgesic therapy for geriatric patients. Among hospitalized elders with acute pain, an opioid is also often needed for optimal pain control.
- Delirium is common in elders and has significant adverse outcomes. Consider undertreated pain as a possible cause.

Suggested Reading

Benzon RM. Essentials of Pain Medicine and Regional Anesthesia. In: Benzon RM, Essentials of Pain Medicine and Regional Anesthesia. Philadelphia: Elsevier; 2005: 18–40.

Casteldon CM, Pickles H. Suspected adverse drug reactions in elderly patients reported to the Committee on Safety of Medicine. Br J Clin Pharmacol. 1988;26(4):347–53.

Chau DL, Walker V, Pai L, Cho Lwin. Opiates and elderly: Use and side effects. Clin Interv Aging. 2008; 3(2):273–8.

Cooper B. Assessment and management of chronic pain in the older adult. Journal of American Pharmacits Association. 2010; 89–101.

Collett B, O'Mahoney S, Schofield P, Closs SJ, Potter J. The assessment of pain in older people. Clin Med. 2007;7(5):496–500.

Gagliese L, Jackson M, Ritvo P, Wowk A, Katz J. Age is not an impediment to effective use of patient-controlled analgesia by surgical patients. Anesthesiology. 2000;93(3):601–10.

Gagliese L, Katz J. Age differences in postoperative pain are scale dependent: a comparison of measures of pain intensity and quality in younger and older surgical patients. Pain. 2003; 103—(1-2):11–20.

Gibson SJ, Farrell M. A review of age differences in the neurophysiology of nociception and the perceptual experience of pain. Clin J Pain. 2004;20(4):227–39.

Gloth FM, 3rd. Pain management in older adults: prevention and treatment. J Am Geriatr Soc. 2001;49(2):188–99.

Greenblatt DJ, Allen MD, Harmatz JS, Shader RI. Diazepam disposition determinants. Clin Pharmacol Ther. 1980;27:301–12.

Herr K. Pain Assessment in the Nonverbal Patient: Position Statement with Clinical Practice Recommendations. American Society for Pain Management Nursing. 2006;44–52.

Jackson SH. Pharmacodynamics in the elderly. J R Soc Med. 1994;87(suppl 23);5–7.

Krulewitch H, London MR, Skakel VJ, Lundstedt GJ, Thomason H, Brummel-Smith K. Assessment of pain in cognitively impaired older adults: a comparison of pain assessment tools and their use by nonprofessional caregivers. J Am Geriatr Soc. 2000;48(12):1607–11.

Macintyre PE. Safety and efficacy of patient-controlled analgesia. Br J Anaesth. 2001;87(1):36–46.

McCleane G. Current Therapy in Pain: Pain in the Elderly. Chapter 50. Saunders Elsevier; 2009: 382–5.

Morrison RS, Magaziner J, Gilbert M, et al. Relationship between pain and opioid analgesics on the development of delirium following hip fracture. J Gerontol A Biol Sci Med Sci. 2003;58(1):76–81.

Rudberg MA, Pompei P, Foreman MD, Ross RE, Cassel CK. The natural history of delirium in older hospitalized patients: a syndrome of heterogeneity. Age Ageing. 1997;26(3):169–74.

Sawyer P, Bodner EV, Ritchie CS, Allman RM. Pain and pain medication use in community-dwelling older adults. Am J Geriatr Pharmacother. 2006;4(4):316–24.

Smith M. Pain assessment in nonverbal older adults with advanced dementia. Perspect Psychiatr Care. 2005;41(3):99–113.

Verdu E, Ceballos D, Vilches JJ, Navarro X. Influence of aging on peripheral nerve function and regeneration. J of Periph Nerv Syst. 2008;5(4):191–208.

Warden V, Hurley AC, Volicer L. Development and psychometric evaluation of the Pain Assessment in Advanced Dementia (PAINAD) scale. J Am Med Dir Assoc. 2003;4(1):9–15.

Chapter 11
Chronic Pain in Geriatric Patients

Vijay Thillainathan, Adam Young, and Asokumar Buvanendran

Introduction

Acute pain is triggered by injury or illness and generally subsides within weeks, while chronic pain lasts for a prolonged period that follows initial onset and often is defined as lasting 3 months or more. In cross-sectional surveys of a geriatric population, over 50% the reported chronic pain and of patients with pain, almost 30% received no analgesics regularly. Thus, it is clear that pain in older patients is both common and undertreated.

Undertreated pain may have serious consequences, such as depression, sleep disturbance, cognitive impairment, malnutrition, and decreased socialization and quality of life (QoL). The extent to which pain interferes with daily activities has been shown to increase incrementally with age up to the oldest age group. For example, the negative impact of postherpetic neuralgia (PHN) on QoL can resemble that resulting from life threatening diseases in the very elderly patients.

Decisions regarding the treatment of chronic pain are complicated because the phenomenon is not uniform. Chronic pain in older adults can be of many types, including pain associated with musculoskeletal disorders, such as degenerative spine conditions and osteoarthritis (OA); nighttime leg pain arising from muscle cramps, restless legs, or other conditions; pain from claudication; pain from cancer and cancer treatment; and neuropathic pain secondary to disorders such as diabetes mellitus and infections such as herpes zoster. Chronic pain can be categorized into four main types: nociceptive, neuropathic, inflammatory, and pain associated with central augmentation. In reality it is often difficult to specify which of these, alone or in combination, may be present in elderly patients in a practice setting.

V. Thillainathan, MD (✉) • A. Young, BS, MD • A. Buvanendran, MD
Department of Anesthesiology, Rush University Medical Center,
1653 W. Congress Parkway, 7th floor Jelke 7, Chicago, IL 60612, USA
e-mail: vthillai5@gmail.com

S.R. Barnett (ed.), *Manual of Geriatric Anesthesia*, DOI 10.1007/978-1-4614-3888-5_11,

Another challenge in the diagnosis and treatment of pain in older patients arises from the complexities of advanced age. Older patients may have atypical manifestations of pain, due to one or more chronic illness, and are frequently on multiple medications. Furthermore older patients may be reluctant or unable to report pain in part because they believe that pain is a normal part of aging. The aging process itself also can affect pharmacokinetics and pharmacodynamics, influencing decisions about treatment.

Assessment of Chronic Pain in the Elderly

Evaluation and treatment of the patient with persistent pain begins with a comprehensive history and physical examination. Obtaining a medical history in an older patient can be difficult and complicated by comorbid conditions such as memory loss, dementia, and neurological or psychiatric illness. Having a caregiver present at the time of evaluation can be useful. During the history, careful attention should be paid to pain symptoms such as onset, location, duration, intensity, quality, palliative or provocative factors, radiation, temporal features (e.g., continuous or intermittent), treatments received and their outcomes, sleep disturbances, presence of psychiatric comorbidities, psychosocial evaluation, and assessment of function. The patient's past medical and surgical history, medication profile, social history, and family history should also be documented along with a complete review of systems.

An objective assessment of the perceived pain is critical, and there are several tools at the clinician's disposal in the evaluation of pain. Intensity of pain can be measured and assessed on subsequent evaluations using a numeric rating scale (NRS) or visual analog scale (VAS). In addition an evaluation for depression may be warranted as patients with persistent pain have been shown to have coexisting depressive symptoms 22–78% of the time. The Beck Depression Inventory (BDI) is an instrument that can be used as a screening tool for depression and means to evaluate efficacy of treatment at follow-up.

Following collection of historical data, the physical examination is typically focused on that which ails the patient. The patient's general appearance should be noted along with any mobilization aids. Complete examination of the musculoskeletal, neurological, and integumentary systems, along with psychiatric evaluation, should follow. The musculoskeletal exam includes a peripheral pulse exam, assessing symmetry of joints and limbs, assessing muscle tone and strength, and demonstrating range of motion (both active and passive). A pain-focused exam may or may not include joint evaluation for erythema, edema, or crepitus; palpation of muscle groups for trigger points; performing a straight leg raise test in the setting of low back pain or radicular symptoms; performing a flexion adduction internal rotation (FAIR) test to assess for piriformis muscle impingement; examining the shoulder for impingement in cases of suspected rotator cuff injury; performing an Adson's test when thoracic outlet syndrome is suspected; and assessing for presence of deformities (such as Charcot joints). A neurological examination consisting of cranial nerve testing, cerebellar function (gait, balance, and coordination), deep tendon reflexes, and sensation (including light touch, vibratory with a 128-Hz tuning fork, and pinprick) should be completed. Additional investigations include presence or absence of pronator drift or Babinski sign, thermal testing [commonly accomplished with dysesthesias (a non-painful stimulus is perceived abnormally but not painful)], hyperalgesia (a painful stimulus is perceived as producing more pain than it normally would), and allodynia (a non-painful stimulus is perceived as pain). Small fiber neuropathy can be tested for using thermal testing. This is accomplished by placing a tuning fork in warm or cold water followed by direct placement onto the patient's skin, assessing for a painful response and comparison to the contralateral limb. Chronic pain can also be accompanied by signs of autonomic dysfunction; this may be manifested as altered sudomotor activity, hair growth or hair loss, change in skin color, trophic or dystrophic changes of the skin, thickening or striation of nails, and varying temperatures between limbs. To complete a thorough skin examination, presence of ulceration or breakdown, signs of physical abuse, and signs of substance abuse such as needle marks, palmar erythema, or spider angiomata should be noted. If there is a need to assess mental status, a mini-mental status exam (MMSE) can be initiated with a psychologist.

Following history and physical, a basic chemistry is frequently recommended and allows the practitioner to assess baseline renal and liver function, prior to prescribing medications that maybe renally excreted. Further investigations should be judiciously chosen based on the patient's history and examination and may include some of the following tests. Plain radiographs of the painful body part may reveal occult fracture, presence of foreign body, or degenerative changes. Nuclear scans are of value when there is concern for a neoplastic process as the cause of pain. Computed tomography scans are of use when the patient has metal implants, is unable to remain still for long periods of time, has a history of claustrophobia, or MRI is unavailable. MRI is the imaging test of choice when the pain is thought to originate from the spine or spinal cord and its roots, for example, for chronic low back pain. Electrodiagnostic studies (nerve conduction studies and electromyelography) evaluate the physiologic health of the nerves and muscles they innervate. Although invasive, these tests can help diagnose injuries to myelin, axons, or the neuromuscular junction. The information they provide includes location of injury and extent of injury and can suggest age of injury. Similarly tissue diagnosis with skin or nerve biopsy can aid in the diagnosis, but are invasive means and should be pursued only when necessary.

General Principle in Management

Physiological Changes

The treatment of chronic pain in the elderly is different from treating pain in the younger population, mainly due to physiological changes that occur with aging. In regard to body composition, skeletal muscle mass decreases and fat content increases. The increase in fat to lean body weight ratio will increase volume of distribution for fat-soluble drugs and resulting in longer half-life for these drugs. In addition total body water decreases, thereby accounting for skeletal muscle mass decrease and adipose tissue increase. As expected albumin level also decreases, especially with malnutrition, but studies have shown minimal effect on protein binding and drug delivery. From a central nervous system (CNS) standpoint, starting at the age of 50 years old, there continues to be a progressive decline in brain mass and associated decrease in neurotransmitter function. The decline in CNS function may make management of persistent pain difficult in an outpatient setting because the patient may not be able to physically take the medication or able to understand which medications to take for his or her pain. The cardiovascular system undergoes wide array of changes during the aging process. Sympathetic outflow increases and parasympathetic outflow decreases which accounts for an elevated resting heart rate. It is also thought that there is alteration in α-receptor responsiveness. These changes can most certainly change the efficacy of medications that specifically target certain receptors to treat pain. The major changes that occur in the pulmonary system include chest wall stiffness, decrease in elasticity of the lung, and loss of muscle tone particularly in the upper airway. These changes will affect the way certain medications, such as opioids, are used that can cause respiratory depression therefore adjuvant therapy becomes useful in managing chronic pain in the elderly.

Non-opioid Adjuvant Therapy

Acetaminophen

Because of its effectiveness and safety, acetaminophen (APAP) is recommended as a first-line and ongoing therapy for chronic pain in older patients, particularly musculoskeletal pain, such as OA and low back pain (LBP). Because some opioids are formulated with APAP, and APAP is available without a prescription, clinicians should educate patients that the maximum safe daily dose is <4 g per day from all sources. Liver failure is an absolute contraindication to APAP use, and relative contraindications include hepatic insufficiency and chronic alcohol abuse or dependence. Transient elevations of alanine aminotransferase in patients on long-term APAP treatment do not appear to indicate liver failure or hepatic dysfunction as long as maximum recommended doses are avoided.

Nonsteroidal Anti-inflammatory Drugs

The 2009 guidelines introduce significant changes in recommendations regarding nonsteroidal anti-inflammatory drugs (NSAIDs). NSAIDS have benefits over APAP, including better effectiveness in chronic inflammatory pain (e.g., rheumatoid arthritis), but in older persons, adverse events associated with NSAIDs include gastrointestinal

(GI) toxicity (often more severe with age), cardiovascular risks, and problems with blood pressure control, renal function, and heart failure management. The protection offered by COX-2 selective agents against GI bleeding is not complete, and other NSAID-related toxicities are the same with COX-2 inhibitors. The 2009 guidelines recommend that both nonselective NSAIDs and COX-2 selective inhibitors be used rarely and with extreme caution in only highly selected patients. Candidates for NSAIDs include those for whom other safer therapies have failed, therapeutic goals are not being met, and risks and complications are outweighed by benefits. Older patients receiving nonselective NSAIDs, or a COX-2 selective inhibitor with cardioprotective doses of aspirin, should take a proton pump inhibitor or misoprostol for GI prediction. Patients should not take more than one NSAID, nonselective or otherwise, for pain control. Aspirin for cardioprophylaxis should not be combined with ibuprofen. Routine assessment is required for all patients taking NSAIDs, with particular attention to GI and renal toxicity, hypertension, heart failure, and drug–drug and drug–disease interactions.

Antidepressants

Four classes of antidepressants have been studied in the treatment of neuropathic pain. Of the four classes, the two which are considered first-line medications will be discussed here: tricyclic antidepressants (TCAs) (desipramine, nortriptyline, and amitriptyline) and serotonin norepinephrine reuptake inhibitors (SNRI) (duloxetine and venlafaxine). Over 20% of chronic pain patients have concomitant depression so adding an antidepressant is very relevant. Although TCAs have not been proven effective in all types of neuropathic pain, they are the most efficacious of all antidepressants. Initial dosing is 10 mg desipramine, amitriptyline, or nortriptyline at bedtime and titrating up, as recommended by the AGS. The dose can be increased by 10 mg every 3–5 days until there is a decrease in pain or maximal dose is reached (100 mg). TCAs are associated with sedation, blurred vision, constipation, dry mouth, urinary retention, orthostatic hypotension, and prolonged QT interval. Relative contraindications for TCA use are cardiac conduction defects and benign prostatic hypertrophy. An EKG should be ordered prior to initiation of therapy with a TCA to evaluate for cardiac conduction abnormalities. Side effects of SNRIs are nausea, somnolence, dizziness, and constipation. Venlafaxine has shown dose-related increases in heart rate and blood pressure.

Anticonvulsants

Anticonvulsants available for pain relief include gabapentinoids: gabapentin and pregabalin. The gabapentinoids have been shown to be effective in the treatment of several chronic pain states. Gabapentin works via the modulation or binding to the $\alpha 2\delta$ subunit of the presynaptic voltage-dependent calcium channel

(VDCC). Gabapentin is thought to act at these VDCC by inhibiting calcium influx and subsequently the release of excitatory neurotransmitters involved in nociception[78]. Gabapentin has a half-life of 5–7 h. Common side effects include dizziness, somnolence, ataxia, and fatigue. Pregabalin works in a similar manner to gabapentin by modifying the VDCC[78]. Pregabalin has greater solubility than gabapentin and therefore moves more readily across the blood–brain barrier. Common side effects include somnolence, dizziness, ataxia, diplopia, and weight gain.

Muscle Relaxants

The class of muscle relaxants contains a range of medications that have been historically prescribed for muscle-related pain, although they produce many other effects—not all of which are well understood. Sensory and muscle spindle afferent signals are modulated in the dorsal root ganglia and ventral horn of the spinal cord. Further modulation of the efferent signals comes in the form of descending pathways from the brainstem and cortex. Changes in the complex homeostatic mechanisms involved in muscle tone can result in spasticity and pain. *Baclofen (Lioresal®)* is a $GABA_B$ receptor agonist. Its onset of action is 3–4 days with a variable duration of action. Baclofen is eliminated unchanged in the urine. Dosing should begin at 5 mg three times a day and titrated up without exceeding 30–40 mg a day total dose. Side effects include drowsiness, slurred speech, weakness, and urinary retention. When used in conjunction with antidepressants, short-term memory loss can occur. In the event of discontinuation, baclofen must be tapered as to avoid CNS excitability and withdrawal symptoms. Caution is warranted in the geriatric population and those with renal insufficiency. *Clonazepam (Klonopin®)* interacts with the $GABA_A$ receptor via the benzodiazepine subunit, thereby enhancing the effects of GABA. Peak serum levels are achieved 1–4 h after ingestion, with a 30–40 h half-life. Hepatic metabolism via cytochrome P450 CYP3A results in acetylated, hydroxylated, or glucuronidated metabolites which are renally cleared. Dosing should begin at 0.25–0.5 mg at bedtime. Sedation, fatigue, and memory problems can occur with clonazepam. Routine monitoring with complete blood counts are necessary as blood dyscrasias can occur. Similar to baclofen, clonazepam must be slowly tapered prior to discontinuation to avoid withdrawal symptoms.

Tizanidine (Zanaflex®) is a centrally acting α-2 adrenergic agonist. Onset of action is 2 weeks, with a variable duration of action. Cytochrome P450 CYP1A2 is responsible for metabolizing tizanidine to water soluble compounds that are renally excreted. The usual dose for elders is 2 mg, up to three times daily. The practitioner should monitor patients on tizanidine for sedation, weakness, urinary function, orthostasis, and cognitive effects.

Opioid Therapy

Morphine

The American Geriatric Society (AGS) states "patients with moderate to severe pain should be considered for opioid therapy." Morphine is the oldest medication in the opioid family and is still widely used today. Morphine exerts its effects by binding to and stimulating μ-receptors. The analgesic effects arise from central stimulation, whereas most side effects result from peripheral stimulation. Following oral administration, peak serum concentrations of morphine are reached after 30 min. The duration of analgesia with morphine is 4–6 h. Morphine has extensive first-pass metabolism by the liver, up to 50%. Phase II metabolism is accomplished by glucuronidation with UDP-glucuronosyl transferase-2B7 (UGT2B7) in the liver which makes the molecule more water soluble and allows for renal excretion. The two metabolites, morphine-3-glucuronide (M3G) and morphine-6-glucuronide (M6G), can accumulate in patients with renal failure and are responsible for some of the unwanted side effects of morphine. The half-life of M6G is prolonged (89–136 h) in renal failure and accumulation is thought to be responsible for narcosis (e.g., obtundation, respiratory depression). With M3G, half-life is prolonged to 41–141 h in renal failure; M3G has been implicated in having neuroexcitatory properties and associated with dose-dependent myoclonus and seizures. Morphine, like all opioids, can cause constipation, nausea and vomiting, pruritis, urinary retention from relaxation of the ureter and bladder, alterations of mood, sedation, and respiratory depression. There are immediate release and sustained release formulations of morphine which are recommended in the treatment of chronic pain in the elderly. Immediate release (MSIR®, Roxanol®) dosing ranges from 2.5 to 10 mg every 4 h. In addition to a tablet form, there is a liquid preparation which may be beneficial in patients who have difficulty swallowing pills. Sustained release (Avinza®, Kadian®, MSContin®, and Oramorph SR®) dosing is 15 mg every 8–24 h and is particularly useful in elderly patients with continuous pain. Short-acting opioids should be used to treat breakthrough pain in patients receiving long-acting opioid preparations. In general sustained release formulations should be used with caution in the geriatric population as there can be increased absorption secondary to decreased GI transit time.

Fentanyl

A synthetic opioid analgesic, fentanyl, has a relative potency of 100 times that of oral morphine. It was first synthesized by Paul Janssen in 1960. Like morphine, its site of action is the μ-receptor. CYP3A4 enzymes metabolize fentanyl to norfentanyl in the liver. Inhibitors of CYP3A4 include azole antifungal agents, macrolide antibiotics, nefazodone, aprepitant, amiodarone, diltiazem, verapamil, and grapefruit juice; these drugs can prolong the half-life of fentanyl. Fentanyl is more lipophilic than morphine and has a much faster onset of action when given parenterally. For chronic pain, fentanyl comes in transdermal (Duragesic®) and transbuccal (Actiq® or Fentora®) formulations. Onset of action with fentanyl transdermal is 12 h due to the creation of a subdermal reservoir from which fentanyl is continuously released; duration of analgesia can last 48–72 h. Increased rates of absorption can occur in the setting of a fever or when patches are placed in areas of skin breakdown. Dosage forms are patches that release a given amount of fentanyl per hour (e.g., 12.5, 25 mcg/hr) and should be replaced every 72 h. Transdermal fentanyl should be used cautiously use in elderly cachectic or debilitated patients who may have altered pharmacokinetics due to poor fat stores, muscle wasting, or altered clearance. Transdermal fentanyl should not be used in the setting of acute pain or in opioid naïve patients. Transbuccal fentanyl comes as lozenges or in the form of a lollipop and has been studied in the treatment of cancer pain. The manufacturers of transbuccal fentanyl recommend titrating dosages as needed with the following initial dosages: Actiq® 200 mcg every 4 h as needed and Fentora® 100 mcg every 4 h as needed. Transbuccal fentanyl bypasses the GI tract and the first-pass metabolism. This increased bioavailability allows for transbuccal fentanyl to be used in the treatment of breakthrough pain; onset is within minutes and the analgesic effect can last up to several hours. As with transdermal fentanyl, transbuccal fentanyl should be administered to those already receiving chronic opioid therapy. Side effects of fentanyl are similar to those of morphine.

Hydromorphone

Hydromorphone, μ-receptor agonist, when given by mouth is 3–5 times more potent than morphine and when given parenterally is 5–7 times more potent than morphine. The effective analgesic effect last 3–4 h. The metabolite produced is hydromorphone-3-glucoronide which lacks any analgesic properties and the risk of accumulation is less particularly in renal insufficient patients, but this metabolite may be responsible for other side effects such as sedation, pruritis, nausea, and vomiting.

Methadone

Administering methadone to the elderly patient can be particularly challenging mainly because of its unpredictable half-life ranging from 8 to 80 h and the difficulty in establishing adequate steady-state levels. The potency of methadone, in comparison to morphine, can range from 1:1 to 1:4. The benefit of methadone is seen in the renally compromised patient where there is no accumulation. The most recent advisory alert issued by the FDA is the incidence of cardiac dysrhythmias, such as QT prolongation and Torsades de pointes, especially when given in combination with drugs that inhibit cytochrome P450. It is recommended that a baseline EKG is obtained prior to initiation of methadone therapy followed regular EKG follow-up by a primary care physician.

Propoxyphene

Propoxyphene is the second most commonly prescribed analgesic after APAP in nursing home residents. Caution is advised when dosing as many older patients may have renal insufficiency and are at risk for toxicity from propoxyphene. Advanced age can lead to significant prolongation and accumulation risks of the metabolites and the parent drug. Elderly patients may be more likely to develop constipation, vomiting, and abdominal pain from propoxyphene than younger patients. Elderly patients taking propoxyphene do not appear more likely to develop dizziness or somnolence than younger patients, but the consequences in elderly patients who experience these effects may be more serious if the CNS effects result in falls and hip fractures. Data from several studies suggest that in both community dwelling and nursing home patients there may be a significant increase in risk of hip fracture in those taking propoxyphene compared with patients not taking analgesics. Propoxyphene use has also been significantly associated with adverse health outcomes (i.e., hospitalizations, emergency department visits, or deaths).

Oxycodone

Synthesized by Freund and Speyer in 1916, oxycodone has a relative potency of 1.5 times that of morphine. Oxycodone has μ-receptor-binding properties but may also exert its effects via κ_2b receptor agonism. The additional κ_2b activity may be of benefit in treating visceral pain. Onset of action is 30 min with the peak plasma level occurring at 1 h, the duration of action is 3–6 h, and oxycodone undergoes hepatic metabolism by cytochrome P450 CYP3A *N*-demethylation, with some contribution by CYP2D6 *O*-demethylation. Excretion is accomplished renally and caution is urged when prescribing oxycodone to patients with liver disease or renal insufficiency. Drugs that inhibit CYP3A4 activity include macrolide antibiotics, azole antifungal agents, and protease inhibitors. Rifampin, carbamazepine, and phenytoin induce CYP450 which results in lower plasma levels of oxycodone. The AGS recommends oxycodone (OxyIR®) dosing to start at 2.5–5 mg every 4–6 h. Sustained release formulations of oxycodone (Oxycontin®) should be dosed beginning at 10 mg every 12 h, although 24 h dosing may be necessary in frail patients. Oxycodone/acet-aminophen (Percocet®) contains the added effects of an aniline analgesic. Dosing for oxycodone/acetaminophen should start at 2.5–5 mg every 4–6 h. Additional precautions should be taken with this formulation as acetaminophen has a 4 g maximal dose every 24 h in patients with normal hepatic function. Side effects of oxycodone are similar to those of other narcotics. Oxycodone should not be initiated in opioid naïve patients.

Hydrocodone

Hydrocodone is a synthetic opioid. A pure agonist of the μ-receptor, it is five times more potent than morphine. Following an oral dose, the onset of action is 30–60 min with a duration of analgesia between 3 and 6 h. Hydrocodone undergoes hepatic metabolism; this is accomplished by cytochrome P450 CYP2D6 via *O*-demethylation and *N*-demethylation. The metabolites include norhydrocodone, and hydromorphone, the latter of which is a more potent analgesic compound than its progenitor. Clearance is achieved renally. AGS recommended dosing begins at 5 mg every 6 h. Formulations of hydrocodone typically include a non-opioid analgesic, including ibuprofen (Vicoprofen®) or acetaminophen (Norco®, Vicodin®). Maximal safe doses of acetaminophen or NSAIDs should not be exceeded when using these combination agents. An elixir (Lortab®) is also available and may be of benefit in geriatric patients with dysphagia. AGS states that hydrocodone is "useful for acute, recurrent, episodic, or breakthrough pain." Unlike some of the aforementioned narcotic agents, hydrocodone can be safely initiated in opiate-naïve patients. Side effects are similar to those associated with all opioid medications. Additional safety concerns with hydrocodone arise based on the compound with which it has been formulated (i.e., acetaminophen or ibuprofen), and patients should be monitored for side effects of these medications as well.

Management of Specific Disease Processes

Low Back Pain

Low back pain is a common problem that affects the majority of the population as they age. Common etiologies are radicular low back pain, lumbar facet syndrome, and discogenic pain. Radicular back pain is characterized as pain, paresthesia, and numbness that follow a dermatomal distribution accompanied by objective physical exam findings. Radicular pain is described as traveling as a narrow band, with a sharp, shooting, and lancinating quality. Objective signs include weakness, diminished reflexes, and positive straight leg raise. Causes of radicular low back pain include herniated dics, intervertebral disc lesions, spinal metastasis, and vertebral body fracture. A herniated disc leads to inflammation in the spinal canal. The inflammatory response is a result of the herniated nucleus pulposus releasing cytokines and other inflammatory mediators leading to a chemical radiculitis. MRI is typically the preferred method of confirming the location of the lesion, although a thorough physical exam can usually provide the clinician with a relatively close approximation. Treatment for low back pain includes bed rest, medications (appropriately dosed NSAIDs, or COX-2 inhibitors, muscle relaxants, and anticonvulsant), and epidural steroids injections (interlaminar vs. transforaminal approach). Epidural steroid injections (ESI) have an anti-inflammatory effect, most likely due to inhibition of phospholiapse-A2 activity, which helps to treat different forms of back pain. There are two approaches to ESI, interlaminar and transforminal. Multiple studies have shown that the transforaminal approach has a better rationale and better efficacy than interlaminar approach. It is advised that ESI be performed under fluoroscopic guidance in order to confirm the correct level of pathology as well as visualize contrast medium within the epidural space. Typically ESIs are performed in a series of three to four injections 2–3 weeks apart within a 6-month time period. There is no benefit of performing more than 3–4 ESI within a 6-month period; when this is exceeded the risks may outweigh the benefits. Complications of ESI include needle trauma, infection, and impaired blood glucose control in diabetes mellitus. Usually the steroid of choice is methylprednisone at 80 mg which can suppress plasma cortisol levels and the ability to secrete cortisol for up to 3 weeks.

Patients with low back pain originating from lumbar facet joints typically describe pain in the low back that radiates to ipsilateral posterior thigh and does not extend past the knees. Physical examination findings will include paraspinal tenderness and reproduction of pain with extension and rotational maneuvers of the lumbar spine. The key component in diagnosing facet syndrome is to have a compatible history, physical exam findings, and positive diagnostic facet block or medial branch blocks. Relief from facet blocks may vary between 3 and 6 months. Facet joints typically have a small volume and only require 1–1.5 mL of injectate, any more may cause severe damage to the facet joint. Similar to ESI, facet injections can be performed 2–3 weeks apart in a 6-month time period and recommended to be performed under fluoroscopic guidance. The complications are similar to ESI and can be avoided with appropriate needling techniques and well-understood knowledge of the anatomy and fluoroscopy.

Buttock Pain

Sacroiliac (SI) joint pain arises from inflammation secondary to dissymmetry of the right and left sacroiliac joints resulting in a misaligned sacrum. The prevalence of SI joint pain is 10–38%. Muscle, ligament, or nerve involvement may also play a role in this pain syndrome. Symptoms can range from low back pain to buttock, groin, or leg pain. Reliable physical exam tests are a Gaenslen test and thigh thrust test. The Gaenslen test involves positioning the patient in the supine or lateral recumbent position followed by maximal flexion of the thigh (on the affected side) and simultaneous extension of the opposite. A thigh thrust test involves the patient flexing at the thigh on the affect side to 90° with the practitioner placing downward stress (towards the spine). With both maneuvers, a positive test reproduces the pain. Local anesthetic infiltration of the SI joint with resolution of the pain was once considered diagnostic, but this has come under controversy recently as there is no published validity of the test. MRI is non-diagnostic for SI joint pathology, but can be of use if alternative diagnoses are possible. Conservative management of SI joint pain typically improves pain in over 90% of patients. Mainstays of therapy involve oral anti-inflammatory medications, SI joint injections, and possibly radiofrequency lesioning.

Piriformis Syndrome

Piriformis Syndrome (PS) is a controversial diagnosis that has been used to explain "sciatica of unclear etiology." In patients with low back pain and sciatica, piriformis syndrome is thought to be the cause in 6–8% of cases. Entrapment of the sciatic nerve or injury of the piriformis muscle is thought to be the cause of this disease. To understand this syndrome, one must recall the anatomy of the sciatic nerve and its fibular (lateral) and tibial (medial) branches, the piriformis muscle, and the pelvis. Exiting the pelvis, the path of the sciatic nerve passes through the sciatic notch and underneath the piriformis muscle the majority of the time (90%). Alternate pathways in a smaller subset of patients include the fibular division of the sciatic nerve passing through the piriformis muscle, or the tibial division passing under while the fibular division passes above the piriformis muscle or the sciatic nerve passes directly through the piriformis muscle. The piriformis muscle externally rotates the hip when the thigh is extended and abducts the hip when the thigh is flexed. The piriformis tendon connects to the superior border of the greater trochanter, along with the tendon of the obturator internus and gemelli. Trauma to the sciatic or gluteal region is thought to be the most common initiating factor, but other factors that have been associated with development of PS include prolonged sitting (immobile patients) and repetitive rotation at the hip. For unknown reasons, PS is more common in women with a ratio of 6:1. Symptoms include a deep, aching buttock pain associated with a limp and sitting intolerance on affected side. Squatting, climbing stairs, walking, or prolonged sitting worsen symptoms. The most common signs of PS are pain on palpation of the sciatic notch and pain with flexion, adduction, and internal rotation of the hip. Additional signs include weakness of ankle dorsiflexion and plantarflexion, weakness with inversion of foot, weakness of toe extension/flexion, decreased ankle jerk reflex, paresthesias, and pain in distribution of the sciatic nerve. PS is considered a clinical diagnosis, and imaging modalities can have nonspecific results but may be useful to exclude other possibilities. Initial therapy for PS is nonoperative and includes oral anti-inflammatory medications (NSAIDs), muscle relaxants, or neuropathic medications (e.g., gabapentin, nortriptyline, or carbamazepine). Physical therapy is another mainstay of conservative therapy which aims to stretch and relax the piriformis muscle. Heat and ultrasound massage have also been suggested as conservative therapies. If conservative therapy fails, therapeutic injections are the next line of therapy. Alleviation of pain with injection was once considered both a diagnostic and therapeutic modality; it is performed with local anesthetic (such as lidocaine) and corticosteroid. Addition (or substitution) of botulinum toxin (BoTox®) may prolong the duration of analgesia following injection. Surgical release of the sciatic nerve should be considered the last resort for patients with PS. If the patient is not a surgical candidate, pain control with intrathecal therapy or spinal cord stimulation should be considered.

Diabetic Peripheral Neuropathy

Diabetic peripheral neuropathy (DPN) is a long-term complication of diabetes. The pathophysiology of DPN is based on few different theories, which include the polyol pathway, microvascular theory, and end-glycosylation theory. The polyol pathway theory postulates that high blood glucose levels leads to an increase in nerve glucose concentrations. The polyol pathway converts glucose into sorbitol and fructose levels also become elevated. The elevated sorbitol and fructose levels lead to activation of aldolase reductase pathway which reduces nitric oxide and glutathione. Reduction in nitric oxide inhibits vasodilation, contributing to ischemia. Neuronal ischemia and infarction are also a part of the microvascular theory and state that the thickened basement membrane and hyperplasia of endothelial cells prevent adequate blood supply to the nerves. The theory of end-product glycosylation is based on the idea that the end products of glucose metabolism are deposited around the nerves which prevents axonal transport. Common symptoms of DPN include pain described as burning, deep aching, electrical, or stabbing sensations usually worse at night. The lower extremities are usually involved with decreased sensation to vibration, pressure, pain, and temperature. Diagnosis of DPN usually based on history and clinical findings, but there are other tests that can help identify the severity of peripheral neuropathy. Nerve conduction studies and electromyography can help determine the characteristics of the neuropathy (axonal, demyelinating) and localization. Typical nerve conduction studies include measurement of the speed of motor and sensory conduction. A nerve biopsy can also be taken, usually the sural nerve, to help determine the stage of neuropathy (mild, moderate, or severe), but with nerve conduction studies and EMG, this is rarely needed. The key component in the management of DPN involves tight glucose control and regular follow-up with primary care physician and/or endocrinologist. Antidepressants and anticonvulsants have been shown to be effective in the management of DPN. Serotonin and norepinephrine reuptake inhibitors (SNRI) such as duloxetine have been shown to be as efficacious as TCAs with a better side effect profile. The anticonvulsants shown to be effective for DPN include pregabalin and gabapentin. The combination of opioids and these agents also improves the efficacy.

Herpes Zoster

Herpes zoster results from reactivation of the varicella virus within the dorsal sensory or cranial nerve ganglia. The acute episode of vesicular rash and pain in a dermatomal distribution can be followed by a syndrome of neuropathic pain in that area which has been termed postherpetic neuralgia (PHN). This disease typically affects the elderly and immunocompromised patients. A prodrome of herpes zoster has been described that consists of flu-like symptoms (fatigue, headache, fever, or nausea), pruritis, or pain in a unilateral dermatomal pattern. Replication of the virus in the dorsal root ganglia, causing inflammation and nerve destruction, has been hypothesized as the cause of the prodromal pain. This prodrome precedes the rash by 3–7 days. The rash is of grouped vesicles on an erythematous base. It is thought that viral replication in the skin is responsible for the necrotic appearance of the epidermis. The vesicular lesions progress to a pustular rash in 7–10 days. These lesions scab over and are cleared by 3 weeks. Variants of herpes zoster include herpes zoster ophthalmicus (involving the ophthalmic branch of cranial nerve V), herpes zoster oticus (with possible involvement of cranial nerves V, VII, IX, and X), and zoster sine herpete (pain in a unilateral dermatomal distribution without rash). Diagnosis of herpes zoster is based on exam findings of the rash in a unilateral dermatomal pattern and pain. Laboratory testing can be used to confirm the diagnosis, but is often unnecessary before initiating therapy. Viral culture is a tedious process and can take weeks to receive the results; direct immunofluorescence assays are much faster (hours) and cost-effective, but the lesions must be in the vesicular stage; viral DNA testing takes at least 24 h and is more expensive than immunoassays. Biopsy is seldom necessary and should be "reserved for difficult to diagnose cases." Therapy for herpes zoster involves antiviral medications. Antiviral medications have been shown to decrease the acute and chronic effects of herpes zoster. Ideally they should be instituted within 72 h of the rash. Antiviral medications are renally excreted and this should be taken into account in patients with renal insufficiency. Acyclovir 800 mg five times a day is recommended to be continued for 7–10 days. Analgesic medication is likely necessary and can range from acetaminophen and NSAIDs to opioids depending on the patient's pain level. If oral medications are unsuccessful in treating the pain associated with herpes zoster, a pain specialist may perform sympathetic blocks or continuous neuraxial analgesia. Immunization from varicella in children and herpes zoster in adults appears to be the most efficacious treatment. Vaccination for herpes zoster decreases the incidence in the geriatric population less than in the general population, but it has a greater effect of reducing the severity of the illness in the elderly. Varicella zoster immune globulin is another therapy used to treat herpes zoster, but is typically reserved for the immunocompromised.

Cancer Pain

In the USA, the majority of cancer and cancer-related deaths occur in person over the age of 65 years. Significant pain is present in 25% of patients undergoing active treatment and up to 90% in patients with cancer that has further metastasized. The origin of cancer pain can be somatic, visceral, or neuropathic, and this variation responds to different forms of therapy. Somatic pain can be divided into superficial or deep. Superficial somatic pain arises from skin, subcutaneous tissue, and mucousal membranes, which is characterized as being sharp, throbbing, or burning sensation. Deep somatic pain arises from muscles, tendons, joints, or bones and is characterized as dull, aching in quality, and generally less localized. Usually somatic pain is responsive to opioids, NSAIDs, COX-2 inhibitors, as well as neural blockade. Visceral pain is a result of a disease process affecting the thoracic, abdominal, or pelvic region. True visceral pain is described as dull, diffuse, and usually midline and can be associated with nausea, vomiting, sweating, and changes in blood pressure and heart rate. Visceral pain responds well to sympathetic blocks. Typically neuropathic pain is effectively treated with a combination of anticonvulsants, opioids, and tricyclic antidepressants. A multidisciplinary approach to management of cancer pain, regardless of the origin, is the most efficacous. This approach involves pharmacologic management, non-pharmacological (interventional) management, antineoplastic therapy, behavioral and psychosocial therapy, and finally hospice care. The antineoplastic therapy, behavioral aspect, and hospice care are equally important but extend beyond the scope of this text. From a pharmacologic standpoint, opioids are considered the mainstay of treatment, but combining other medications (anticonvulsants, antidepressants, NSAIDs, etc.) can improve QoL. Interventional procedures such as intrathecal pumps, neurolytics blocks, vertebroplasty, and kyphoplasty can considerably help to relieve some pain. These procedures should be considered as adjuvant to pharmacologic management.

Key Points

- Chronic pain is very common in the elderly population.
- When prescribing medication in older patients, age- and disease-related changes in pharmacokinetics and pharmacodynamics may require a reduction in doses.
- Acetaminophen is considered the first-line treatment for elderly patients with noncancer chronic pain.
- NSAIDs should be used cautiously if at all as older patients have a higher risk of developing side effects such as gastrointestinal bleeding and renal impairment.

- A thorough history and physical examination is required to appropriately diagnose the underlying cause of pain.
- Depression is very commonly associated with chronic pain and initial pain evaluations should include an assessment for depressions.
- Lower back pain is one of the most common causes of chronic pain in older patients.
- Treatment of chronic back pain with repeated epidural steroid and facet joint injections should not exceed 3 or 4 injections in a 6-month period.
- Neuropathic pain from diabetes or other causes may respond to the antidepressant and antiseizure medications as well as traditional analgesics.

Suggested Reading

American Geriatrics Society Panel on the Pharmacological Management of Persistent Pain in Older Persons. Pharmacological Management of Persistent Pain in Older Persons. Journal of the American Geriatric Society. 2009;57(8):1331–1346.

Benzon HT, Hurley RW, Deer TR. Chronic Pain Management. In: Barash PG, Cullen BF, Stoelting RK, Cahalan MK, Stock MC, eds. Clinical Anesthesia. 6th Ed. Philadelphia, Pa: Lippincott, Williams, & Wilkins; 2009: 1505–1531.

Dworkin RH, Turk DC, Farrar JT, et al. Core Outcome Measures for Chronic Pain Clinical Trials: IMMPACT Recommendations. Pain. 2005; 113(1-2):9–19.

Dworkin RH, Turk DC, Wyrwich KW, et al. Interpreting the Clinical Importance of Treatment Outcomes in Chronic Pain Clinical Trials: IMMPACT Recommendations. Journal of Pain. 2008; 9(2):105–121.

Gloth, III FM. Pain Management in Older Adults: Prevention and Treatment. Journal of The American Geriatric Society. 2001; 49:188–199.

Irving G, Squire P. Medical Evaluation of the Chronic Pain Patient. In: Fishman SM, Ballantyne JC, Rathmell JP, eds. Bonica's Management of Pain. 4th Ed. Philadelphia, Pa: Lippincott, Williams, & Wilkins; 2010: 210–224.

Katz N, Mazer NA. The Impact of Opioids on the Endocrine System. Clinical Journal of Pain. 2009; 25:170–175.

McGuirk BE, Bogduk N. Chronic Low Back Pain. In: Fishman SM, Ballantyne JC, Rathmell JP, eds. Bonica's Management of Pain. 4th Ed. Philadelphia, Pa: Lippincott, Williams, & Wilkins; 2010: 1106–1123.

Oxman MN, Levin MJ, Johnson GR, et al. For the Shingles Prevention Study Group. A Vaccine to Prevent Herpes Zoster and Postherpetic Neuralgia in Older Adults. New England Journal of Medicine. 2005; 352:2271–2284.

Peura DA. Gastrointestinal Safety and Tolerability of Non-Selective Non-Steroidal Anti-Inflammatory Agents and Cyclooxygenase-2-Selective Inhibitors. Cleveland Clinic Journal of Medicine. 2002; 69(Supplement 1):SI31–39.

Rupert MP, Lee M, Manchikanti L, et al. Evaluation of Sacroiliac Joint Interventions: A Systematic Appraisal of the Literature. Pain Physician. 2009;12(2):399–418.

Thakur R, Kent JL, Dworkin RH. Herpes Zoster. In: Fishman SM, Ballantyne JC, Rathmell JP, eds. Bonica's Management of Pain. 4th Ed. Philadelphia, Pa: Lippincott, Williams, & Wilkins; 2010: 339–357.

Trescot AM, Datta S, Lee M, Hansen H. Opioid Pharmacology. Pain Physician. 2008; 11(Supplement 2): S133–153.

Williams BS, Buvanendran A. Nonopioid Adjuvants in Multimodal Therapy for Acute Perioperative Pain. Advances in Anesthesia. 2009; 27:111–142.

Chapter 12
The Elderly Patient and the Intensive Care Unit

Steven J. Schwartz and Frederick Sieber

At least 20–50% of all ICU admissions occur in patients older than 65 years of age, and geriatric patients account for almost 60% of all ICU days. Unfortunately, many older patients' final days are spent in the ICU; 40% of Medicare patients who die are admitted to an ICU during their terminal illness, accounting for 25% of all Medicare expenditures. Additionally, of those who survive, many are discharged to a subacute facility with persistent organ failure where they will eventually die. Furthermore, those discharged to a subacute care facility have a higher mortality rate compared to those discharged home (31 vs. 17%). The decision to admit an elderly patient to an ICU should be based not only on their comorbidities, acuity of illness, and prehospital functional status, including quality of life, but also on their preference for the use of life-sustaining treatments if it is known. The underlying disease process is not altered despite the use of invasive procedures in terminally ill patients, and potential harm or discomfort can occur if invasive procedures are used inappropriately. To avoid such unintended consequences and enhance optimal end-of-life decision making, healthcare providers need to identify, explain, and negotiate consensus therapeutic goals.

In 2005, spending by Medicare for those older than 65 years totaled $342 billion, representing 17.1% of the total of $2 trillion spent nationwide for health care. Intensive care consumes 4% of national healthcare expenditures. During the last 6 months of their lives, 11% of Medicare recipients spend 8 or more days in the ICU; various studies documenting ICU occupancy by those older than 65 years old note that this ranges from one quarter to one half of the available beds. These statistics alone show the profound financial burden that must be borne to provide a medically sound and appropriate depth of care, a significant portion of which will be provided in the ICU.

S.J. Schwartz, MD(✉)
Department of Anesthesiology and Adult Critical Care, Johns Hopkins Hospital,
4940 Eastern Avenue, Baltimore, MD 21220, USA
e-mail: sschwa27@jhmi.edu

F. Sieber, MD
Department of Anesthesiology and Adult Critical Care, Johns Hopkins Bayview
Medical Center, 4940 Eastern Avenue, Baltimore, MD 21220, USA

S.R. Barnett (ed.), *Manual of Geriatric Anesthesia*, DOI 10.1007/978-1-4614-3888-5_12,

Cardiovascular Illness in the Critical Care Setting

Cardiovascular disease may be either the primary or secondary problem for elderly patients receiving critical care. The therapeutic options targeted at the cardiovascular system in the critical care setting range from medical management with the goal of symptom relief and comfort care to invasive therapies such as invasive monitoring, percutaneous coronary intervention (PCI), intraaortic balloon pump therapy, and cardiac surgery. Age alone is not a contraindication for invasive therapies, however, the goals such as symptom relief, improvement of quality of life, and survival benefit of any therapy should be clearly established for individual patients. End-of-life issues deserve special consideration in the elderly, as these are often challenging issues that will likely be more frequently encountered in critical care settings as science and technology advance. The number of potential cardiac issues encountered in the ICU is vast; some of the common issues are listed in Table 12.1 with some of the possible therapies that might be offered.

Acute Coronary Syndrome

Acute Coronary Syndrome (ACS) is a clinical spectrum of acute coronary artery vascular events: unstable angina, non-ST-elevation myocardial infarction (MI) and

Table 12.1 Common CV problems experienced by the elderly in critical care settings

CV problem	Possible acute therapies
Unstable angina/NSEMI	ASA, β-blocker, heparin, LMWH, nitroglycerin, glycoprotein IIb/IIIa platelet inhibitor, cardiology consultation
STEMI	Percutaneous coronary intervention, fibrinolytic therapy, ASA, β-blocker, heparin, LMWH, nitroglycerin, cardiology consultation
Systolic dysfunction with heart failure	Diuretics, nitroprusside, nesiritide, nitroglycerin, inotropic agents
Diastolic dysfunction with heart failure	Diuretics, nesiritide, nitroglycerin
Atrial fibrillation—rate control	β-blockers: metoprolol, esmolol Calcium antagonists: verapamil, diltiazem Other: digoxin, amiodarone
Atrial fibrillation—rhythm control	Amiodarone, ibutilide, electrical cardioversion
Atrial fibrillation—embolic prophylaxis	Heparin, LMWH, warfarin, ASA
Ventricular fibrillation	Advanced life support protocol
Ventricular tachycardia	Advanced life support protocol, electrical cardioversion, amiodarone
Aortic stenosis	Diuretics, arrhythmia management, inotropic agents, endocarditis prophylaxis, cardiology consultation
Mitral regurgitation	Diuretics, nitroprusside, nitroglycerin, arrhythmia management, inotropic agents, intraaortic balloon pump, endocarditis prophylaxis, cardiology consultation

ST-elevation MI. The incidence of ACS, as well as its morbidity and mortality, markedly increase with age. Compared with patients who experience ST-elevation MI, those with unstable angina/non-ST-elevation MI are more likely to be elderly, have a higher incidence of diabetes, hypertension, and known coronary artery disease, and have a worse prognosis.

The indicated medical therapy of aspirin, β-blockers, angiotensin-converting inhibitors (ACE-I), and nitroglycerin does not differ for the elderly patient. The elderly derive the same survival benefits as younger adults do with aspirin and β-blockers post-infarction, although the survival benefit associated with ACE-I post-infarction in the very elderly is less clear. There is evidence that 30-day mortality maybe 10% lower than for placebo in patients 65–74 years of age treated with ACE-I postinfarction, but no survival benefit has been demonstrated in patients ≥75 years of age. The elderly clearly do obtain survival benefit from ACE-I therapy when the clinical syndrome of heart failure (HF) or left ventricular systolic dysfunction is present. It is important to note that there may be more complications from the usual medical therapy seen in the elderly compared with younger adults. These complications include a greater risk of renal dysfunction with ACE-I therapy postinfarction and more gastrointestinal bleeding with aspirin therapy.

In the setting of unstable angina/non-ST-elevation MI, unfractionated or low-molecular weight heparin is indicated in addition to the basic medical therapy. Current data suggest that glycoprotein IIb/IIIa platelet inhibitors are of benefit to acute non-ST-elevation MI patients with high-risk markers, including elderly patients. High-risk markers include elevated biochemical markers, dynamic ST changes, and continuing ischemic symptoms, particularly in those patients likely to undergo percutaneous coronary intervention (PCI). The increased risk of bleeding complications from oral antiplatelet agents (aspirin and clopidogrel), heparin and glycoprotein IIb/IIIa platelet inhibitors, and possible bradycardia and hypotension associated with the use of β-blockers and nitrates, must always be considered for each individual patient's risk profile.

Reperfusion therapy is the optimal treatment for acute ST-elevation MI regardless of age and gender. The highest risk patients, such as the elderly and those with anterior MI, derive the greatest benefit. Absolute contraindications to fibrinolytic therapy are hemorrhagic stroke, intracranial neoplasm, active internal bleeding, or suspected aortic dissection, all of which have a higher incidence in the elderly.

In-hospital mortality among patients with acute MI is primarily caused by cardiogenic shock or one of the mechanical complications of acute MI, and both are more common in the elderly. Life-threatening complications include ventricular septal defect, free wall rupture and papillary muscle rupture. Patients experiencing these complications have a mean age of 66 years and mortality is high, 90% or greater, when medical therapy alone is employed. Although survival is improved with urgent surgical treatment, mortality remains quite high: 50% surgical mortality for ventricular septal defect and a 40–90% surgical mortality for papillary muscle rupture.

Surgical Revascularization

Revascularization accomplished by coronary artery bypass surgery (CABG) needs careful consideration in the elderly, especially in those ≥75 years of age, because CABG mortality rises rapidly beyond this age. The goal of surgical therapy should always be clearly defined; is it indicated for symptom relief or to prolong survival? If the only indication is for symptom relief, all attempts to manage symptoms medically or with PCI should be made before considering surgical intervention, as its morbidity and mortality may obviate any benefit. CABG may be appropriate for elderly patients who have high-risk clinical markers associated with ACS and those with chronic severe angina who have failed medical therapy. High-risk markers include resting dynamic ECG changes uncontrolled with medical therapy, three-vessel coronary artery disease (CAD), impaired left ventricular function, left main or proximal left anterior descending disease, previous MI, and diabetes. Surgical revascularization can be expected to prolong survival in patients who have left main disease or its equivalent, or three-vessel disease with diminished left ventricular systolic function.

Age alone is not a contraindication, but the presence of comorbid illnesses increases with age, and an overall risk profile must be carefully considered. Mortality related to CABG can be estimated to be 30% or higher in the elderly with multiple comorbid conditions.

Heart Failure

Ventricular dysfunction with its clinical syndrome of HF is a major public health problem in the United States. There are two major categories of ventricular dysfunction that can lead to HF, systolic dysfunction, and the commonly termed diastolic dysfunction. The primary mechanism leading to systolic dysfunction is the impairment of ventricular contractility leading to increased ventricular volumes. The primary mechanism for diastolic dysfunction is the impairment of compliance or the inability to increase ventricular end-diastolic volumes and stroke volume. Current evidence suggests that diastolic dysfunction is the cause of the HF syndrome in at least 50% of the elderly with HF, and that the proportion increases with advancing age. Elderly HF patients, with either systolic or diastolic dysfunction, have high morbidity, frequent hospitalizations, and a high incidence of comorbid conditions including stroke, MI, renal dysfunction, and pulmonary disease. Critically ill elderly patients with HF have a poor prognosis, and their management can be complicated. Predictors of mortality include age, male gender, recent hospitalization, diabetes, left ventricular dilatation, systolic dysfunction, coronary artery disease, renal insufficiency, hyponatremia, reduced peak oxygen consumption, and increased minute ventilation.

Identification of the clinical syndrome of HF can be challenging, especially in the elderly patient who may be critically ill from other problems. Older patients may present with atypical symptoms of HF, such as fatigue, failure to thrive, somnolence, weakness, and confusion. In both diastolic and systolic dysfunction patients commonly experience symptoms of congestion. On physical examination, a laterally or inferiorly displaced apical impulse with an S3 supports systolic dysfunction rather than diastolic dysfunction. Rales, an elevated jugular venous pressure, hepatomegaly, ascites, edema, and evidence of low cardiac output may be found in either. An ECG, chest radiograph, and echocardiogram are essential diagnostic tests. An abnormal ECG highly correlates with the presence of CV disease, and an enlarged cardiac shadow or pulmonary vascular congestion on chest radiograph supports cardiac dysfunction. Ventricular systolic function, ventricular hypertrophy, valvular dysfunction, chamber size, and some assessment of hemodynamics can be made by echocardiography. The measurement of B-type natriuretic peptide levels may also aid in the identification of ventricular dysfunction and the syndrome of HF.

The management goals can be multiple, including relieving of symptoms, maintaining adequate perfusion and vital organ function, controlling volume status, identifying the underlying causes of ventricular dysfunction, identifying the type of ventricular dysfunction (systolic versus diastolic), and initiating appropriate long-term therapy such as ACE inhibitors. The symptoms most likely to be experienced by critically ill elderly are congestion related. Diuretic therapy, hormonal therapy, or other vasodilator therapies are essential approaches for managing congestive symptoms. In cases of systolic dysfunction, low cardiac output, or hypotensive states, inotropic therapy may be appropriate. Appropriate inotropes include dobutamine and milrinone. In patients with the HF syndrome and hypertension, it is absolutely essential to control blood pressure.

A very important issue facing critical care physicians taking care of elderly patients with HF is the high 1-year mortality in these patients, which can be as high as 25–50%. End-of-life issues are often poorly addressed in this group of patients, and the discussion of end-of-life issues may need to begin in the critical care setting, especially for patients who do not respond to optimal therapy.

Implantable Cardioverter-Defibrillator (ICDs) and the ICU

ICDs are becoming more common in elderly patients, and there are at least two clinical scenarios in which the disarming of ICD tachycardic therapy should be considered in the elderly ICU patient with an ICD. The first is when the ICD is being activated inappropriately, either because of self-limited ventricular arrhythmias or because of rapid atrial arrhythmias that the ICD identifies incorrectly. The second is when the patient is expected to die, and ICD discharges may only prolong the dying process or cause unnecessary discomfort. Included are "Do Not Resuscitate" patients who are receiving comfort-only care. In all such cases, the decision to deactivate the tachycardic therapy mode must be fully discussed with the patient or his or her next of kin and documented in the medical record. It is also appropriate to respect a patient's decision of not wanting to disarm the device.

Pulmonary Issues in the Elderly in the Critical Care Setting

The term "chronic obstructive pulmonary disease" (COPD) describes a category of respiratory conditions characterized by inflammatory damage to small and large airways, destruction of lung parenchyma, and limitation of expiratory airflow. The range of clinical symptoms related to COPD is broad, from mild end expiratory wheezing to respiratory failure requiring mechanical ventilation.

Smoking is the primary etiologic factor for most patients with COPD, who may present with clinical manifestations of chronic bronchitis, emphysema, or a combination of these two disorders. Chronic bronchitis is defined by the presence of chronic cough in patients who experience airway mucus hypersecretion, increased risk of bronchial infections, and expiratory airflow limitation. Emphysema denotes the presence of irreversible lung damage with destruction of alveolar tissue that causes impaired respiratory gas exchange and expiratory airway collapse with airflow limitation.

Elderly patients with moderate to severe COPD experience acute exacerbations of their airway disease, each of which presents a risk for acute respiratory failure. Although definitions of acute exacerbations vary, recent consensus statements define exacerbations by the presence of one or more of the cardinal symptoms of increased dyspnea, increased sputum volume, and increased sputum purulence (Table 12.2).

Bronchial infections are important causes of acute exacerbations with bacterial, atypical bacterial and viral pathogens being the most commonly identified microbes. Ten to 20% of patients with acute exacerbations have infections with two or more pathogens. Among atypical pathogens, *Chlamydia pneumoniae* has been estimated to account for 5–10% of acute exacerbations but up to 18% of exacerbations that result in admission to the ICU. Viral bronchitis is found in 30–40% of patients with acute exacerbations but only 16% of those who require ICU admission (Table 12.3).

Pharmacologic Management of Acute Exacerbation of Airway

Elderly patients with an acute exacerbation of airway disease experience increased resistance to expiratory airflow and increased work of breathing, which can cause respiratory muscle fatigue. Most therapeutic recommendations for managing elderly

Table 12.2 Criteria for grading the severity of an acute exacerbation of chronic bronchitis

American College of Chest Physicians–American College of Physicians/American Society of Internal Medicine Guidelines
Mild exacerbation: presence of any one of the cardinal symptoms of increased dyspnea, increased sputum volume, or increased sputum purulence with the addition of an upper respiratory infection within the past 5 days, fever with no other cause, increased wheezing or cough, or a 20% rise over baseline in respiratory rate or heart rate
Moderate exacerbation: presence of any two of the three cardinal symptoms of an exacerbation
Severe exacerbation: presence of all three of the cardinal symptoms of an exacerbation

Table 12.3 Common infectious causes of acute exacerbations of chronic bronchitis

Bacterial
Nontypable *Haemophilus influenzae*
Moraxella catarrhalis
Streptococcus pneumoniae
Haemophilus parainfluenzae
Staphylococcus aureus
Pseudomonas aeruginosa and other Gram-negative bacilli (occurs more commonly with FEV1 < 50% predicted)
Atypical bacterial
Mycoplasma pneumoniae
Chlamydia pneumoniae
Viral
Parainfluenzae virus
Rhinovirus
Influenzae virus
Coronavirus
Respiratory syncytial virus
Adenovirus

patients in the ICU with acute exacerbations of COPD derive from expert consensus because of the paucity of large prospective randomized trials. Initial management includes supplemental oxygen by nasal cannula or through a face mask that controls oxygen flow. Oxygen flows are titrated with goals of achieving oxygen saturation between 90 and 92% and a partial pressure of arterial oxygen between 60 and 64 mm Hg. Oxygen flow is monitored to prevent hypercapnia, which can result from the effects of supplemental oxygen on increasing dead-space ventilation and ventilation-perfusion mismatching.

Inhaled bronchodilators promote bronchodilation that can achieve a 15–29% increase in FEV_1 and FVC within 1–2 h. Randomized trials support the conclusion that short-acting β-agonists (albuterol, levalbuterol, pirbuterol, bitolterol, fenoterol, metaproterenol, terbutaline) and anticholinergic-type inhaled bronchodilators (ipratropium bromide) have similar efficacy for managing acute exacerbations, and both are more effective than parenteral bronchodilators. The faster onset of action of β-agonists and the lower frequency of adverse effects with anticholinergic drugs determine drug selection for individual patients. Initial therapy for critically ill patients is usually with a nebulizer, as these patients may experience difficulties using meter dose inhalers. Data does not support the use of parenteral aminophylline for critically ill elderly patients hospitalized in the ICU with acute exacerbations of COPD.

The role of bacterial infections in causing exacerbations of airway disease supports the use of antibiotics, although most studies of antibiotic efficacy for acute exacerbations were performed before the era of multidrug resistant bacteria, and the appropriate selection of antibiotics for critically ill patients remains unclear. Critically ill patients and patients with risk factors for poor outcomes (baseline

Table 12.4 Principles for initiating noninvasive positive pressure ventilation

Identify appropriate patient
Review the equipment with the patient and explain care
Fit an appropriate-sized mask
Adjust ventilator initially at a low pressure (8–10 cm H_2O inspiration; 4–5 cm H_2O expiration) with the patient holding the mask in place
Ask the patient to report comfort level and adjust ventilator pressures accordingly
Adjust oxygen flow rates to meet target oxygen saturation levels
Adjust the mask to avoid leaks
Monitor patient frequently and coach breathing patterns
Gradually increase inspiratory pressures for maximal relief of dyspnea

$FEV_1 < 50\%$ predicted, comorbid conditions, three or more exacerbations during the last 12 months) benefit from newer fluoroquinolones (levofloxacin, moxifloxacin) because of the risk of Gram-negative organisms. If *Pseudomonas aeruginosa* is suspected (baseline $FEV_1 < 35\%$ predicted, underlying bronchiectasis, multiple courses of antibiotics), ciprofloxacin is the preferred antibiotic.

Prospective, randomized controlled trials demonstrate that systemic corticosteroids improve outcome for patients with acute exacerbations, as demonstrated by more rapid improvement in measured airflow, gas exchange, and respiratory symptoms with decreased treatment failure rates and relapse rates. Hyperglycemia is the major complication of corticosteroid therapy for hospitalized patients with acute exacerbations.

Ventilatory Support for Patients with Acute Exacerbation

Positive pressure ventilation unloads respiratory muscles and prevents or treats respiratory muscle fatigue. Ventilatory support can be provided by a tight-fitting face mask in the form of noninvasive positive pressure ventilation (NIPPV) or by tracheal intubation with mechanical ventilation (Table 12.4).

All hospitalized elderly patients who present with respiratory distress from acute exacerbations should be evaluated for NIPPV. Patients admitted with even mild respiratory acidosis may benefit from NIPPV. Unfortunately, only 20% of hospitalized patients are candidates for NIPPV. Poor candidates for NIPPV include patients with cardiovascular instability, respiratory arrest, limited ability to clear increased airway secretions, poor airway control, agitation or severe encephalopathy (Glasgow Coma Scale < 10), uncooperability, upper gastrointestinal bleeding, upper airway obstruction, high risk for aspiration, and facial features that interfere with proper fitting of a face mask. Recent studies demonstrate that the use of NIPPV does not require more nursing or respiratory therapist time compared with intubation and mechanical ventilation.

Patients with severe respiratory failure who are not candidates for NIPPV require intubation and mechanical ventilation. Ventilatory support provides an increased minute ventilation to correct abnormalities in gas exchange, and unloads respiratory muscles to allow recovery from respiratory muscle fatigue. Patients with acute respiratory failure have increased airflow limitation, which slows expiratory airflow and delays alveolar emptying.

Weaning from Mechanical Ventilation

Most patients intubated for respiratory failure due to COPD improve within the first 72 h of care and undergo successful weaning and early extubation. Goals for these patients are to reverse bronchospasm, rest fatigued ventilatory muscles, prevent dynamic hyperinflation, and avoid oversedation, which is associated with increased risks for nosocomial pneumonia and delayed weaning.

Prognosis and Outcome

COPD is a progressive disease characterized by a long preclinical phase and a gradual decline in lung function over years after patients become symptomatic. Some patients experience an abrupt and permanent loss of lung function during acute exacerbations. The mortality of patients hospitalized for an acute exacerbation is 3–4%, but mortality climbs to 11–24% for patients who require ICU admission. Disabling symptoms of dyspnea are the most important factors decreasing quality of life.

Neurological Disease and the Elderly Patient

Stroke: Incidence and Risk Factors

Stroke is the third leading cause of death and the leading cause of disability in the elderly. Approximately 500,000 individuals in this age group suffer strokes annually in the United States, corresponding to one event every 45 s and leading to one death every 3 min. Among those 55 years and older, the incidence of stroke doubles with each additional decade of life, despite a decline in the United States, Canada, and Western Europe through the later part of the twentieth century to the present, attributable to improved management of modifiable risk factors. Among these factors, hypertension is by far the most powerful; aggressive blood pressure control can reduce the risk of stroke by 40%. Coronary atherosclerosis, left ventricular hypertrophy, and atrial fibrillation contribute to stroke risk. Diabetes mellitus may increase likelihood of stroke by a factor of two to four; tight glucose control significantly reduces this risk, and may postpone such vascular complications as retinopathy and nephropathy.

Acute Phase of Stroke (ICU Admission to 48 h)

Management of the acute phase involves, first and foremost, ensuring airway and hemodynamic stability. Thereafter, the goals of care are (1) identification of the stroke as ischemic or hemorrhagic, (2) initiation of thrombolytic therapy when indicated, and (3) recognition and therapy of medical or neurologic complications. The first goal is most easily achieved by obtaining a noncontract-enhanced CT scan of the brain as quickly as possible when stroke is suspected. Hemorrhage is usually obvious on this scan, although early in the course of ischemic stroke there may be no visible abnormality. Early CT may reveal one of the many mimics of stroke: subarachnoid hemorrhage, subdural hematoma, neoplasm, or hydrocephalus. Contrast enhancement may improve yield if tumor or infection are likely. Recall that comorbid conditions abound in the elderly; cardiac arrhythmias or infarction may provoke or result from a cerebrovascular event, mandating 12-lead electrocardiogram (ECG) and continuous cardiac monitoring in all stroke patients. Questions of the numerous other causes of altered mental status in the geriatric patient must be investigated and settled quickly. Current recommendations for management include initiation of intravenous thrombolytic therapy with recombinant tissue plasminogen activator (rt-PA) as soon as possible, within 180 min of onset of stroke, in the absence of contraindications. Use of rt-PA appears to improve outcome from stroke at 3 months. There is a relative paucity of data documenting treatment of older patients, however, that while there may be poorer outcome from stroke in the elderly population, there is no increased likelihood of rt-PA-induced severe intracranial hemorrhage. A number of stroke scales, including the National Institutes of Health Stroke Scale (NIHSS), have been devised to assist in quantification of severity of stroke-related symptoms, as a guide to optimal management.

Infectious Disease

Each year in the United States nearly 2,500 cases of sepsis occur per 100,000 persons aged 85 years or older, with older persons being much more likely to acquire sepsis and bacteremia than younger persons. Comorbidities, institutionalization, and instrumentation all place older persons at high risk for bacteremia and sepsis. Increasing age is associated with a high risk of death due to bacteremia and sepsis, although recent evidence suggests that many older patients do respond well to treatments of proven efficacy (Table 12.5).

Elderly patients are more likely than younger patients to experience infections due to gram-negative organisms. In a study comparing young and old patients with community-acquired bacteremia, *Escherichia coli* was the most frequently isolated pathogen among older patients and, *Staphylococcus aureus* was the most common pathogen among younger adults.

Age-related differences in the microbiology of bacteremia and sepsis are, in part, a result of differences in the source infections leading to these disorders among

Table 12.5 Disorders

Disorder	Definition
Infection	A pathologic process caused by the invasion of normally sterile tissue or fluid or body cavity by pathogenic or potentially pathogenic microorganisms
Bacteremia	Presence of bacteria in the blood
SIRS	The systemic inflammatory response (SIR) to a variety of clinical insults exhibited by at least two of the following: (1) temperature >38 °C or <36 °C, (2) heart rate >90 beats/min, (3) respiratory rate >20 breaths/min with a $PaCO_2$ <32 mm Hg, and (4) WBC >12,000/mm^3 or <4,000/mm^3 or >10% immature (band) forms
Sepsis	SIRS and documented or suspected infection
Severe sepsis	Sepsis complicated by organ dysfunction
Septic shock	Sepsis complicated by hypotension (i.e., SBP <90 mm Hg or MAP <60 mm Hg) despite adequate fluid resuscitation

older patients when compared with younger patients. For example, urinary tract infections, which are typically due to gram-negative organisms, are more frequently the source of bacteremia and sepsis in older patients than in younger patients.

Both short- and long-term institutionalization carry with them multiple risks for infection. Hospitalized patients as well as those residing in long-term care facilities are at high risk for complications, such as decubitus ulcers (a common source of bacteremia), and for colonization or infection with antibiotic-resistant organisms. Age per se does not appear to be an independent risk factor for MRSA infection. However older patients are more likely to be exposed to multiple factors that are independently associated with MRSA infection, including nursing home residence hospitalization in the past 6 months, antimicrobial use in the past 3 months, and indwelling urinary catheters.

Older patients are also at increased risk for colonization with gram-negative organisms that may lead to bacteremia and sepsis. Nursing home residence, hospitalization, respiratory disease and poor functional status are associated with oropharyngeal colonization with gram-negative bacilli.

Older patients with bacteremia or sepsis often present a diagnostic challenge to clinicians because nonspecific clinical manifestations of infection are common. Common non specific signs and symptoms include altered mental status, tachypnea, anorexia, malaise, generalized weakness, falls, and urinary incontinence. Clinicians should have a heightened suspicion for infection when evaluating older patients with such symptoms. Older patients are less likely to develop fever than younger patients to develop a fever with bacteremia or sepsis.

Prognostic Differences Between Older and Younger Patients

Although the severity of illness (as indicated by organ dysfunction and acute physiologic abnormalities) has more prognostic importance than age, older patients are at higher risk of death due to bacteremia and sepsis than are younger patients. Factors

Table 12.6 Association of acute physiology score and age with 28-day mortality in patients with sepsis

Parameter	Number	28-day mortality (%)	ARLL	Confidence interval
Acute physiology score				
0–40	152	12	1.0	1.0
41–60	330	22	1.99	1.14–3.45
61–80	348	36	4.27	2.48–7.37
101–120	75	64	15.67	7.90–31.08
120+	72	85	42.93	21.25–86.71
Age, years				
0–44	184	26	1.0	1.0
45–54	116	34	1.33	0.75–2.36
55–64	203	33	1.59	0.97–2.62
65–74	315	35	1.61	1.01–2.55
75–84	285	41	2.31	1.45–3.70
85+	100	42	2.29	1.27–4.11

independently associated with increased mortality were severe sepsis, shock, infection with a gram-positive organism, and a poor prognosis of preexisting disease. The urinary tract as the source of bacteremia appears to be associated with improved survival (Table 12.6).

Despite the increasing incidence of bacteremia and sepsis in older patients and the high risk of death associated with these infectious disorders, many elderly patients respond remarkably well to appropriate therapy. Clinicians must maintain a high index of suspicion to quickly diagnosis bacteremia or sepsis in older patients and initiate appropriate interventions in a timely manner.

Quality of Life and Decision Making in Geriatric Critical Care

Whenever an intervention such as a tracheostomy is considered in the ICU patient, it is necessary to have a discussion about the patient's desire for his or her quality of life, their projected prognosis, and the optimal timing in the natural progression of their disease.

Of utmost importance is preservation of the quality of life. What this means may differ widely from patient to patient. In the setting of terminal illness, this discussion naturally extends into the topic of the quality of dying as well. Patients and their families are often concerned about the potential limitations that tracheostomy and eventual ventilator dependence will place on the patient's quality of life. Often, there are concerns that tracheostomy serves to prolong life without contributing significantly to quality of life. Additionally, for most patients, a tracheostomy implies an impending change in swallowing and speech function. It is necessary for the physician to address these fears, to present possible options for voice and swallowing preservation, and to discuss realistic outcomes for the individual patient before proceeding.

Table 12.7 Indications for percutaneous endoscopic gastrostomy tube placement

Feeding
Malignant dysphagia
Esophageal cancer
Head and neck cancer
Lung cancer
Brain metastasis with neurologic dysphagia
Benign dysphagia
Radiation-induced strictures
Neurologic or neuromuscular dysphagia
Decompression
Benign conditions
Gastroparesis
Diffuse gut motility disorder
Malignant conditions
Diffuse peritoneal carcinomatosis
Malignant gastric outlet obstruction

Table 12.8 Indications for percutaneous endoscopic cecostomy tube placement

Decompression
A. Malignant colonic obstruction
Colon cancer
Pelvic malignancies
B. Benign colonic obstruction
Colonic pseudo-obstruction (Ogilvie syndrome)
Neurogenic bowel
C. Fecal incontinence
Antegrade irrigation

Common reasons for placement of a tracheostomy include airway obstruction, chronic aspiration, or the need for pulmonary toilet or prolonged ventilation from general deconditioning, an acute neural insult, or progressive neuromuscular decline. Loss of control of any one of the closely coordinated functions of the upper aerodigestive tract (respiration, deglutition, or speech) often may result in difficulties with the others.

Percutaneous endoscopic gastrostomy (PEG) tubes are most commonly placed for feeding purposes with the intention of maintenance or improvement in nutritional status. The primary indications for PEG tube placement are listed in Table 12.7. PEG tube placement is generally very well -tolerated, with complication rates ranging from 2 to 15%. Complications largely consist of pain, bleeding, infection, and peritonitis. PEC tube placement is performed primarily for relief of colonic obstruction or antegrade irrigation for colonic motility disorders (Table 12.8). There are several ethical considerations involved in placement of PEG or PEC tubes, and the decision

Table 12.9 Common scoring systems for patients with severe sepsis or septic shock

Scoring system	Description
ICU scoring systems	
Acute Physiology and Chronic Health Evaluation (APACHE) II Online calculators: http://www.icumedicus.com/icu_scores/apache.php http://www.sfar.org/scores2/apache22.html	Developed as mortality prediction tool consists of variables including temperature, MAP, heart rate, respiratory rate, oxygenation, arterial pH, serum sodium, serum potassium, serum creatinine, hematocrit, white blood count, GCS, age, chronic health APACHE IV is recommended except for sepsis patients, in whom APACHE II is more appropriate; APACHE II score ≥25 indicates rhAPC administration is appropriate
Simplified Acute Physiology Score (SAPS) II online calculators: http://www.icumedicus.com/icu_scores/saps.php http://www.sfar.org/scores2/saps2.html	Introduced in 1994 includes variables similar to APACHE
Sequential Organ Failure Assessment (SOFA) online calculators: http://www.icumedicus.com/icu_scores/sofa.php http://www.sfar.org/scores2/sofa2.html	Developed to describe severity of organ dysfunction includes questions regarding cardiovascular, neurologic, renal, liver, respiratory, and coagulation function
Multiple Organ Dysfunction Score (MODS) Online calculators: http://www.icumedicus.com/icu_scores/mods.php http://www.sfar.org/scores2/mods2.html	Developed to describe severity of organ dysfunction. Includes questions regarding cardiovascular, neurologic, renal, liver, respiratory, and coagulation function

to place these devices should be made after thorough discussion with the patient or decision maker regarding the goals, benefits, risks, and expected outcomes of the procedure and the underlying disease.

Scoring Systems

Scoring systems provide an aggregate quantitative indicator of several patient characteristics, including organ dysfunction and vital signs, to assess condition severity, prognosis, or progression. Descriptions of commonly used scoring systems are included in Table 12.9. Web-based tools to calculate patient scores are available for many of these scoring systems. Physiologic scoring systems have been applied to therapeutic decision support, outcomes and evaluation research, quality care analysis, and benchmarking. In clinical decision processes, scoring systems have been used to determine illness severity and predict mortality risk.

Nutritional Issues in the Elderly ICU Patient

Malnutrition or undernutrition is a complicating factor in the efficient and successful management of an elderly ICU patient. The natural decline in energy expenditure

Table 12.10 Undernutrition in the elderly: common causes

Functional decline and social isolation from family and other support systems
Anorexia associated with older age—the so-called anorexia of aging—or chronic illness
Anatomic or gustatory impediments to mastication or swallowing
Abuse or neglect
Insufficient financial resources

with age begins at about age 30 and accompanies the age-related increase in body fat-to-protein ratio. The prevalence of undernutrition in hospitalized, geriatric patients is relatively high and is often unrecognized. Malnutrition at the onset of critical illness portends poor outcome, as does insufficient nutritional support during the course of the illness. Mortality is considerably higher in the malnourished elderly patient, compared to those who are nutritionally replete (Table 12.10).

Identification of malnutrition in the elderly patient may be facilitated by the routine employment of easily used physical examination and laboratory screening tools as part of an organized, proactive nutrition screening program.

Undernutrition imposes a considerable burden on the marginally compensated geriatric patient. The condition known as protein-energy malnutrition (PEM) and micronutrient deficiency complicate the treatment of several conditions seen in the ICU. These include the contribution of gastrointestinal tract nonintegrity to multiorgan system failure and other common cardiovascular, pulmonary, and infectious issues. Wound healing is impeded by a poor nutritional state in particular, development of decubitus ulcers is more common in malnourished elderly individuals, and successful management is decidedly more difficult. Patients with PEM are at increased risk for serious complications while in the hospital, with slower recovery, poorer functional status at discharge, and higher rates of mortality after discharge. Nutritional deficiency is found in 35–65% of elderly hospitalized patients.

Obtaining the patient's weight immediately on admission is an obvious step in assessing nutritional condition. Because of the various types of body habitus found in ICU patients, a calculation of the Quetelet body mass index (BMI) is helpful to standardize weight to height, providing a relatively standardized estimate of body fat: BMI = weight (kg)/by height (in m^2). In the geriatric population, a BMI less than 20 is predictive of nearly 50% 1-year mortality; indeed, it may be a stronger predictor of mortality than is diagnosis. Similar results have been found among critically ill adults with a BMI less than or equal to the 15th percentile. Such data suggests that the optimal BMI may be higher in the elderly than in the general population. Misguided hypocaloric feeding, directed at mobilizing excess fat stores in the obese, but malnourished, elderly patient may worsen the situation by leaving the ongoing catabolic protein breakdown associated with critical illness uncorrected.

Several easily measured laboratory parameters are reflective of nutritional status on admission, and some can be followed periodically to assess the success of nutritional support. Albumin is a product of hepatic metabolism, synthesized ultimately from ingested or infused nitrogenous precursors in the presence of adequate caloric support. Although it is held that the serum albumin level is reflective of the nutritional state, various factors influencing serum albumin levels make it only vaguely reflective of overall nutritional status. Serum albumin level does decline somewhat with age—0.8 g/L per decade for individuals older than 60 years of age—but generally remains within the numerical normal range. Significantly reduced albumin concentration, therefore, should be attributed to disease processes and be aggressively investigated. A substantial decline in serum albumin concentration is accurately predictive of mortality and worse outcome among the elderly. However, the half-life of albumin, 18–19 days, limits the applicability in monitoring acute metabolic and synthetic functions, in which rapid change is significant. Alternatives to albumin include prealbumin and retinol-binding protein. The former has a half-time of 2 days and is not affected by age but is elevated with steroid use. The latter has a half-time of 12 h, decreases slightly with age, and is elevated in the setting of acute liver injury. The serum level of renally excreted retinol binding protein is artificially elevated in renal failure, which may falsely suggest nutritional integrity in patients with reduced renal function.

Total energy expenditure (TEE) may rise to as high as 40–50 kcal/kg/day in critically ill, septic, or trauma patients, and repletion is difficult without correcting the underlying inciting process. The farther behind the patient starts, the more difficult is the recovery of positive nitrogen balance. Catabolic processes characteristic of critical illness are not reversible by nutrient supplementation alone; they are incited by inflammatory mediators rather than by pre-existing deficiency or inadequate repletion and are thus not forestalled by aggressive nutritional support. Traditional guidance recommends 25 kcal/kg/day of nutritional support, with an additional protein supply of 1.2–1.5 g/kg/day, based on usual body weight. Obese individuals warrant feeding based on ideal, rather than usual, body weight: men: IBW (kg) = 50 + 2.3 kg per inch over 5 ft and women: IBW (kg) = 45.5 + 2.3 kg per inch over 5 ft, where IBW is ideal body weight.

Greater accuracy can be achieved using the Harris-Benedict equations to determine the estimated resting energy expenditure (REE) as a guide to calculation of nutritional needs:

$$\text{Men: REE} = 66.5 + (13.75 \times \text{weight in kg}) + (5.003 \times \text{height in cm}) - (6.775 \times \text{age in years})$$

$$\text{Women: REE} = 655.1 + (9.563 \times \text{weight in kg}) + (1.850 \times \text{height in cm}) - (4.676 \times \text{age in years})$$

Enthusiastic overprovision of macronutrients in a misguided and vain attempt to thwart and correct inflammatory catabolism, on the other hand, leads to a host of complications and considerable morbidity for which the geriatric patient may be unable to compensate. Furthermore, the confounding factor of obesity sometimes seen in the nutritionally deficient geriatric patient makes the recipe that provides optimal nutritional support frustratingly difficult to determine. In general, most, although not all, studies show that enteral nutrition is preferred because of the purported preservative effects on intestinal mucosal integrity, cost issues, and a lesser degree of risk exposure to the patient, both infectious and mechanical, associated with placement of flexible nasointestinal feeding tube versus central line for parenteral nutrition.

Outcome After a Critical Illness in the Geriatric Population

Life expectancy is greater at any given age now than it was even 15 years ago, and there is an increasing percentage of elderly patients overall requiring medical care. Given current healthcare constraints objective evaluation must be made of the appropriateness—and likelihood of successful outcome—of aggressive critical care medical services that are provided to patients, including the elderly. At present, geriatric patients represent between 25 and 50% of all ICU admissions. In 2000, ICU costs represented 13.3% of hospital costs, 4.2% of healthcare expenditures, and 0.56% of the U.S. gross domestic product. The enormous expense associated with ICU care has prompted some analysts to raise the subject of limits on expenditures for the elderly. Meaningful discussions addressing the more philosophical issues of critical care such as the correct level of aggressiveness of care and appropriateness of withdrawal of care, to say nothing of the financial issues, simply cannot be addressed in any rational way without an accurate picture of what critical care accomplishes in these elderly patients.

A successful ICU admission is defined within cultural and social, as well as personal, contexts. Although the family member's "do everything for Granddad" dictum is familiar, it often represents an unrealistic appraisal of the possible benefit from certain modalities of care that can be done, but possibly should not be done. Although the ICU is designed as a temporary environment that allows support of body functions during recovery, the complicated technology and meticulous attention to detail that characterizes that environment is not the basis for such "magical" accomplishments as saving the life of a patient who has a lethal condition, despite the expectations and exhortations of some. Nonetheless, death can often skillfully be forestalled with polished and professional ICU care to such a degree that it may occur immediately after a de-escalation of such care, or later while the patient is on the general ward, in a step-down unit or rehabilitation facility, or after returning home (either early or late) to a life with varying similarity to that prior to the original serious medical occurrence. Meaningful discussions with elderly patients and their families, whether prior to complex morbid surgical procedures or as an ICU stay extends past the first few days, must include accurate outcome data, so as to facilitate informed decisions regarding the specifics and suitability of continued care. Studies addressing outcome in the critically ill geriatric population have produced various results that vary with the metric employed, the duration over which the outcome is monitored, and broad intrapopulation patient variability. The latter category highlights differences in age, premorbid physical status, statements of preference regarding aggressiveness of long-term medical care, and patient and family declarations addressing such subjective concepts as posthospitalization quality of life. The term outcome must be specifically defined as to the depth of support required by the post-ICU elder and its correspondence with that autonomous person's preferences, which, again, may vary widely, based on cultural, religious, national, and other parameters. Although some elders may prefer a less aggressive care regimen designed around end-of-life comfort at the expense of duration of remaining life, others may desire life extension in the face of critical illness by use of complex technology despite a vanishingly small or nonexistent expectation of recovery. Furthermore, the clinician's perceptions of the patient's desires may not be accurate, and thus may lead to withdrawal of care or withholding of a modality of treatment in a manner that would not be considered in the care of a younger patient. It is important to remember that while age may be associated with worse outcome from critical illness; numerous investigations have demonstrated that age, in and of itself, is less a factor than is the severity of the specific condition that warrants intensive care or the general medical condition of the patient prior to the institution of intensive care. Quality of life (QOL) in the post-ICU elder is not necessarily inferior to that of younger individuals; indeed, overall QOL has been demonstrated to be similarly good across age groups ranging from middle-aged to very old (above 80 years). While years of living bring elderly patients with the most complex illnesses and comorbid conditions to the door of the hospital and intensive care unit, it is to be remembered that the elderly can recover fully, or almost so, from profoundly serious illness despite numerous worrisome impediments that would discourage all but the most optimistic clinician. Although a substantial percentage of the elderly cannot be brought back to an independent level of functioning, every effort should be expended to achieve accurate diagnosis and expeditious treatment, providing full intensive support to conditions that are correctable and recognition when reasonable limits have been reached. It should be stressed that every effort should be made to honor the patients autonomy and that their wishes should be addressed early and in a timely fashion.

Key Points

- At least 20–50% all ICU admissions occur in patients older than 65 years of age, and geriatric patients account for almost 60% of all ICU days.
- The decision to admit an elderly patient to an ICU should be based not only on their comorbidities, acuity of illness, and prehospital functional status, including quality of life, but also on their preference for the use of life-sustaining treatments if it is known.
- Reperfusion therapy is the optimal treatment for acute ST-elevation MI regardless of age and gender. Absolute contraindications to fibrinolytic therapy are hemorrhagic stroke, intracranial neoplasm, active internal bleeding, or suspected aortic dissection, all of which have a higher incidence in the elderly.
- Mortality related to CABG can be estimated to be 30% or higher in the elderly with multiple comorbid conditions.
- Current evidence suggests that diastolic dysfunction is the cause of the heart failure syndrome in at least 50% of the elderly with heart failure, and that the proportion increases with advancing age.
- In the event of increasing respiratory failure, positive pressure ventilation unloads respiratory muscles and prevents or treats respiratory muscle fatigue. Ventilatory

support can be provided by a tight-fitting face mask in the form of noninvasive positive pressure ventilation (NIPPV) or by tracheal intubation with mechanical ventilation.

- Elderly patients are more likely than younger patients to experience infections due to gram-negative organisms.
- Malnutrition or undernutrition is a complicating factor in the efficient and successful management of an elderly ICU patient.
- The prevalence of undernutrition in hospitalized, geriatric patients is relatively high and is often unrecognized.
- Mortality is considerably higher in the malnourished elderly ICU patient, compared to those who are nutritionally replete.
- Wound healing is impeded by a poor nutritional state in particular, development of decubitus ulcers is more common in malnourished elderly individuals, and successful management is decidedly more difficult.

Suggested Reading

Alsarraf AA, Fowler R. Health, economic evaluation, and critical care. J Crit Care. 2005;20:194–197.

Angus DC, Kelley MA, Schmitz RJ, et al. Committee on Manpower for Pulmonary and Critical Care Societies (COMPACCS). Caring for the critically ill patient. Current and projected workforce requirements for care of the critically ill and patients with pulmonary disease: can we meet the requirements of an aging population? JAMA. 2000;284:2762–2770.

Antman EM, Anbe DT, Armstrong PW, et al. American College of Cardiology/American Heart Association Task Force on Practice Guidelines (Writing Committee to Revise the 1999 Guidelines for the Management of Patients With Acute Myocardial Infarction). ACC/AHA guidelines for the management of patients with ST-elevation myocardial infarction–executive summary: a report of the American College of Cardiology/American Heart Association Task Force on Practice Guidelines (Writing Committee to Revise the 1999 Guidelines for the Management of Patients With Acute Myocardial Infarction). Circulation. 2004;110(5):588–636.

Aurigemma GP, Gaasch WH. Clinical practice. Diastolic heart failure. N Engl J Med. 2004;351:1097–1105.

Bach RG, Cannon CP, Weintraub WS, et al. The effect of routine, early invasive management on outcome for elderly patients with non-ST-segment elevation acute coronary syndromes. Ann Intern Med. 2004;141(3):186–195.

Brucks S, Little WC, Chao T, et al. Contribution of left ventricular diastolic dysfunction to heart failure regardless of ejection fraction. Am J Cardiol. 2005;95:603–606.

CDC/National Center for Health Statistic. Cardiovascular disease in the elderly. www.cdc.gov/nchs/. Accessed April 1, 2007.

Crispell KA. Common cardiovascular issues encountered in geriatric critical care. Crit Care Clin. 2003;19:677–691.

Martin GS, Mannino DM, Moss M. The effect of age on the development and outcome of adult sepsis. Crit Care Med. 2006;34:15–21.

Rice DP, Fineman N. Economic implications of increased longevity in the United States. Annu Rev Public Health. 2004;25:457–473.

Helpful Websites and Calculators

Acute Physiology and Chronic Health Evaluation (APACHE) II Online calculators: http://www.icumedicus.com/icu_scores/apache.php http://www.sfar.org/scores2/apache22.html
Simplified Acute Physiology Score (SAPS) II Online calculators: http://www.icumedicus.com/icu_scores/saps.php http://www.sfar.org/scores2/saps2.html
Sequential Organ Failure Assessment (SOFA) Online calculators: http://www.icumedicus.com/icu_scores/sofa.php http://www.sfar.org/scores2/sofa2.html
Multiple Organ Dysfunction Score (MODS) Online calculators: http://www.icumedicus.com/icu_scores/mods.php http://www.sfar.org/scores2/mods2.html

Chapter 13
Trauma and the Geriatric Patient

Suresh Agarwal and Ruben J. Azocar

Traumatic injuries to patients over the age of 65 are a major public health concern. In 2007, the Center for Disease Control and Prevention found that accidental injuries are the fifth overall cause of death in all age groups and the ninth leading cause of death in older adults. For geriatric patients there are important issues to be considered that may not apply to younger victims of traumatic injury.

Trauma following accidental injury in the older patient may lead to different sequelae than younger counterparts. This is due to the combined effect of preexisting comorbidities commonly found in older adult patients and underlying age-related changes in basic physiology. Preexisting comorbidities have the most significant impact upon the outcome of elderly patients in terms of mortality, morbidity, and disposition. As with any trauma patient, cardiopulmonary disorders, particularly with concomitant anticoagulation use, are ominous predictors of outcome. In 1997, elderly patients accounted for 25% of all trauma fatalities: over 36,000 deaths.

In certain circumstances, outcomes between older and younger patients may be similar, for example, in those with severe injuries in which few are expected to survive; age may not make a major difference. However the impact of aging can be a critical factor in the outcomes of patients with less severe injuries, and the older patient may succumb to injuries that would have been considered survivable in a younger patient. Regardless of age, it is important to attempt to quantify the injuries sustained by trauma victims, and there are multiple scales that can be used to quantify the severity of injury in trauma patients. One of the most commonly used classifications is the Injury Severity Scale (ISS). This scoring system takes into account the severity of injury in up to

S. Agarwal, MD, FACS, FCCM (✉)
Chief, Trauma, Acute Care Surgery, Burn, and Surgical Critical Care,
University of Wisconsin Hospital and Clinics,
G5/335 Clinical Science Center, 600 Highland Avenue, Madison, WI 53792-3236, USA
e-mail: agarwal@surgery.wisc.edu

R.J. Azocar, MD
Department of Anesthesiology, Boston Medical Center, Boston University School of Medicine,
88 East Newton Street, Boston, MA 02118, USA

S.R. Barnett (ed.), *Manual of Geriatric Anesthesia*, DOI 10.1007/978-1-4614-3888-5_13,

three different regions of the body and allows one to predict outcome of patients based upon trauma to each of those regions: the higher the score, the greater the mortality. One of the shortcomings of this scoring system for elderly patients is that preexisting comorbidities are not taken into consideration. The common presence of age-related comorbidities partly explains why geriatric patients tend to have higher mortalities across the scale compared to younger patients.

The paradigm of resuscitating trauma patients is not different for older vs. younger patients. The cornerstone of management of all trauma victims relies on the "ABC's" of evaluation, management, and resuscitation applied in a systematic manner to identify and treat potentially life-threatening issues rapidly and effectively. As can be seen from the table from the Advanced Trauma Life Support Course of the American College of Surgeons, there are multiple comorbid conditions in older patients that significantly modify the response of older patients to the evaluative and resuscitative process. Although the definition of the older patient classically involves all patients greater than the age of 65, the evidence suggests that individuals sustaining a traumatic injury over the age of 45 may be at higher risk compared to those under 45 years and those above the age of 75 years represent a particularly vulnerable population when involved in a trauma.

The primary survey of the trauma patient—ABCDE—begins with systematic assessment of the Airway, Breathing, Circulation, Disability of the neurologic system, and finally Exposure. Normal physiological age changes and common preexisting comorbidities can negatively impact the physiologic reserve in each of these areas. Nevertheless, the evaluation process of the trauma patient is systematic and regimented to prevent missing and delaying the treatment of injuries that may otherwise have dire consequence. The goal of the primary survey is to identify and treat *immediately* life-threatening injuries. The secondary survey is a rapid head to toe assessment of the patient to identify and treat *potentially* life-threatening injuries.

Primary Survey

Airway

As with all trauma patients, non-intubated geriatric patients should be provided with supplemental oxygen upon arrival to the trauma bay. Patency of the airway should be rapidly assessed with a heightened suspicion of obstruction. Sleep apnea and a susceptibility to airway obstruction are common in the older adult. Elderly patients can have relative macroglossia, and the supine position and ligamentous laxity increase the risk of the tongue falling back and causing an airway obstruction. Trauma patients presenting in the supine position, on a backboard and in a cervical stabilization collar, are also at increased risk of aspiration—particularly if they have a full stomach. A history of gastroesophageal reflux or the presence of lower esophageal sphincter tone are frequent preexisting conditions in the elderly patients, and in addition, aging is associated with reduced pharyngeal protective reflexes. These conditions predispose the older patients to aspiration.

Table 13.1 Glasgow coma scale for head injury

Eye opening	
Spontaneous	4
To voice	3
To pain	2
None	1
Verbal response	
Oriented	5
Confused, disoriented	4
Inappropriate words	3
Incomprehensible sounds	2
None	1
Best motor response	
Follows commands	6
Localizes pain	5
Withdraws from pain	4
Decorticate posturing	3
Decerebrate posturing	2
None	1
Add together scores for all three categories (3–15)	
Severe traumatic brain injury	3–8
Moderate traumatic brain injury	9–12
Mild traumatic brain injury	13–15

Indications for placement of a definitive airway can be divided into two categories: airway protection and/or ventilation. When patients can be managed without endotracheal intubation, the oropharynx should be examined to rule out obstructive causes contributing to respiratory distress. In the elderly patient, dentures are common and these should be removed prior to intubation; slipped or broken prostheses may be the cause of obstructive symptoms. As mentioned there is a high incidence of sleep apnea in geriatric patients, and airway obstruction is not uncommon in the sedated or semiconscious patients. A chin tilt and jaw thrust may be effective in relieving the obstruction caused by a large tongue or upper airway collapse in the geriatric patient.

Trauma patients frequently require ventilatory support. Potential causes of respiratory insufficiency are multiple and include apnea from paralysis either from medication administration or neuromuscular injury, an altered level of sensorium as a result of their traumatic injury, and chest wall injuries. Even in the absence of complete respiratory failure, patients with inadequate respiratory efforts as manifested by tachypnea, hypoxia, hypercarbia, or cyanosis should have an airway established. In addition, patients with decreased responsiveness associated with traumatic brain injury may need ventilatory support in order to hyperventilate if signs of impending cerebral herniation exist. Typically, this is for patients with a Glasgow Coma Score (GCS) of less than or equal to eight (see Table 13.1).

Several additional factors may contribute to a potentially challenging airway in elderly patients that require intubation. As mentioned before, dentures should be sought for and removed prior to intubation. Due to decreased saliva production, the nasopharynx is more fragile than in younger patients and is more likely to bleed or be significantly injured; this may make the visualization of the airway more difficult, especially if repeated attempts at intubation are required. Many older patients with cardiovascular disease may also be taking anticoagulants and antiplatelet medication which may predispose to bleeding. As with all trauma patients, midline cervical stabilization should be performed and maintained throughout the intubation process. Aging is associated with changes in bone calcification and ligament rigidity, and preexisting conditions such as rheumatoid arthritis, ankylosing spondylitis, thoracic kyphosis, and temporomandibular joint degeneration may contribute to a difficult airway. During all trauma intubations, it is important to have appropriate equipment and personnel on hand.

Breathing

Older patients have a reduced respiratory reserve due to anatomic and physiologic changes associated with aging. In addition there is an increased incidence of lung diseases such as chronic obstructive pulmonary disease. Older patients with severe or end-stage pulmonary disease may be dependent on supplemental home oxygen or dependent on a "hypoxic respiratory drive" to maintain adequate ventilation. These patients must receive supplemental oxygen following a trauma, and no patient should be allowed to remain hypoxic in the face of injury. Oxygen can be delivered using a nonre-breathing mask, a simple face mask, or nasal cannula; the choice will depend on the patient's presenting condition. As stated above, consideration should be given to early intubation, particularly if there is an elevated partial pressure of carbon dioxide on capnometry or measured by arterial blood gas. Elderly patients in general have reduced physiological reserve; therefore, interventions to stabilize pulmonary and cardiovascular function should be instituted earlier than might be considered in an otherwise fit younger patient with similar injuries.

Due to increased osteoporosis and decreased cartilage in the thoracic cage, older patients are more likely to experience fractures of their ribs. Rib fractures are an independent predictor of mortality in the elderly, particularly when associated with pulmonary contusions, hemothorax, or pneumothorax. Additional pulmonary complications such as pneumonia, atelectasis, and subsequent respiratory failure are common in the elderly population. Judicious management of fluid resuscitation is important as even healthy elderly patients are susceptible to pulmonary edema due to age- and disease-related diastolic dysfunction.

Circulation

The goals of resuscitation of the elderly patient are the same as for all trauma patients, to restore homeostasis. In the geriatric population caution regarding the interpretation of normal is advised with respect to acceptable physiological endpoints. A "normal" blood pressure and heart rate in an elderly patient with underlying hypertension and ischemic heart disease may be defined differently than in a younger otherwise healthy patient. The elderly hypertensive vasculopathic patient may require a higher blood pressure to maintain vital organ perfusion than a younger patient. In addition elderly patients are frequently on medications that affect their cardiovascular and renal systems and impact their baseline physiologic responses. An example is the use of beta blockers in an older patient; these patients may present with a falsely reassuring slow heart rate and the beta blocker may block a compensatory tachycardia during impending shock. Similarly, the regular use of diuretics is associated with chronic mild volume contraction and possible depletion of electrolytes, including sodium, potassium, and magnesium. These issues may contribute to blood pressure lability frequently encountered in older patients.

From a laboratory standpoint one of the main endpoints of a successful resuscitation is the clearance of end products of acidosis, and this applies to all ages of victims. Common markers of acidosis include lactate, base deficit, and mixed venous saturation. Trauma is frequently associated with substantial blood loss, and the optimal hemoglobin in the elderly patient population remains controversial. Current consensus recommends maintaining a hemoglobin of >10 g/dL in patients >70 years of age; however, studies examining this endpoint are currently ongoing.

Preexisting anticoagulant therapy, including platelet inhibitors and warfarin, may complicate the management of geriatric trauma patients. There are multiple comorbidities common to the geriatric patient that require thromboprophylaxis, including atrial fibrillation, prior cerebrovascular accidents or myocardial infarction, cardiac stents, prior pulmonary emboli, and mechanical heart valves. Thus, it is not uncommon for an elderly patient to be on these medications. Rapid correction of antithrombotics with platelets and fresh frozen plasma is an essential corollary to operative intervention in these patients. A ratio of 1:1:1 of packed red blood cells, fresh frozen plasma, and platelets is recommended for the resuscitation of patients with ongoing hemorrhage requiring resuscitation.

Although the use of pulmonary artery catheters has lost favor in the critical care community, there is good evidence for early use of invasive monitoring in elderly patients. Unlike in other patient populations, there appears to be a mortality benefit when aggressive, monitored resuscitation is performed in the geriatric patient. As with all trauma patients, delaying source control of bleeding portends a worse outcome regardless of the monitoring strategy.

Polypharmacy and multiple comorbidities can alter the resuscitative efforts in elderly trauma patients. A thorough history, including past medical history of cardiovascular disease, diabetes mellitus, and chronic renal insufficiency, will be required. An accurate medication list should be sought from family members and medical records, this can provide important information about underlying comorbidities as well as possible drug interactions. Although cardiovascular medications such as beta blockers, calcium channel blockers, and diuretics are among the most commonly prescribed for the elderly patients, psychotropics are also common in the elderly population. A full knowledge of medications can help to improve outcome and help to plan necessary tests and procedures.

Deficits

Neurologic disease is common in the elderly population and a major challenge encountered when treating the elderly trauma victim is establishing whether a neurologic deficit is new or part of a preexisting condition. Irrespective of the baseline conditions, elderly trauma victims are more susceptible to a central neurologic event due to age- and disease-related changes. Thin venous walls of bridging veins in the dura are more likely to tear and cause a subdural hematoma. Atherosclerotic plaques in the arterial system are more likely to dissect or dislodge resulting in cerebrovascular accidents. During the assessment, confusion in geriatric patients should not be attributed solely to "old age," and any evidence of a decreased sensorium, confusion, or new weakness should be carefully examined and evaluated. Non-contrast computed tomography of the brain and cervical spine should be performed, and magnetic resonance imaging may be necessary to assist with the diagnosis. Many elderly patients have benign age-related cortical atrophy, and a new neurological finding may present in a more subtle fashion than in the younger patient. In addition, the older patient is much more likely to have preexisting underlying cervical and lumbar disc disease that predisposes them to herniation of their cervical and lumbar discs after trauma with consequent spinal cord impingement. There may be a delay in presentation of spinal cord damage in the geriatric patient after an injury. It is therefore imperative that these patients are monitored continuously when there is any suspicion of cord instability. In the older patient, the mechanism of injury may be subtle, such as fall from standing or a simple trip on a side walk, and a higher index of suspicion should be maintained for neurological injury in patients older than 70 years of age following minor accidents.

Exposure

The older patient's ability to thermoregulate is significantly hampered by extensive changes in their skin, connective tissue, and vasculature as well as an age-related declining basal metabolic rate. Older patients have altered ability to detect and respond to declined ambient temperatures. In addition the older patient has reduced ability to vascoconstrict effectively in the face of lower temperatures, and shivering is less effective at increasing heat production. These changes place the geriatric patients at a higher risk for the development of hypothermia and potential infection. Early and aggressive measures should be undertaken to maintain normothermia. Older patients may also have reduced immune systems be more susceptible to developing significant infections following trauma. In addition to appropriate wound cleaning, and antibiotics as indicated, simple measure such as tetanus immunization should not be overlooked in this population.

Secondary Survey

Once the primary survey has been completed, a thorough secondary survey should be undertaken. This includes a complete head to toe examination to assess for associated injuries that are not immediately life threatening.

Osteoporosis is common in the elderly patients, and they are more susceptible to hip fractures, pubic fractures, humeral fractures, rib fractures, and spinal column injuries compared to younger victims. A full skeletal survey, including range of motion examination, is recommended to assess for fractures and other soft tissue injury. At a minimum, any site that has a visible or palpable deformity or decreased range of motion should be X-rayed to rule out bony injury. Immobilization of these areas should be performed with caution, as age- and disease-related changes to the soft tissue and connective structures predisposed to the development of skin breakdown and ulceration. Prolonged inactivity and disuse can also lead to worsened functional outcomes and may impact survival in the long term.

As with all trauma victims, the secondary survey includes a complete systematic examination of the patient that should include a careful physical examination of the chest, abdomen, and pelvis. Clinical examination may be supplemented with rapid ultrasonographic examination of the pericardium and abdominal cavity, also known as FAST or focused abdominal sonography for trauma.

When working with older trauma victims, practitioners should also vigilant of signs of elder abuse, especially in an older patient with significant cognitive impairment. Signs of abuse may include poor hygiene, dehydration, and evidence of multiple healing previous injuries. Should abuse be suspected, a careful and thorough history and physical examination must be performed in a safe environment. If there is a suspicion of abuse, this should be reported through appropriate social service channels for further investigation and follow-up.

Summary

Overall, the goals of resuscitation and management of the geriatric patient involved in trauma remain the same as those for any victim of injury. A thorough primary exam with focus on the ABCDE's of trauma (Airway, Breathing, Circulation, Deficit, and Exposure) is followed by a complete secondary survey that provides information regarding the immediately and potentially life-threatening injuries that patients may experience. In the older patient, an understanding of anatomic and physiologic changes, a thorough history of comorbidities and medications, and assiduous monitoring will result in optimal outcomes.

Key Points

Comorbidities in trauma patients are predictive of worsened outcome and mortality.

- Cardiopulmonary disease, particularly with associated anticoagulation use, portends a worsened outcome.
- Assessment of elderly patients, as with any trauma patient, should be done in a systematic fashion in accordance with the American College of Surgeon's Advanced Trauma Life Support Course.
- Systematic approach should include a primary survey, in which immediately life-threatening problems are identified, and a secondary survey, in which potentially life threatening of morbidity increasing injuries are identified.
- Utilizing the ABCDE system of Airway, Breathing, Circulation, Deficit, and Exposure enhances the systematic and timely review of patients.
- Older patients may have physiologic and anatomic changes that impact each element of the ABCDE's.
  - Dentures, increased risk of aspiration, and conditions such as ankylosing spondylitis add to the challenge of intubation during airway assessment and treatment.
  - Hypoxia should not be tolerated in a trauma patient, regardless of history of chronic obstructive pulmonary disease.
  - Endpoints of resuscitation should include measurements of lactate, base deficit, and mixed venous oxygen saturation. Pulmonary artery catheterization should be considered early during the resuscitation of elderly patients.
  - Confusion, obtundation, and agitation should be diagnoses of exclusion: their etiology should not be attributed to a patient's age or intoxication.
  - Great care should be made to prevent hypothermia.
- Due to osteoporosis and other comorbidities, elderly patients are more likely to suffer fractures and other musculoskeletal injuries.
- Awareness and suspicion of elderly abuse should be considered in all assault patients and in those who have a distinct history of trauma recidivism.

Suggested Reading

American College of Surgeons: Advanced Trauma Life Support Program for Doctors. Chicago: 2007.

Asensio JA, Trunkey DD. Current Therapy of Trauma and Surgical Critical Care. Philadelphia: 2008.

Feliciano DV, Mattox KL, Moore EE. Trauma. New York: 2008.

Flint L, Meredith JW, Schwab CW, et al. Trauma: Contemporary Principles and Therapy. Philadelphia: 2008.

Part IV
Specialist Areas

Chapter 14
Cardiovascular Aging and Anesthesia

John D. Mitchell

Age-related cardiovascular changes are inevitable and cardiovascular diseases are common in many older patients. Thus, in order to effectively treat geriatric patients, anesthesiologists should be able to recognize the contributions of both normal aging and overt disease to decreased cardiovascular reserve as well as understand the impact of anesthesia on cardiovascular homeostasis in the elderly.

Endurance, Response to Work, and Functional Capacity

Physiologic reserve is reduced with aging, as is the ability to mount a compensatory response to episodic hemodynamic instability. With age, the heart becomes less responsive to sympathetic stimuli, but responses to parasympathetic stimuli remain unchanged. There is a decrease in resting parasympathetic tone, which makes the response to parasympathetic withdrawal less dramatic. This leads to attenuated increases in heart rate and contractility during exercise and a decrease in maximal attainable heart rate. The reduced heart rate response to provocative stimulation cannot be reversed with conditioning. Therefore, in order to preserve cardiac output, older patients exhibit a compensatory increase in left ventricular end-diastolic volume (LVEDV).

Like maximum heart rate, peak oxygen consumption and aerobic capacity also decline with age. Longitudinal studies have demonstrated that this decline is much more marked with aging than suggested by earlier cross-sectional studies. Endurance training does appear to reduce the negative impact of aging on maximal oxygen consumption, diastolic filling parameters, and stiffening of the arteries.

J.D. Mitchell, MD (✉)
Department of Anesthesia, Critical Care and Pain Medicine, Beth Israel Deaconess Medical Center, Harvard Medical School, 110 Deaconess Road, CC-470-C, Boston, MA 02139, USA
e-mail: jdmitche@bidmc.harvard.edu

S.R. Barnett (ed.), *Manual of Geriatric Anesthesia*, DOI 10.1007/978-1-4614-3888-5_14,

Age-Related Physiologic Changes

Cellular Changes

Aging induces alternations in gene expression and transcription. Mechanisms for this include oxidative injury, nonenzymatic glycosylation, apoptosis, and inflammation. In mammals, reactive oxygen species (ROS) production increases and cellular sensitivity to ROS is enhanced, resulting in increased cellular damage and reduced mitochondrial functioning. An example of age-related cell level changes is reduced translation of an ATPase in the sarcoplasmic reticulum, resulting in prolonged relaxation in the myocytes.

Structural Cardiac Changes

Myocytes are terminally differentiated by adulthood and therefore cannot regenerate. Apoptosis (programmed cell death) and cell necrosis lead to a decreased number of cardiac myocytes with age. This effect is even more prominent in men compared with women. To compensate for decreases in the total number, myocytes increase in size (hypertrophy) during normal aging. While myocytes decrease, fibroblasts remain active and produce collagen; thus, the heart becomes more fibrous and less compliant with age.

Sinoatrial (SA) node function and the conduction system may become compromised with age. The SA node undergoes a decline in cell number with concomitant fibrosis and fat deposition. This suggests a possible etiology for increasing arrhythmias (e.g., tachy-brady, sick sinus syndrome). In addition, amyloid deposits generally accumulate in the heart with age. One form of amyloid primarily deposits in the atria, and another accumulates throughout the heart. It is possible that these deposits interfere with myocardial conduction and increase the risk of atrial fibrillation. Notably, neither amyloid type appears functionally nor biochemically related to primary amyloidosis, which can cause a restrictive cardiomyopathy. Fibrosis attacks all cells in the heart and may contribute to conduction block with age. Lastly, the atrial hypertrophy with age likely predisposes to atrial fibrillation.

Valves often undergo annular dilatation and calcification with aging. Valvular calcification was noted in 47% of aortic and 39% of mitral valves in those over 80 years on autopsy. In the aortic position, this frequently manifests as progressive aortic stenosis with advancing age. In the mitral valve, senile calcification often remains confined to the annulus but may progress to involve the valve leaflets as well, with resulting mitral stenosis.

Myocardial Function

Compensatory mechanisms (below) allow for preservation of resting cardiac output in the healthy elderly adult. Resting systolic function is likewise preserved in the

Table 14.1 Functional changes in the aging cardiovascular system

Overall preserved resting left ventricular ejection fraction	
Increase with age	Decrease with age
Left ventricular end-diastolic pressure	Response to b-agonists
Duration of myocardial relaxation	Arterial compliance
Myocardial stiffness	Maximum aerobic capacity
Systolic blood pressure	Baroreceptor sensitivity
Ischemic heart disease	Maximal heart rate
Increase in diastolic filling due to atrial contraction	Diastolic relaxation
Increased diastolic dysfunction	Reduced early passive diastolic filling

absence of disease. Animal studies suggest that papillary muscle contractile function is also preserved (Table 14.1).

A decreased rate of diastolic relaxation is due in part to effects of aging on the calcium ATPase in the sarcoplasmic reticulum. Ventricular relaxation requires energy and can be further altered in states of increased energy demand such as hypoxic or ischemic episodes. LVEDP is increased due to prolonged relaxation and increased stiffening of the left ventricle. This shifts the filling profile of the left ventricle from one where most filling occurs early in diastole (young) to one where more filling occurs in late diastole. This later filling results from an active atrial contraction and is vulnerable to disruption if the cardiac rate is too high or the rhythm becomes uncoordinated as with atrial fibrillation. The net result can be sudden onset of heart failure symptoms and helps explain the high (30–40%) incidence of heart failure episodes in the elderly attributable to diastolic dysfunction.

Ventricular and vascular stiffening in the elderly combine to result in increased ventricular pressures in the elderly. Myocardial thickening occurs as a compensatory response to increased pressure work in the ventricle. These changes account in part for increased pressure liability in the elderly. Fluid shifting also can result with exertion, salt intake, or positional changes. Diastolic volume is also increased in the elderly.

Vascular Structure and Compliance (Table 14.2)

With advancing age, there are increases in the amount of lipid, collagen, and minerals deposited in the vascular bed that impair arterial relaxation peripherally. There is thickening of the muscular layer of the media, decreases in elastin, increases in collagen, and increased variability in the size, shape, and direction of endothelial cells. These changes can increase turbulent flow and predispose vessels to the deposition of lipid or disruption/dissection. Older individuals also may have an increased risk of exposure to chronic infections which increase inflammation and are linked with increased atherosclerosis. Endothelial function tends to decline with age, though some of these changes may also be due to disease states such as hypercholesterolemia and hypertension. Reduced production of nitric oxide (NO) by endothelial cells contributes to a decrease in vascular relaxation with age.

Table 14.2 Age-related vascular structural changes and implications

Increase in vascular intimal thickness
Increase in atherosclerosis
Increase in vascular thickness
Increase in collagen cross-linking and elastase activity
Systolic hypertension
Left ventricular wall thickening and hypertrophy
Increase risk of cerebrovascular accident
Increase in atherosclerosis
Changes in vascular tone
Decreased in nitric oxide production and effects
Increased in vascular stiffening and hypertension
Early arthrosclerosis
Reduced physical activity
Frailty and immobility
Deconditioning
Negative impact on hypertension, development of heart failure

Intimal thickening, large artery dilation, and central artery wall stiffening predispose to systolic hypertension, increased pulse wave velocity, and widening pulse pressure, putting elderly patients at an increased risk for cardiovascular disease. Arteries become stiffer and less elastic with reduced compliance over time. These stiffened vessels have reduced distensibility and a higher pulse wave velocity reflected back to the heart during systole, this increases afterload and may lead to worsening left ventricular hypertrophy. Clinically, these changes are manifested as systolic hypertension with a wide pulse pressure. Women maintain aortic compliance better than men until they are postmenopausal but then experience a rapid decline in distensibility unless receiving estrogen supplements.

In general, arterial aging is a risk factor for cardiovascular disease and worsening cardiovascular outcomes. Changes with age are, in turn, worsened by comorbid conditions such as diabetes, hypertension, and end-stage renal disease.

Coronary Blood Flow

Coronary blood flow is reduced due to the change in timing of the pulse wave reflection back toward the heart. In the young, the pulse wave coincides with diastole, augmenting coronary filling, but in the elderly, it occurs during systole increasing afterload and myocardial work.

Autonomic Changes and Orthostasis

Reductions in baroreceptor sensitivity and β-receptor function make the aged heart less responsive to sympathetic stimuli with unchanged responses to parasympathetic stimuli. There are decreased adrenergic effects on calcium transport, reducing the normal contractile response to β-stimulation. Parasympathetic tone is reduced and vagal afferent reflexes are also attenuated. In contrast, sympathetic nervous system activity remains largely unchanged. Norepinephrine levels increase with age secondary to increased production and decreased clearance. Despite elevated levels of catecholamines, the heart response to norepinephrine is decreased in the elderly, in part due to β-receptor desensitization. The decreased beta receptor response plays a critical role in the decline of maximal heart rate responses with aging.

Age-related autonomic dysfunction is characterized by the decline in beta receptor responsiveness and alterations in baroreceptor function, predisposing the elderly patient to orthostasis and increased blood pressure lability. Thirty percent of patients over the age of 75 experience orthostatic hypotension, defined as a decrease of 20 mm Hg or more in systolic (or 10 mm Hg or more diastolic) blood pressure on standing. When hypertensive elderly patients are eliminated from analysis, orthostasis occurs in <7% of those over 75 years.

Underlying Cardiovascular Conditions in the Elderly

There is a marked increase in cardiovascular conditions which impact anesthesia administration and surgery in elderly patients. The following is a brief summary of common cardiovascular comorbidities.

Hypertension occurs commonly in the aged population. Isolated systolic hypertension, as defined by a systolic blood pressure over 160 mm Hg with a diastolic blood pressure <90 mm Hg, and a wide pulse pressure are both related to risk of perioperative cardiac morbidity. Hypertension is also a factor in coronary artery disease development as well as other end-organ damage such as cerebrovascular disease and renal insufficiency. Hypertension, especially if poorly controlled, predisposes patients to increased hemodynamic instability under anesthesia. Chronic hypertension leads to an alteration of the autoregulatory curve such that patients require higher mean arterial pressures to maintain end-organ perfusion. Since the administration of anesthetic agents tends to decrease blood pressure intraoperatively, hypoperfusion and end-organ dysfunction may occur if the hypertension is treated too aggressively prior to induction of anesthesia. In general, if blood pressure is lower than 180 mm Hg systolic and/or 110 mm Hg diastolic without evidence of end-organ dysfunction, treatment is generally not required prior to anesthesia. Pressures higher than this may require intervention with intravenous agents, but usually, the surgery need not be delayed, provided there is no end-organ dysfunction such as visual change or altered mental status. The decision to proceed with surgery should also take into account the consequences of perioperative hypertension, although in the absence of symptoms, no benefit has been shown by delaying surgery. Postoperative hypertension is common in the chronically hypertensive patient and can be challenging to treat especially in ambulatory centers with limited ability for prolonged monitoring. Postoperatively, it is important to rule out common perioperative conditions that may be contributing the development of hypertension such as pain, hypercarbia, and urinary retention. After ruling out other obvious causes leading to hypertension, and if blood pressure is not restored to within 20% of baseline, then treatment with intravenous antihypertensive agents is warranted.

Congestive heart failure (CHF) represents the most frequent source of nonelective hospitalization in those over 65 years of age. While systolic heart failure is still common in the elderly, diastolic heart failure is found in over 1/3 of all older CHF patients. Diastolic dysfunction is largely a diagnosis of exclusion but can also be facilitated by echocardiographic approaches. Diagnosis by echo uses mitral inflow patterns, tissue Doppler, pulmonary inflow patterns, and techniques of propagation velocity to demonstrate signs of impaired diastolic function. Whether systolic or diastolic in origin, symptomatic heart failure in the elderly predicts is a consistent risk factor for worse postoperative outcomes, including death.

Arrhythmias account for a large proportion of cardiovascular diseases in the elderly. Arial fibrillation rates are 10× higher in otherwise healthy adults over age 60 than their younger cohort. "Lone A-fib" (no other underlying cardiac disease) was found in 17% of males and 6% of females aged 70 years or older in the Framingham group. These individuals had a fourfold higher risk of stroke. Therapies for atrial fibrillation include rate control and anticoagulation. In the elderly, rhythm conversion to sinus by chemical or electrical cardioversion, and percutaneous or surgical ablation, may be less of a priority unless patients are symptomatic clinically. Other common arrhythmias in the elderly include sick sinus syndrome and paroxysmal atrial tachycardia. Pacemakers are commonly encountered in elderly patients and reprogramming of pacemakers or use of a magnet is often required during surgery. Appropriate emergency pacing equipment should also be available when managing pacer dependent patients.

While not exclusively a disease of the elderly, the prevalence of myocardial ischemia increases markedly with age. In contrast to patients with unstable angina, controlled or stable angina carries a low risk of perioperative complications. Patients with unstable angina should be triaged based on ACC/AHA guidelines and may need urgent cardiology consultation. Patients with a history of a recent myocardial infarction (MI) carry an increased risk of reinfarction; consideration should be given to postponing elective surgery for 3 months following an acute MI. Patients who have recently undergone percutaneous revascularization using a stent may also need a delay in surgery with the length of the delay is based on the type of stent placed. While anticoagulation has been recommended for 4–6 weeks following bare-metal stent placement and for at least 6–12 months after drug-eluting stent placement, surgery is typically deferred when possible during this interval, or else, antiplatelet therapies continued perioperatively (though this may not always confer protection from stent thrombosis). A 2010 retrospective study of almost 2,000 patients suggested that waiting at least 6 weeks to perform noncardiac surgery reduces risks of complications in patients with either bare-metal or drug-eluting stents. This does not suggest that a 6-week waiting period is safe to use as a decision point for elective surgeries, only that the risk of surgery within the first 4 weeks was significantly (up to four times) higher than in patients operated on after 4 weeks. Perioperative outcomes were also worse in this population if stents had been performed for acute MI rather than chronic ischemia.

Valvular heart disease in the elderly markedly increases the morbidity and mortality in the perioperative period. Aortic stenosis, in particular, increases in frequency with aging, and in general, valve calcification with age is very common. Aortic valve stenosis is progressive in nature and results in left ventricular hypertrophy until the end stages, when the failing left ventricle dilates. A valve replacement is indicated if the valve area <1 cm^2 or symptoms of depressed ventricular function, syncope, angina, or dyspnea are present. Patients with critical aortic stenosis should be considered for valve replacement prior to elective surgery. For patients undergoing surgery with moderate aortic stenosis, rate control, adequate preload, and BP support (to maintain diastolic coronary perfusion) are the key features of management. Other valve lesions in the geriatric population should be managed with the understanding that diastolic dysfunction is often superimposed on the lesion.

Volume depletion. Age-related impairments of salt and water homeostasis combined with a reduced osmotic drive to thirst predispose elderly patients to hypovolemia. This is frequently compounded by concomitant antihypertensive therapies and periods of fasting for surgery. Volume depletion in the perioperative period can be challenging to address, particularly in patients with coexistent diastolic dysfunction and a limited ability to tolerate volume loading.

Anesthetic Implications

The following section will highlight cardiovascular preoperative issues relevant to the elderly patient.

Preanesthetic Evaluation

The preoperative cardiovascular evaluation for elderly patients is a key element of any preanesthetic assessment. Functional capacity is predictive of cardiac morbidity and mortality following surgery and is one of the most important aspects of the preoperative assessment. Questioning patients about metabolic equivalents (METS) as related to daily activities is a useful way to assess the exercise tolerance of those who may not participate in conventional forms of regular exercise. The American College of Cardiology/American Heart Association (ACC/AHA) and European Society of Cardiology guidelines both use a combination of functional capacity and other predictors to establish baseline cardiovascular risks and divide surgical risks into low (<1%), intermediate (<5%), and high (>5%). Advanced age alone is only a minor predictor of outcome, whereas congestive heart failure and valvular heart disease are major predictors of cardiovascular risk. Heart failure symptoms are particularly critical to elicit, as uncompensated congestive heart failure (CHF) is one of the most significant predictors of poor perioperative outcomes. Physical exam in the elderly may point to a number of comorbidities which could impact cardiovascular outcomes. Volume status should be assessed through evaluation for edema, jugular venous distension, hepatojugular reflux, cardiac gallops, rales on pulmonary exam, and mucous membrane examination. Murmurs or rhythm disturbances should also be sought on cardiac evaluation, as should evidence for cardiomegaly such as an apical displacement or a precordial heave. Carotid artery auscultation should be conducted to evaluate for bruits as evidence of carotid stenosis.

Laboratory and imaging studies can prove important in the cardiovascular assessment of the geriatric patient. Given that the incidence of anemia and electrolyte disturbances are higher in the elderly with cardiovascular disease, preoperative laboratory studies such as blood counts and chemistry panels may prove helpful in selected patients to aid in preoperative assessment. In patients on anticoagulant therapy, preoperative assessment of coagulation status is usually indicated in the perioperative period. In elderly patients, brain natriuretic peptide (BNP) levels may prove a useful tool, particularly to screen ambulatory patients for cardiovascular disease, but further studies are still needed. Echocardiography can help provide insight into ventricular function and status of valves and should be considered in patients with significant cardiac comorbidities such as history of myocardial infarction (MI), CHF, or valvular heart disease. While X-ray and electrocardiogram evaluation are often helpful in patient assessment, they are not directly predictive of outcomes in this patient population.

Preoperative Recommendations for Common Cardiovascular Medications

Sixty-six percent of the elderly population are on prescription medications and many take four or more medications, and cardiovascular drugs are among the most commonly prescribed.

Appropriate management of beta-blocker therapy in the perioperative period can be complex. In patients already taking a beta-blocker, administration should be continued in the perioperative period to avoid complications of beta-blocker withdrawal and to reduce perioperative morbidity. Patients at high risk of myocardial ischemia or patients at intermediate cardiovascular risk undergoing high-risk surgery should also be considered for perioperative beta-blockade. The POISE trial demonstrated an increased risk of stroke or mortality in patients with few indications who were newly started on perioperative beta-blockade undergoing moderate or low risk noncardiac surgery. Some methodological issues with this study, including low blood pressures down to 100 mm Hg systolic, relatively high levels of drug dosing, and absence of titration to physiologic endpoints such as blood pressure or heart rate, question its broad applicability. However most current evidence does support the perioperative use of beta-blockers in elderly patients undergoing high-risk surgery, such as vascular bypass surgery. Beta-blockers are not indicated for patients undergoing low- or intermediate-cardiovascular-risk surgery without other clinical indications.

Angiotensin-converting enzyme (ACE) inhibitors and angiotensin receptor blockers (ARBs) improve ventricular function during long-term administration and provide benefits in the management of hypertension and congestive heart failure (CHF). However, they can contribute to significant hypotension on induction of anesthesia. In most cases, this hypotension responds to vasopressors such as phenylephrine, but refractory hypotension has been described. In general it is reasonable to hold these medications the night before surgery.

Diuretic regimens deserve careful thought in the perioperative period. Given the effect of volume depletion on the ability to maintain hemodynamic stability under anesthesia, consideration should be given to withholding diuretics on the day of surgery. This should be balanced, however, by the consideration that urine output may be diuretic dependent in patients with long-standing diuretic use.

Clonidine and other alpha-2 agonists carry significant risks of rebound hypertension if withdrawn. They can cause hypotension and bradycardia in conjunction with anesthetic agents but also result in decreased anesthetic requirements.

Patients on long-standing nitrate therapy for angina have an increased risk of perioperative cardiac complications and death. Results are mixed as to whether these agents confer any decrease in intraoperative ischemic events.

In patients on anticoagulant therapy, preoperative assessment of coagulation status, or planning for a bridge from longer-acting anticoagulants such as Warfarin to shorter-acting analogues (heparin or enoxaparin), may be indicated in the perioperative period. Consideration to continue platelet inhibitors such as aspirin or clopidogrel should be individualized based on type of surgery and indication for the agent.

Intraoperative Monitoring and Management

Blood pressure lability must be anticipated and aggressively managed in the geriatric population. Logical strategies include keeping blood pressure within 20% of baseline or at least within the autoregulatory zone of MAP 50–150. In patients with known or suspected coronary disease, MAP>60 is often suggested to maintain coronary perfusion. Many blood pressure changes in older patients are due to changes in SVR and therefore are usually easily corrected with administration of alpha agonists such as phenylephrine. Conversely, since elevated SVR typically drives hypertension in the elderly, increasing depth of anesthetic is often the most effective first-line approach to managing intraoperative hypertension.

Heart rate typically has a narrower acceptable range in elderly patients. Given the high incidence of LVH (which effectively fixes stroke volume), bradycardia can significantly decrease cardiac output. Conversely, a high incidence of coronary artery disease also makes tachycardia undesirable. Rates of 60–80 beats per minute are therefore typically preferred in this population.

Given stiffening of veins and myocardium, it is difficult for the aged cardiovascular system to manage excess intravascular volume. This volume therefore redistributes into other tissues such as the heart and lungs and ultimately can result in heart failure and/or pulmonary edema. Despite this, higher baseline filling pressures are needed to achieve adequate ventricular filling in the face of reduced diastolic compliance, so that hypovolemia is also poorly tolerated. Difficulties with volume management are often worsened by declining renal function, decreasing urine output, or diuretic dependence which make urine output an unreliable marker of volume status. Given the challenges of volume management, administration of fluids to correct hypotension is only recommended to correct underlying hypovolemia or acute blood loss.

Traditional methods of evaluating volume status and cardiac function in patients at high cardiovascular risk during noncardiac surgery include central venous pressure (CVP) monitoring and analysis of pulmonary artery catheter (PAC) tracings. PAC placement is invasive and time consuming. There is no randomized controlled trial data to support the utility of the PA catheter in patient management and routine use is therefore discouraged. CVP, while still useful for vascular access and trending volume status, has been demonstrated to be a limited and inconsistent marker of the latter. Transesophageal echocardiography has emerged as a useful tool to evaluate volume status, ventricular function, and valve function in the perioperative period but requires expert operators to aid in clinical decision making. While end-diastolic volume on echocardiography correlates with volume status, continuous monitoring is somewhat labor intensive.

Arterial cannulation allows pressure monitoring, blood sampling, and waveform contour and variability analysis, making it a better monitoring choice for higher risk geriatric patients. In mechanically ventilated patients in a sinus rhythm, pulse pressure variability and, to a lesser extent, systolic pressure variability of the arterial line tracing have been shown to be predictive of volume responsiveness during hypotensive episodes in a wide variety of patients. Devices to provide arterial contour analysis for cardiac output estimation are also commercially available and may prove helpful as trend monitors of cardiac function.

Other noninvasive measures of cardiac performance and volume status exist, such as pulse plethysmographic-derived variability indices or measurement of respiratory carbon dioxide rebreathing to calculate cardiac output are commercially available and show promise as less invasive techniques for monitoring cardiac function and volume status.

Choices of Agents

The principle goals in a geriatric population include maintaining homeostasis and avoiding complications. Common solutions include reduced doses, titration of agents, and altered dosing frequency. Comments here focus on cardiovascular and hemodynamic stability.

While premedication with midazolam may have drawbacks from a mental status perspective, it is not a substantial cardiac depressant and has only mild vasodilatory effects when used judiciously. Therefore, from a cardiovascular standpoint, if it is needed to ameliorate anxiety despite preoperative counseling and reassurance, titration of small doses (0.05–0.15 mg/kg) may be useful in the elderly population. Higher doses or infusions coupled with narcotics have long been the mainstay of anesthetic management for the cardiac cripple but are giving way to more balanced techniques in all but the frailest subjects.

Most induction agents can be used if titrated appropriately. Because of its profound vasodilatory effect, propofol should be given in divided doses starting with 50% or less of a standard induction dose. While studies suggest that 80% of standard doses (1.5–1.8 mg/kg) may be indicated, a slow induction using lower doses (0.8–1.2 mg/kg) can often result in unconsciousness with less hypotension. Bradycardia may result during induction, particularly in patients on beta-blockers. In anticipation of the decrease in SVR, it is reasonable to pretreat patients with significant cardiovascular comorbidities with a vasoconstrictor such as phenylephrine to maintain vascular tone during induction. Etomidate represents the induction agent with the least cardiovascular impact, making it an excellent choice in patients with poor ventricular function, hypovolemia, or significant preload dependence (such as severe aortic stenosis). Ketamine produces tachycardia and myocardial depression at induction doses and is therefore a poor choice in patients with cardiovascular disease. Small doses (0.02–0.04 mg/kg), used as part of procedural sedation regimes, may not engender as significant a degree of cardiovascular side effects and be an appropriate adjunct to reduce the use of propofol and benzodiazepines, but further study needs to be undertaken in this regard. Sodium thiopental results in myocardial depression, increased heart rate, and vasodilatation. While these effects can be attenuated through reduced (80% of weight based) and slow dosing, this unfavorable hemodynamic profile makes it undesirable in patients with significant cardiovascular disease.

Inhalational agents are well tolerated in health older adults. Those with cardiovascular disease, however, need careful management with these agents. All volatile anesthetics engender myocardial depression, increased myocardial sensitivity to catecholamies, and significant vasodilatation. Heart rate increases seen in younger patients to compensate for hypotension typically do not occur in elderly patients. Isoflurane and desflurane may be associated with transient tachycardia and hypotension if increased rapidly above 1 minimum alveolar concentration (MAC). Slow, incremental increases in volatile concentration can prevent this response. MAC of volatile agents is significantly lower (decreased by 6% per decade) in the elderly and dosing should be decreased accordingly.

Opioids are relatively cardiac stable and well tolerated in the elderly. The onset of morphine is delayed, but the kinetics of fentanyl and alfentanil remain relatively unchanged. Narcotic dosing requirements decrease by 50% by age 85, primarily due to increased sensitivity of the aged brain.

Muscle relaxants have few cardiovascular side effects. Pancuronium can induce vagolysis with resultant tachycardia and may also promote arrhythmias via this mechanism, so it is unfavorable from a cardiovascular standpoint. Atracurium can cause hypotension due to histamine release if administered rapidly. Cisatracurium, rocuronium, vecuronium, and mivacurium have no clinically significant cardiovascular side effects. Succinylcholine can engender changes in heart rate and rhythm, most commonly bradycardia, which results from activation of acetylcholine receptors in the sinoatrial node.

Anticholinesterase reversal agents are potentially arrhythmogenic. Vagolytic agents such as glycopyrrolate may cause undesirable tachycardia, and consideration should therefore be given to reducing the dose in patients at risk for rate-related demand ischemia. Nevertheless, glycopyrrolate is preferred over atropine since, as a quaternary amine, glycopyrrolate is less able to enter the CNS and increase the risk of delirium. Clinical trials of sugammadex suggest that it has no significant cardiovascular side effects and also obviates the need for administration of anticholinergic agents.

Postoperative Care

Advanced age per se does not require additional postoperative care. ACC/AHA guidelines and European Society of Cardiology guidelines help identify patients at high risk from a cardiovascular standpoint; these patients usually benefit from additional monitoring and careful management in the postoperative period. Most considerations for postoperative care in this age group center around the type of surgery, but factors such as a history of post-op delirium or a baseline history of dementia may suggest the need for increased care. In a study of 544 patients aged 70 and older undergoing noncardiac surgery, multivariate analysis identified ASA status, emergency surgery, and intraoperative tachycardia as predictors of perioperative complications. Negative cardiac outcomes were predicted in this cohort by clinical evidence of CHF. In a multivariate cohort analysis of over 400 patients over age 60 (with 14% age 80 or older), predictors for mortality included a history of coronary artery disease, valvular heart disease, and ASA status, whereas higher serum albumin levels (reflective of better nutritional status) were protective. Overall mortality was 8.2% in this population (mean age 70.8 ± 8.1 years), while morbidity was 15.8%. Notably, when controlled for, pulmonary, heart failure, and thromboembolic risks did not impact mortality. This patient group was quite functional at baseline with only 2% dependent on others for their activities of daily living. Unfortunately, the sample was skewed toward abdominal procedures and therefore may not reflect trends in orthopedic or neurosurgical populations adequately. In cardiac surgical patients, complication rates in those 80 or older were 15% as opposed to 7.6% in those under 80. Neurological dysfunction and associated mortality may be more than twice as high in patients over aged 80. More studies need to be undertaken to look at risks in the very old as this population increases with time.

Key Points

- While many elderly patients maintain good cardiovascular health, the high incidence of comorbid diseases superimposed on the physiologic changes of aging makes it incumbent upon the anesthesiologist to integrate the patient's cardiovascular status with the stress imposed by the surgical procedure.

- Functional capacity is one of the most critical predictors of outcome following noncardiac surgery.
- Cardiovascular reserve is lower in the geriatric population; thus, hemodynamic instability should be anticipated and managed aggressively to keep patients near their baseline blood pressure and heart rate.
- Systemic vascular resistance tends to demonstrate an exaggerated decrease during anesthesia as compared with younger patients, and elderly patients frequently benefit from early pharmacologic intervention to support SVR, for example, with phenylephrine.
- Most anesthetic agents can be used without significant cardiovascular side effects, provided dosing is adjusted downward to reflect the altered pharmacodynamics in the elderly.

Suggested Reading

Alexander KP, Newby LK, et al. Acute coronary care in the elderly, part II: ST-segment-elevation myocardial infarction: a scientific statement for healthcare professionals from the American Heart Association Council on Clinical Cardiology: in collaboration with the Society of Geriatric Cardiology. Circulation. 2007; 115(19): 2570–89.

Alexander KP, Newby LK, et al. Acute coronary care in the elderly, part I: Non-ST-segment-elevation acute coronary syndromes: a scientific statement for healthcare professionals from the American Heart Association Council on Clinical Cardiology: in collaboration with the Society of Geriatric Cardiology. Circulation. 2007; 115(19): 2549–69.

Andrawes WF, Bussy C, et al. Prevention of cardiovascular events in elderly people. Drugs Aging. 2005; 22(10): 859–76.

Barnett S, Jankowski C, et al. A Geriatric Anesthesiology Curriculum. S. f. A. o. G. Anesthesia. 2010.

Cruden NL, Harding SA, et al. Previous coronary stent implantation and cardiac events in patients undergoing noncardiac surgery. Circ Cardiovasc Interv. 2010; 3(3): 236–42.

Das S, Forrest K, et al. General anaesthesia in elderly patients with cardiovascular disorders: choice of anaesthetic agent. Drugs Aging. 2010; 27(4): 265–82.

Ferrari AU, Radaelli A, et al. Invited review: aging and the cardiovascular system. J Appl Physiol. 2003; 95(6): 259–17.

Fleg JL, Morrell CH, et al. Accelerated longitudinal decline of aerobic capacity in healthy older adults. Circulation. 2005; 112(5): 674–82.

Groban L. Diastolic dysfunction in the older heart. J Cardiothorac Vasc Anesth. 2005; 19(2): 228–36.

Groban L, Butterworth J. Perioperative management of chronic heart failure. Anesth Analg. 2006; 103(3): 557–75.

Hutcheon SD, Gillespie ND, et al. B-type natriuretic peptide in the diagnosis of cardiac disease in elderly day hospital patients. Age Ageing. 2002; 31(4): 295–301.

Janczewski AM, Spurgeon HA, et al. Action potential prolongation in cardiac myocytes of old rats is an adaptation to sustain youthful intracellular Ca2+ regulation. J Mol Cell Cardiol. 2002; 34(6): 641–8.

Jani B, Rajkumar C. Ageing and vascular ageing. Postgrad Med J. 2006; 82(968): 357–62.

Kass DA. Age-related changes in venticular-arterial coupling: pathophysiologic implications. Heart Fail Rev. 2002; 7(1): 51–62.

Kregel KC, Zhang HJ. An integrated view of oxidative stress in aging: basic mechanisms, functional effects, and pathological considerations. Am J Physiol Regul Integr Comp Physiol. 2007; 292(1): R18–36.

Lakatta EG. Arterial and cardiac aging: major shareholders in cardiovascular disease enterprises: Part III: cellular and molecular clues to heart and arterial aging. Circulation. 2003; 107(3): 490–7.

Lakatta EG, Levy D. Arterial and cardiac aging: major shareholders in cardiovascular disease enterprises: Part I: aging arteries: a "set up" for vascular disease. Circulation. 2003; 107(1): 139–46.

Lakatta EG, Levy D. Arterial and cardiac aging: major shareholders in cardiovascular disease enterprises: Part II: the aging heart in health: links to heart disease. Circulation. 2003; 107(2): 346–54.

Lakatta EG, Sollott SJ. Perspectives on mammalian cardiovascular aging: humans to molecules. Comp Biochem Physiol A Mol Integr Physiol. 2002; 132(4): 699–721.

Laurent S, Cockcroft J, et al. Expert consensus document on arterial stiffness: methodological issues and clinical applications. Eur Heart J. 2006; 27(21): 2588–605.

Leung JM, Dzankic S. Relative importance of preoperative health status versus intraoperative factors in predicting postoperative adverse outcomes in geriatric surgical patients. J Am Geriatr Soc. 2001; 49(8): 1080–5.

Liu LL, Dzankic S, et al. Preoperative electrocardiogram abnormalities do not predict postoperative cardiac complications in geriatric surgical patients. J Am Geriatr Soc. 2002; 50(7): 1186–91.

Machado AN, Sitta Mdo C, et al. Prognostic factors for mortality among patients above the 6th decade undergoing non-cardiac surgery: cares–clinical assessment and research in elderly surgical patients. Clinics (Sao Paulo). 2008; 63(2): 151–6.

Najjar SS, Scuteri A, et al. Arterial aging: is it an immutable cardiovascular risk factor? Hypertension. 2005; 46(3): 454–62.

Newsome LT, Kutcher MA, et al. Coronary artery stents: Part I. Evolution of percutaneous coronary intervention. Anesth Analg. 2008; 107(2): 552–69.

Newsome LT, Weller RS, et al. Coronary artery stents: II. Perioperative considerations and management. Anesth Analg. 2008; 107(2): 570–90.

Pimentel AE, Gentile CL, et al. Greater rate of decline in maximal aerobic capacity with age in endurance-trained than in sedentary men. J Appl Physiol. 2003; 94(6): 2406–13.

Poldermans D, Bax JJ, et al. Guidelines for pre-operative cardiac risk assessment and perioperative cardiac management in non-cardiac surgery: the Task Force for Preoperative Cardiac Risk Assessment and Perioperative Cardiac Management in Non-cardiac Surgery of the European Society of Cardiology (ESC) and endorsed by the European Society of Anaesthesiology (ESA). Eur Heart J. 2009; 30(22): 2769–812.

Priebe HJ. The aged cardiovascular risk patient. Br J Anaesth. 2000; 85(5): 763–78.

Pugh KG, Wei JY. Clinical implications of physiological changes in the aging heart. Drugs Aging. 2001; 18(4): 263–76.

Rooke GA. Cardiovascular aging and anesthetic implications. J Cardiothorac Vasc Anesth. 2003; 17(4): 512–23.

Sear JW, Higham H. Issues in the perioperative management of the elderly patient with cardiovascular disease. Drugs Aging. 2002; 19(6): 429–51.

Stathokostas L, Jacob-Johnson S, et al. Longitudinal changes in aerobic power in older men and women. J Appl Physiol. 2004; 97(2): 781–9.

Tay EL, Chan M, et al. Impact of combination evidence-based medical therapy on mortality following myocardial infarction in elderly patients. Am J Geriatr Cardiol. 2008; 17(1): 21–6.

Vaes B, de Ruijter W, et al. The accuracy of plasma natriuretic peptide levels for diagnosis of cardiac dysfunction and chronic heart failure in community-dwelling elderly: a systematic review. Age Ageing. 2009; 38(6): 655–62.

Chapter 15
Pulmonary Issues in the Elderly Patient

Anup Pamnani, Cynthia A. Lien, and G. Alec Rooke

The anatomical and physiological changes to the respiratory system that accompany aging pose a unique set of challenges to the anesthesiologist caring for the geriatric patient. In addition, the elderly patient is prone to multiple comorbid conditions that predispose to the development of respiratory failure (Fig. 15.1).

Physiologic Changes Associated with Aging

Significant alterations in compliance of the lung tissue and thoracic wall occur with age. While lung parenchyma loses elastic recoil and becomes more compliant, the chest wall becomes stiffer due to calcification of the thoracic skeleton. Kyphosis of the thoracic spine, frequently the result of osteoporotic disease, and arthritis of the costovertebral joints also decrease the compliance of the thoracic cage. The anteroposterior diameter of the chest increases causing decreased curvature of the diaphragm, which decreases diaphragmatic efficiency and increases the work of breathing (Fig. 15.2). In addition, age-related weakening of the accessory muscles of respiration predisposes to fatigue and ventilatory failure.

Upper airway dysfunction is common in the geriatric patient. Hypotonia of the pharyngeal musculature and poor dentition predispose to airway obstruction.

A. Pamnani, MD (✉)
Department of Anesthesiology, New York Hospital, Weill Cornell Medical Center, 525 East 68th Street, Suite M-303, New York, NY 10021, USA
e-mail: anup.pamnani@gmail.com

C.A. Lien, MD
Department of Anesthesiology, Weill Cornell Medical College, 525 East 68th Street, New York, NY 10065, USA

G.A. Rooke, MD, PhD
Department of Anesthesiology and Pain Medicine, University of Washington Medical Center, 1959 NE Pacific Street, P.O. Box 356540, Seattle, WA 98195-6540, USA

S.R. Barnett (ed.), *Manual of Geriatric Anesthesia*, DOI 10.1007/978-1-4614-3888-5_15,

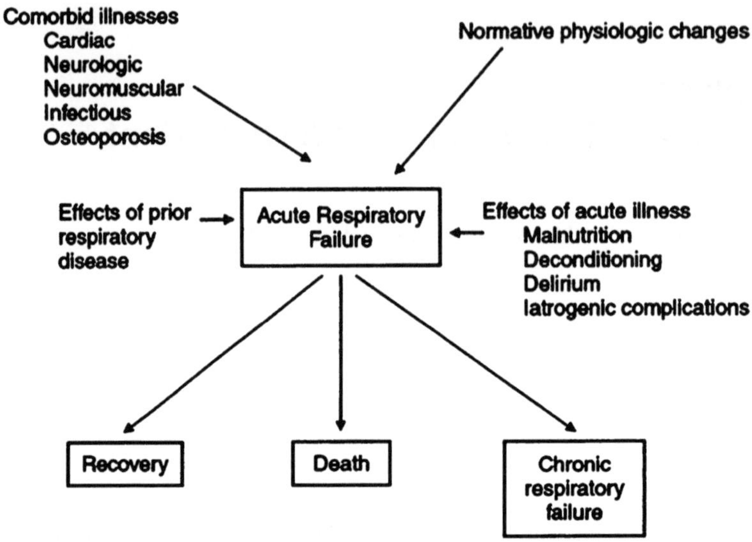

Fig. 15.1 The complex interacting factors that contribute to the development of and recovery from acute respiratory failure in elderly patients (Reprinted from Sevransky JE, Haponik EF. Respiratory failure in elderly patients. Clin Geriatr Med 2003;19(1):207. With permission from Elsevier.)

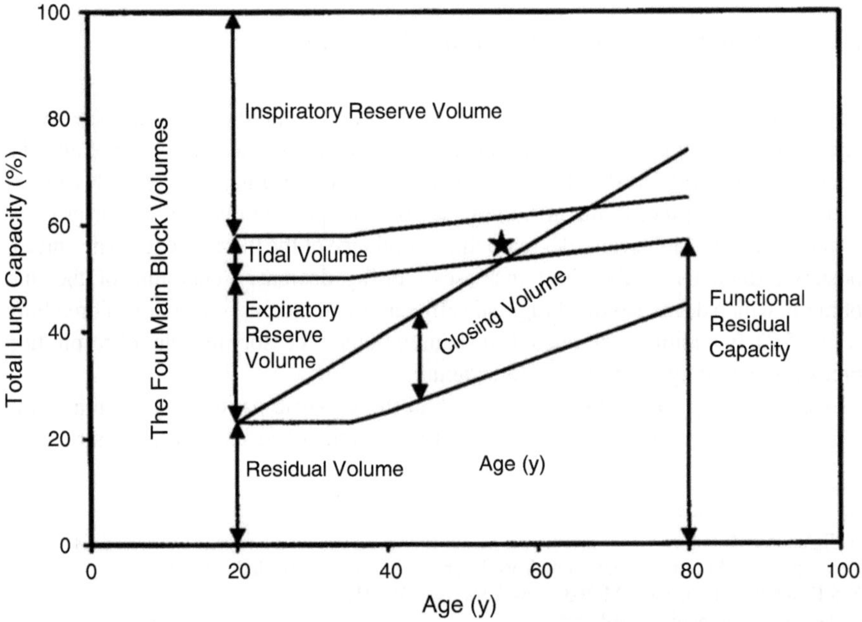

Fig. 15.2 Decreased elastic recoil leads to enlargement of the thorax (*barrel-shaped appearance*) and flattening of the diaphragm. The flatter diaphragm requires more muscle power and, consequently, more energy to develop the same transdiaphragmatic pressure (increased work of breathing). During increased loads on the diaphragm, such as postoperative abdominal distension or increased airway resistance by mucus formation, the flatter diaphragm tends to fatigue and decompensate earlier (Reprinted from Zaugg M, Lucchinetti E. Respiratory function in the elderly. Anesthesiol Clin North Am 2000;18(1): 52. With permission from Elsevier.)

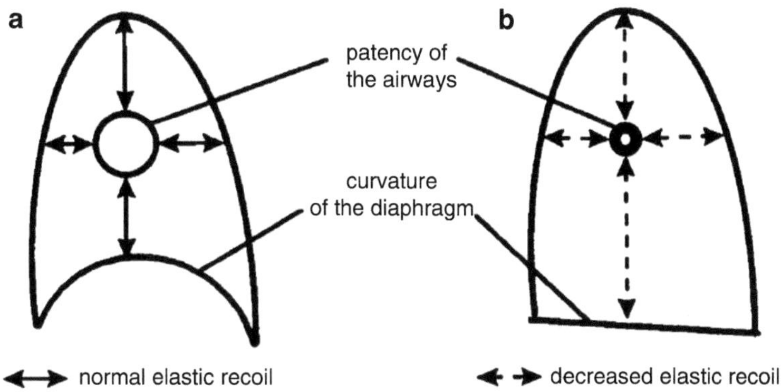

Fig. 15.3 Changes in lung volumes with aging (erect position). Residual volume (RV) and functional residual capacity gradually increase by aging, while expiratory and inspiratory reserve volumes (ERV, IRV) and thus vital capacity decrease. Specific (height-adapted) total lung capacity (TLC) does not change with aging. Forced expiratory volume in 1 s (FEV_1) can be significantly reduced in old people. The loss of elastic recoil results in a narrowing of small airways with a diameter <1 mm and increases the closing volume (CV). The closing capacity (RV+CV) may even be larger than FRC, thus closing the small airways during normal tidal breathing (*star*). This may significantly impair pulmonary gas exchange (Reprinted from Zaugg M, Lucchinetti E. Respiratory function in the elderly. Anesthesiol Clin North Am 2000;18(1): 52. With permission from Elsevier)

Sleep-disordered breathing increases in prevalence with age and obstructive sleep apnea (OSA) is more prevalent than in younger patients.

The elderly patient is highly susceptible to aspiration pneumonia. The etiology of this is multifactorial including age-related dysfunction of the neurologic, pulmonary, and gastrointestinal systems. Hypotonia of the pharyngeal musculature can impair the cough mechanism. Finally, upper esophageal dysfunction and poor oral hygiene have a significant impact on the volume and bacterial load of the aspirate. Additional dysfunction may accompany neurologic disease such as stroke or dementia, predisposing to dysphagia and loss of protective airway reflexes.

Forced expiratory volume in 1 second (FEV_1) declines 10–30 ml per year after age 30. As a result, respiratory rate increases slightly to maintain adequate minute ventilation. Forced vital capacity (FVC) also declines gradually with age but to a lesser extent than the reduction in FEV_1. As a consequence, the ratio of FEV_1 to FVC (FEV_1/FVC) in apparently healthy older patients may be lower (55–65%) compared to younger patients. Closing capacity (CC), the volume at which elastic recoil of the lungs becomes insufficient to support patency of small bronchioles, increases with age. Although FRC increases slightly with age, the increase in CC counteracts this effect. By 60 years of age, CC exceeds FRC in the standing position (Fig. 15.3). Carbon monoxide diffusing capacity (D_LCO) also declines after age 40.

Arterial oxygenation is progressively impaired with increasing age. This is attributable more to ventilation/perfusion (V/Q) mismatch than to the decrease in D_LCO. Conversely, carbon dioxide exchange is unimpaired and the partial pressure of arterial carbon dioxide ($PaCO_2$) is unchanged relative to a younger patient. The ventilatory

Table 15.1 Age-related changes in respiratory function and their relationships to perioperative pulmonary complications

Age-related change in respiratory function	Clinical consequence
↓ Chest wall compliance	↑ Work of breathing
↑ Lung compliance	↓ Ventilatory response to exercise
↑ Respiratory system resistance	
↑ Residual volume	Impaired gas exchange
↑ Small airways closure	
↑ Ventilation–perfusion mismatch	
↓ Respiratory muscle strength	↓ Secretion clearance
↓ Protective cough and swallowing reflexes	↑ Aspiration risk
Altered control of breathing	
↓ Responsiveness to imposed respiratory loads	Hypoventilation
↓ Responsiveness to hypoxemia and hypercarbia	Hypoxemia and hypercarbia
↑ Sensitivity to anesthetic agents and opioids	Respiratory failure in early postoperative period

From: Sprung J, Gajic O, Warner DO. Review article: age related alterations in respiratory function—anesthetic considerations. Can J Anaesth. 2006;53(12):1245. With kind permission from Springer Science+Business Media B.V.
Symbols: ↓—decreased; ↑—increased

response to hypoxia and hypercapnia decreases, by as much as 50 and 40%, respectively. This decreased responsiveness predisposes the geriatric patient to opiate-induced ventilatory depression. Mucociliary clearance and the effectiveness of the cough mechanism may also be diminished, increasing the risk of pulmonary infection in the perioperative period. The age-related changes in respiratory function and their relationship to perioperative pulmonary function are summarized in Table 15.1.

Chronic Obstructive Pulmonary Disease

Chronic obstructive pulmonary disease (COPD) is a syndrome commonly associated with aging that can complicate anesthetic management in the geriatric patient. COPD is common in the elderly population and it is the fourth leading cause of death in the United States. The disease is characterized by progressive development of irreversible airflow limitation. It includes two subtypes: chronic bronchitis, characterized by chronic mucus production and obstruction of small airways, and emphysema which presents with enlarged air sacs, destruction of lung parenchyma, loss of elasticity, and closure of small airways. The risk factors for development of COPD include cigarette smoking, respiratory infection, occupational exposure to certain toxins, and genetic predisposition such as alpha-1-antitrypsin deficiency.

Physical examination of the geriatric patient with severe COPD typically reveals tachypnea and a prolonged expiratory phase to airflow. In addition, breath sounds may be diminished and expiratory wheezing is frequently heard on auscultation. Sputum production can be significant in the patient with chronic bronchitis. Because of this, signs of pulmonary infection may be obscured in these patients. Frequently, changes in the degree of sputum production and its discoloration may be the only clues to an underlying pneumonia.

Pulmonary function testing may be indicated in those patients with severe disease and poor exercise tolerance. A preoperative chest radiograph can help assess for signs of acute pulmonary infection or establish a baseline for comparison should postoperative pulmonary complications occur. Hyperlucency and evidence of bullae are diagnostic of emphysema. Arterial blood gas (ABG) testing is particularly helpful in patients with end-stage disease to assess the degree of CO_2 retention. An electrocardiogram (EKG) should be obtained in patients with evidence of COPD. Signs of right heart disease on physical exam or EKG should prompt a search for evidence of cor pulmonale via additional tests such as echocardiography.

Medical management of COPD revolves around encouraging smoking cessation, use of supplemental oxygen when indicated, and bronchodilators. The benefit of smoking cessation in patients with COPD has been well established. In the Lung Health Study, a randomized trial of smoking cessation in patients with mild and moderate COPD, smoking cessation reduced the rate of decline in lung function and decreased mortality in the long term. Use of supplemental oxygen, particularly in patients with significant baseline hypoxia, has also been associated with slowing the progression of disease. Such therapy is typically initiated when baseline PaO_2 is <55 mmHg and oxygen saturation (SpO_2) is $<88\%$. Supplemental oxygen is provided at least 18 h a day at flow rates that raise the SpO_2 to $>90\%$. By improving arterial oxygenation, pulmonary vascular resistance is decreased and progression of right heart dysfunction can be delayed. In addition, oxygen therapy may improve functional status which is a strong predictor of morbidity and mortality in the elderly patient with COPD.

The elderly patient is particularly susceptible to acute exacerbations of COPD and chronic bronchitis. Older patients with acute exacerbations of chronic bronchitis are also more susceptible to infection by drug-resistant organisms. Inhaled beta agonists and anticholinergics form the mainstay of therapy for both acute exacerbations of COPD and of chronic bronchitis. Typically, inhaled anticholinergic medications are more effective than beta agonists. The addition of inhaled steroid therapy can be particularly helpful at alleviating symptoms and reducing the incidence of exacerbations. The use of systemic steroids has also been shown to be particularly effective in those cases where treatment failure is evident. Medical management of acute exacerbations of COPD and of chronic bronchitis should take into account the frequent presence of comorbidities in the elderly patient. The use of inhaled beta agonists can exacerbate underlying coronary artery disease and oral steroid therapy may precipitate delirium. Antibiotic therapy is frequently used to treat acute exacerbations of chronic bronchitis and may necessitate special consideration in the geriatric patient. Dosing and selection of antibiotics should take into account the pharmacokinetic and pharmacodynamic changes associated with aging. Choice of antibiotic therapy should also take into account the prevalence of drug-resistant organisms in the elderly.

Perioperative management of COPD is targeted at maintaining oxygenation, decreasing the incidence of disease exacerbation, and avoiding ventilatory depression in the postoperative period. Patients that are hypoxemic should receive oxygen supplementation, and the elderly are indeed more likely than younger patients to require oxygen and for a longer duration. Inhaler therapy should be continued in the perioperative period. Aggressive pulmonary rehabilitation is associated with significantly fewer respiratory complications.

Regional anesthesia is a useful modality in patients with COPD since it avoids the need to instrument the airway which can potentially exacerbate obstructive symptoms. In addition, regional techniques can be used to provide effective postoperative analgesia which may decrease the incidence of respiratory failure.

If general anesthesia is employed, care must be taken to optimize ventilatory management to account for the obstructive nature of the patient's disease. Typically, low respiratory rates with long expiratory times are employed to prevent air trapping. Patients with bullae and hyperinflated lungs should be closely monitored for the occurrence of pneumothorax. Nitrous oxide and significant amounts of PEEP are best avoided in these patients.

Episodes of symptom exacerbation are common in the perioperative period. Severe episodes often due to infections have an adverse effect on outcomes and can cause permanent loss of lung function. Presentation in the older patient is often subtle making an underlying pneumonia difficult to diagnose. Cultures are frequently nonconfirmatory and systemic signs of inflammation, such as elevated white blood cell count, fever and tachycardia, are common in the perioperative patient. If infection is thought to be the underlying etiology, antibiotic therapy should be promptly. Choice and duration of antibiotic therapy should be guided by culture data, if available, with expert consultation. Bronchodilator therapy may also be useful to help relieve dyspnea and clear secretions. Severely symptomatic patients in whom underlying infection is not a concern may benefit from being initiated on intravenous corticosteroid therapy.

Anesthetic Management of the Aging Pulmonary System

Although COPD is common in older patients, most elderly do not have chronic lung disease, at least not severe disease. Nevertheless, the aging process, plus possible subclinical disease, makes perioperative pulmonary complications more common than even cardiac complications. Thus, it is important to employ a wide variety of strategies in the perioperative period to minimize the risk of pulmonary complications in the geriatric patient (Fig. 15.4).

Preoperative Assessment

Preoperative evaluation and optimization of respiratory function is of critical importance in the elderly patient due to the significant morbidity and mortality associated

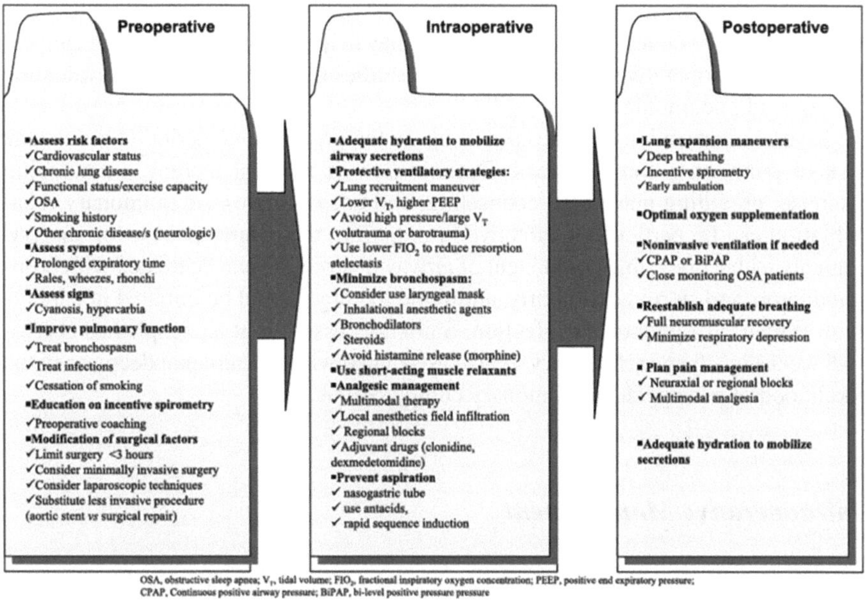

Fig. 15.4 Perioperative strategies used to minimize pulmonary complications (From: Cartin-Ceba R, Sprung J, Gajic O, Warner DO. In: Mcleskey et al. Geriatric Anesthesiology. 2nd ed. New York, NY: Springer; 2008: p. 156. With kind permission from Springer Science+Business Media B.V.)

with pulmonary complications. The risk of respiratory failure is more closely associated with the severity of underlying disease than age. Thus, comorbid pulmonary diseases should be carefully assessed in the context of the planned surgical procedure. The preoperative period also presents an opportunity to aggressively optimize underlying pulmonary disease.

The history should focus on evaluation of respiratory symptoms, risk factors for aspiration (neurological disease, impaired swallow and gag function, increased intraabdominal pressure, esophageal disease, history of reflux), nutritional status, and severity of existing pulmonary and cardiac disease. Evaluation of exercise tolerance and functional status are of particular importance as they are highly predictive of cardiopulmonary risk. Physical examination should focus on auscultation of the lungs, examination of the airway, and evaluation for signs of cardiac, particularly right heart, dysfunction.

A chest radiograph and electrocardiogram are indicated in symptomatic patients and those with evidence of acute pulmonary or cardiac disease. Chest X-rays should not, however, be performed routinely in asymptomatic patients. The use of such screening X-rays is of little diagnostic value and may lead to further tests that often cause more harm than good. Pulmonary function tests (PFTs) may be indicated in patients who are symptomatic or have poor exercise tolerance and from whom adequate history cannot be elicited. In addition, PFTs may help predict the need for postoperative ventilation in patients with significant pulmonary disease scheduled to undergo pneumonectomy. Patients with a history of severe COPD and poor exercise tolerance are prone to chronic hypercarbia and hypoxia. Thus, establishing baseline $PaCO_2$ and PaO_2 values an arterial blood gas may help guide ventilatory management during the perioperative period. Laboratory studies should also focus on evaluation for signs of pneumonia.

Several interventions can be carried out in the preoperative period to reduce the risk of pulmonary complications. Optimization of medical therapy, encouraging exercise, providing nutritional counseling, and use of aggressive pulmonary rehabilitation can be particularly effective in preparing the elderly patient for surgery. Patients with a reversible component of airway obstruction can be treated with bronchodilators and steroids. Similarly, antibiotic therapy should be initiated in patients with evidence of pulmonary infection. Smoking cessation, if accomplished at least 6–8 weeks in advance of surgery, is also associated with a significant decrease in the likelihood of perioperative pulmonary complications.

Intraoperative Management

Numerous strategies can be employed in the anesthetic management of the geriatric patient to reduce the risk of intraoperative and postoperative pulmonary complications. The goals are to maintain effective ventilation in spite of altered lung mechanics, prevent bronchospasm, and mucus plugging in susceptible patients and prevent respiratory failure.

If preoperative sedation is employed, it should be carefully titrated to minimize the risk of cognitive dysfunction and respiratory depression. Benzodiazepines, in particular, may be associated with an increased risk of delirium and should be used with caution. Similarly, polypharmacy may lead to significant respiratory complications in the postoperative period and should, whenever possible, be avoided. Induction and maintenance of anesthesia should take into account the altered pharmacokinetics of medications in the elderly patient. Overmedication may lead to significant levels of residual anesthetic thus increasing the risk of postoperative respiratory failure. Likewise, long-acting neuromuscular blockers and opiates are best avoided.

Intraoperative ventilatory management should be directed by the elderly patient's lung mechanics. Such management should also be carefully tailored to the physiology of underlying pulmonary disease. Preoxygenation might take longer in the geriatric patient than a younger patient since FRC tends to be increased. Administration of inhaled beta agonists and ipratropium may help decrease airway resistance and decrease mucus production in patients with obstructive disease. Provided the patient is not at risk for aspiration, use of a laryngeal mask airway (LMA) should be considered to minimize the risk of bronchospasm. Additional measures to prevent exacerbation of obstructive disease include the use of inhaled anesthetics, such as sevoflurane, and intravenous agents such as propofol. In patients with significant mucus production, adequate hydration and frequent suctioning will prevent inspissation of secretions. Patients with prolonged exhalation while awake (e.g., obstructive disease) will most certainly have slow exhalation during anesthesia and will require increased expiratory time. Low tidal volumes may be useful in patients with restrictive disease. Hyperventilation should be avoided in the patient with chronic, compensated hypercapnia as this may lead to impaired oxygen delivery due to a left shift of the hemoglobin oxygen dissociation curve. If intraoperative hypoxemia is thought to be due to atelectatic alveoli, the use of occasional recruitment maneuvers may be an alternative to significant levels of PEEP which can predispose to decreased preload and accompanying hypotension.

Regional anesthesia may be of particular benefit in the elderly patient. By avoiding general anesthesia and endotracheal intubation, exacerbation of COPD may be avoided. In addition, certain regional techniques may allow for earlier mobilization and decreased respiratory splinting. Neuraxial anesthesia is often well accepted by elderly patients and avoids some of the problems with general anesthesia. Nevertheless, care must be taken to avoid high levels of blockade that could impair coughing or even respiration. Neuraxial opiates must be used carefully to avoid respiratory depression. Peripheral nerve blocks may be particularly beneficial in the geriatric patient. Their use is associated with a low incidence of respiratory depression. In addition, complications associated with neuraxial techniques, such as epidural hematoma and CNS infection, can be avoided. It is worth noting that if sedation is employed in conjunction with regional anesthesia, it may potentiate the risk of perioperative complications such as delirium and aspiration pneumonia.

Postoperative Management

Postoperative management of the geriatric patient with compromise of pulmonary function should focus on maintaining effective gas exchange, counteracting the effects of residual anesthesia and neuromuscular blockade, preventing aspiration, reducing the risk of pulmonary infection and prophylaxis against deep venous thromboembolism.

As mentioned previously, the intraoperative use of short-acting medications is a particularly effective strategy for reducing the risk of ventilatory failure in the postoperative period. All drug dosing should take into account the altered pharmacokinetics and pharmacodynamics in the elderly patient. Generous supplemental oxygen reduces the frequency of hypoxic episodes. Deep venous thromboembolism (DVT) and subsequent pulmonary emboli (PE) are a significant cause of morbidity and mortality in the elderly. Aggressive prophylaxis with sequential compression devices, anticoagulation, and early mobilization should be employed as prevention.

Postoperative delirium, an acute confusional state characterized by cognitive dysfunction and disturbed sleep–wake cycles, has a significant impact on pulmonary morbidity and outcome after surgery. Risk factors include age, preoperative cognitive dysfunction, poor functional status, alcohol use, and polypharmacy. Avoidance of precipitating factors including alterations in sleep–wake cycles, malnutrition, physical restraints, bladder catheters, and other iatrogenic factors can significantly decrease the incidence of this complication. Further, interventions such as frequent visits from family members, regular orientation to time and location, and use of sensory aids, such as eyeglasses and listening devices, can be particularly effective in limiting its manifestations.

Adequate pain control in the geriatric patient is associated with significantly fewer pulmonary complications. However, the benefits of adequate postoperative pain control should be weighed carefully against the risk of respiratory depression due to opiate medications. When appropriate, adjunctive pain medications should be utilized to maximize the efficacy of postoperative pain control while reducing the risk of opioid-related respiratory depression. Regional anesthetic techniques are particularly efficacious at achieving effective postoperative pain control. When used appropriately, such techniques may decrease the likelihood of respiratory depression. Further, their use may aid in earlier mobilization, thus reducing the risk of DVT and subsequent PE.

In contrast to the intraoperative period, atelectasis contributes significantly to postoperative hypoxemia and other pulmonary complications. This is particularly true of patients that have undergone major abdominal and thoracic procedures. Early mobilization, upright positioning, incentive spirometry, and chest physiotherapy are particularly effective strategies for recruiting atelectatic lung units. When aggressively employed, these methods can significantly reduce the incidence of pulmonary complications in the elderly patient.

Noninvasive positive pressure ventilation (NIPPV) may also have a significant role in improving ventilatory mechanics in the immediate postoperative period. Beneficial effects include prevention of reduction in lung volume, decreased incidence of atelectasis, and decreased work of breathing. NIPPV may be of significant utility in those patients with marginal ventilatory status. The use of NIPPV in the immediate postoperative period in susceptible patients can reduce the incidence of respiratory failure leading to reintubation. Substantial benefit may also be derived from the use of perioperative NIPPV in patients with a history of obstructive sleep apnea (OSA). Institution of this modality is associated with fewer episodes of apnea and hypoxia in the patient at risk for OSA. NIPPV may also be of significant benefit in the critically ill elderly patient in respiratory failure. NIPPV use has the benefit of avoidance of intubation-related trauma, preservation of airway defense mechanisms, and a reduction in the incidence of nosocomial pneumonia. The benefits of this therapy have been demonstrated in elderly patients with respiratory failure due to pulmonary edema, acute exacerbations of COPD, and pneumonia. NIPPV should not be initiated in patients that lack the ability to protect their airway. Disadvantages of NIPPV include a higher risk of aspiration when compared to endotracheal intubation and the potential for facial injury from mask application.

Prevention of pneumonia in the postoperative period merits special attention as this complication is associated with significant morbidity and mortality in the elderly patient. Aspiration and respiratory failure leading to mechanical ventilation are the leading causes of pulmonary infection in the postsurgical period. Management of these complications has been discussed in more detail elsewhere in this chapter. Once pulmonary infection is suspected, it should be aggressively managed. Pulmonary secretions should be sent for laboratory testing and culture. Antibiotic management, tailored to the susceptibility of cultured organisms, should be instituted immediately once pneumonia is suspected.

Prevention of Aspiration Pneumonia in the Elderly

Aspiration pneumonia is a serious complication that accounts for significant morbidity and mortality in the elderly patient in the perioperative period. As previously mentioned, physiologic and pathologic alterations of the neurologic, pulmonary, and gastrointestinal system predispose the elderly to an increased risk of aspiration. Further, the use of anesthetic, neuromuscular blocks, and analgesic medications in the perioperative period can exacerbate underlying risk factors. Prevention in the preoperative period may require coordination among a variety of health-care professionals including pulmonologists, clinical dieticians, oral hygienists, respiratory and physical therapists, and nurses.

Oropharyngeal flora such as *Staphylococcus aureus* and aerobic Gram-negative bacilli are the most common pathogens implicated in aspiration pneumonia. The risk of aspiration is high in patients with degenerative neurologic disorders and a history of cerebrovascular disease. The progressive decline of the elderly immune system combined with the reduction in mucociliary clearance and decreased respiratory muscle strength also predispose the elderly to a higher risk of aspiration. In addition, decreased gastric acid secretion predisposes the elderly patient to colonization of gastric contents by pathogenic organisms such as *Clostridium perfringens* which can increase the risk of pneumonia after aspiration.

Measures aimed at preventing aspiration in high-risk elderly patients should be undertaken throughout the perioperative period. Gastric emptying agents, such as metoclopramide, when administered sufficiently in advance of anesthesia, are effective at reducing the volume of gastric fluid. Rapid sequence induction followed by endotracheal intubation is indicated in patients with risk factors for aspiration.

Should intraoperative regurgitation occur, it should be treated with aggressive suctioning of the pharynx, head-down position and endotracheal intubation, if necessary, to guarantee adequate oxygenation. Fiberoptic bronchoscopy may be utilized to aspirate large particulate matter. As with younger patients, prophylactic antibiotics are not indicated unless the aspirate is feculent. Similarly, steroid therapy is controversial and should not be employed prophylactically. Bronchospasm secondary to aspiration pneumonitis can be treated with inhaled and intravenous bronchodilating agents as necessary. If hypoxemia develops, it can be treated with PEEP and oxygen supplementation. Severe cases of aspiration can lead to the development of acute respiratory distress syndrome (ARDS). These patients are prone to significant hypoxia and decreased lung compliance necessitating complex ventilatory management.

In the postoperative period, a multidisciplinary approach is also effective in preventing aspiration in the high-risk geriatric patient. In at-risk patients, the swallowing mechanism should be clinically evaluated by a specialist. Dietary modifications should be tailored to the findings of such a clinical evaluation. Food consistency, as well as size and frequency of meals, should be altered based on the patient's ability to swallow. There does not appear to be any clear data suggesting that placement of feeding tubes offers protection against aspiration pneumonia. However, tube feeding may be indicated in patients when severe dysfunction of the gag and swallow mechanism is present. Whenever artificial feeding is employed, it should be used as a short-term bridge until the ultimate goal of rehabilitating the patient's swallow and gag function is achieved. Prior to considering placement of a feeding tube, every attempt should be made to preserve oral intake. This can be accomplished by addressing common reversible interacting factors such as delirium and use of sedative agents.

Oral hygiene is also of particular importance. Poor dental and oral hygiene predispose the elderly patient to an increased incidence of colonization of the oropharynx with Gram-negative organisms. This is associated with an increased frequency and severity of pneumonia in the elderly. Aggressive oral care reduces colonization with potentially pathogenic organisms and decreases the bacterial load of the oropharyngeal cavity. Improvement in oral hygiene has been associated with a significantly reduced risk of aspiration and improved morbidity and mortality.

Thoracic Surgery in the Geriatric Patient

Lung cancer is the most prevalent diagnosis in the geriatric patient presenting for thoracic surgery. Unlike younger patients, the goals of therapy may often be the relief of symptoms and improvement of quality of life rather than long-term survival. Several anesthetic considerations are relevant to the geriatric patient presenting for thoracic surgery. Age by itself is a poor predictor of perioperative risk and outcome after surgery. Individual patients may have vastly different functional limitations independent of their age. In fact, functional status is the single most important determinant of perioperative risk in the geriatric patient presenting for a thoracic procedure.

Thoracic surgery is typically considered to be of intermediate cardiovascular risk in the younger patient based on American College of Cardiology/American Heart Association (ACC/AHA) guidelines. In the elderly, however, thoracic procedures may represent a high risk for cardiovascular and pulmonary complications. Pneumonectomy, in particular, is associated with a significantly higher risk of in-hospital mortality in the geriatric patient. A preoperative echocardiogram can be helpful in diagnosing unsuspected pulmonary hypertension, particularly if an elderly patient is scheduled for a significant resection.

Testing of predicted postsurgical pulmonary function may also be valuable in the geriatric patient presenting for a thoracic procedure. Such testing may be of particular benefit in the patient presenting for pneumonectomy. A predicted postresection FEV_1 of greater than 40% is associated with a higher likelihood of extubation in the operating room at the end of the procedure. Assessment of lung parenchymal function and cardiopulmonary reserve add to the predictive value of pulmonary function testing. Lung parenchymal function can be assessed by arterial blood gas analysis and measurement of D_LCO. PaO_2 values of <60 mmHg and $PaCO_2$ values of >45 mmHg have been associated with poorer outcomes. Additionally, a predicted D_LCO of <40% has been associated with increased respiratory complications and cardiac complications independent of FEV_1. Cardiopulmonary reserve can be assessed by evaluating functional capacity. The ability to climb more than three flights of stairs is associated with decreased morbidity and mortality whereas an inability to achieve two flights represents high risk. If a quantitative assessment of cardiopulmonary function is needed, maximal oxygen consumption (VO_2max) can be measured. A VO_2max of >15 ml/kg/min is associated with very low risk.

Intraoperative management of the elderly thoracic patient is similar to that of a younger patient. The type of lung isolation technique used varies based on patient size, gender, type of surgery, and underlying pathology. Age is typically not a factor when deciding which lung isolation technique to employ. The physiologic challenges that exist during one-lung ventilation are also similar to those found in younger patients. However, the geriatric patient may be prone to a greater degree of V/Q mismatch (with resultant hypoxia) at baseline. In addition, an obstructive pattern of ventilation may be noted even in patients who do not carry a diagnosis of COPD. Hypoxic pulmonary vasoconstriction (HPV) does not appear to be influenced by age. As with younger patients, the reflex is inhibited by certain agents such as volatile anesthetics and intravenous vasodilators.

Pulmonary Issues in the Critically Ill Geriatric Patient

Patients aged 65 or older account for as much as 48% of intensive care admissions in the United States. Respiratory complications are one of the leading causes of admission of the geriatric patient to the intensive care unit. A significant proportion of these patients, up to 40%, require mechanical ventilation. The physiologic changes associated with aging necessitate adjustment of the typical ventilatory management strategies employed.

Chronic Respiratory Failure

Chronic ventilator dependency, defined as the need to mechanically ventilate a patient more than 6 h a day in excess of 21 days, affects a disproportionate number of elderly patients. Since prolonged respiratory failure is associated with considerable mortality (up to 40%), it is of significant concern. Complications common in the elderly ICU patient, such as ventilator associated pneumonia (VAP), malnutrition, cardiac dysfunction and airway injury, make weaning from mechanical ventilation more difficult.

Traditional weaning parameters do not typically apply to the elderly patient dependent on chronic mechanical ventilation. Measurement of ventilatory parameters such as minute ventilation, vital capacity, negative inspiratory force, and rapid shallow breathing index, which may be of significant utility in younger patients, should not be solely relied on to predict suitability for extubation. Instead, weaning from mechanical ventilation can be a complicated process with frequent setbacks.

The approach to extubation should be multidisciplinary and focused on optimizing the function of all organ systems. Hemodynamic stability is an essential component of any weaning strategy. The geriatric patient should require minimal or no vasopressor support and be free of any unstable arrhythmias. Adequate nutrition is also of vital importance since the increased work of breathing imposed by spontaneous ventilation consumes significant energy. Nutritional supplementation, if necessary, should be aggressively instituted with the goal of improving respiratory muscle strength. Sedative drugs, frequently employed to increase tolerance to mechanical ventilation, should be gradually titrated off prior to weaning. Prevention and treatment of delirium, a common cause of respiratory failure in elderly ICU patient, should be vigorously pursued.

Acute Respiratory Distress Syndrome in the Elderly

Acute respiratory distress syndrome (ARDS) is another source of significant mortality in the critically ill elderly patient. ARDS is characterized by diffuse inflammatory injury to the lung with hypoxemic respiratory failure. The acute phase of ARDS is defined by hypoxemia resistant to supplementary oxygen therapy, diffuse pulmonary infiltrates similar in appearance to cardiogenic pulmonary edema, and a PaO_2 to FIO_2 ratio (PaO_2/FiO_2) of <200. Once lung injury manifests, an underlying cause should be sought and aggressive treatment instituted. Sepsis is the most common cause of progression of ALI to ARDS in the critically ill elderly patient.

The management of ARDS may be particularly complex in the geriatric patient. Therapy is directed at utilizing PEEP to improve oxygenation while minimally compromising cardiovascular stability. Every attempt should be made to reduce inspired oxygen concentration so as to minimize the risk of pulmonary oxygen toxicity. The use of low tidal volumes during positive pressure ventilation has displayed significant benefit in multiple studies of critically ill patients. It should be noted, however, that the benefit of low tidal volume ventilation strategies is not as well defined in the elderly patient with ARDS. This may be due to the fact that the lungs of the elderly patient require greater expansion to prevent atelectasis and ventilator-associated pneumonia.

Pulmonary Infection in the Elderly ICU Patient

Lung infection is another significant source of mortality and morbidity in the critically ill geriatric patient. Pulmonary infections are a frequent cause of sepsis, which can rapidly progress to multiorgan system dysfunction and death. In addition, age-related compromise of the immune system renders the elderly hospitalized patient particularly vulnerable to nosocomial infection. Ventilator-associated pneumonia (VAP) is a frequent complication in elderly patients that are mechanically ventilated.

Numerous strategies can be employed as prophylaxis against this complication. The use of "VAP bundles," checklists of routine preventive measures, has been shown to be particularly effective at reducing morbidity from VAP. Such checklists establish a standardized protocol for interventions such as sedation holidays, head up positioning, chest therapy, oral care, and aspiration prophylaxis, which maximizes their combined efficacy. Management of pulmonary infection is similar to that of a younger critically ill patient. Antibiotics, pulmonary rehabilitation, and mechanical ventilation, if necessary, should be aggressively employed.

Key Points

- Significant physiologic and anatomic changes occur to the pulmonary system of the geriatric patient necessitating alterations in ventilatory management during the perioperative period.
- Chronic obstructive pulmonary disease (COPD) is a syndrome primarily associated with aging that significantly affects anesthetic management in elderly patients.
- The elderly patient is prone to hypoxia since arterial oxygenation is progressively impaired with increasing age. This is attributable primarily to ventilation/perfusion mismatch. Postoperative supplemental oxygen may be needed more often and for longer periods than in young patients.
- Preoperative risk assessment in the geriatric patient presenting for thoracic surgery correlates more closely with the severity of underlying pulmonary pathology than age itself.
- Perioperative pulmonary considerations for the geriatric patient include maintaining effective ventilation in spite of altered lung mechanics, preventing bronchospasm and mucus plugging in susceptible patients and prevention of respiratory failure in the postoperative period.
- Early mobilization, upright positioning, incentive spirometry, and chest physiotherapy are particularly effective strategies in the postoperative period for reducing the incidence of pulmonary complications in the elderly patient.
- Supplemental oxygen therapy may significantly improve functional status in the elderly patient with severe COPD. In patients with significant baseline hypoxia, this therapy also been associated with slowing the progression of disease.
- Physiologic and pathologic alterations of the neurologic, pulmonary, and gastrointestinal system predispose the elderly to an increased risk of aspiration pneumonia. An aggressive multidisciplinary approach should be employed to prevent aspiration pneumonia in the geriatric patient.
- Adequate pain control in the geriatric patient may help prevent pulmonary complications. However, the benefits of adequate postoperative pain control should be weighed carefully against the risk of respiratory depression.
- Respiratory complications are one of the leading causes of admission of the geriatric patient to the intensive care unit. Chronic ventilator dependency is associated with considerable mortality in the critically ill, elderly patient. The approach

to weaning chronically ventilator dependent elderly patients should be multidisciplinary and focused on treatment of underlying pathology. Traditional weaning parameters may not apply to these patients.
- Prevention of ARDS and ventilator-associated pneumonia in the critically ill geriatric patient is associated with significantly decreased mortality and morbidity.

Suggested Reading

Albertson TE, Louie S, Chan AL. The Diagnosis and Treatment of Elderly Patients with Acute Exacerbations of Chronic Obstructive Pulmonary Disease and Chronic Bronchitis. J Am Geriatr Soc. 2010;58:570–579.

Cartin-Ceba R, Sprung J, Gajic O, Warner DO. In: Mcleskey, et al. Geriatric Anesthesiology. 2nd ed. New York, NY: Springer; 2008:149–164.

Castillo MD, Heerdt PM. Pulmonary resection in the elderly. Curr Opin Anaesthesiol. 2007;20(1):4–9.

Eachempati SR, Hydo LJ, Shou J, Barie PS. Outcomes of acute respiratory distress syndrome (ARDS) in elderly patients. J Trauma. 2007;63(2):344–50.

El Solh AA, Ramadan FH. Overview of respiratory failure in older adults. J Intensive Care Med. 2006;21(6):345–51.

Epstein CD, El-Mokadem N, Peerless JR. Weaning older patients from long-term mechanical ventilation: a pilot study. Am J Crit Care. 2002;11(4):369–377.

Gatti G, Cardu G, Lusa AM, Pugliese P. Predictors of postoperative complications in high-risk octogenarians undergoing cardiac operations. Ann Thorac Surg. 2002;74(3):671–7.

Griffith KA, Sherrill DL, Siegel EM, Manolio TA, Bonekat HW, Enright PL. Predictors of loss of lung function in the elderly: The Cardiovascular Health Study. Am J Respir Crit Care Med. 2001;163(1):61–68.

Hardie JA, Mørkve O, Ellingsen I. Effect of body position on arterial oxygen tension in the elderly. Respiration. 2002;69(2):123–8.

Kleinhenz ME, Lewis CY. Chronic ventilator dependence in elderly patients. Clin Geriatr Med. 2000;16(4):735–756.

Kurup V. In: Hines RL, Marschall KE eds. Stoelting's Anesthesia and Coexisting Disease. 5th ed. Philadelphia, Pa: Churchill Livingstone; 2008:161–197.

Liu LL, Wiener-Kronish JP. Perioperative anesthesia issues in the elderly. Crit Care Clin. 2003;19(4):641–56.

Marik PE, Kaplan D. Aspiration pneumonia and dysphagia in the elderly. Chest. 2003;124(1): 328–336.

Marik PE. Management of the critically ill geriatric patient. Crit Care Med. 2006;34 (9 Suppl): S176–82.

Niewoehner DE. Clinical practice. Outpatient management of severe COPD. N Engl J Med. 2010; 362(15):1407–16.

Rosenthal RA, Kavic SM.Assessment and management of the geriatric patient. Crit Care Med. 2004;32(4 Suppl):S92–105.

Sevransky JE, Haponik EF. Respiratory failure in elderly patients. Clin Geriatr Med. 2003;19(1):205–224.

Silvay G, Castillo JG, Chikwe J, Flynn B, Filsoufi F. Cardiac anesthesia and surgery in geriatric patients. Semin Cardiothorac Vasc Anesth. 2008;12(1):18–28.

Slinger P. Update on anesthetic management for pneumonectomy. Curr Opin Anaesthesiol. 2009; 22(1):31–7.

Smetana GW. Preoperative pulmonary assessment of the older adult. Clin Geriatr Med. 2003;19(1): 35–55.

Sprung J, Gajic O, Warner DO. Review article: age related alterations in respiratory function—anesthetic considerations. Can J Anaesth. 2006;53(12):1244–1257.

Solh AA, Ramadan FH. Overview of respiratory failure in older adults. J Intensive Care Med. 2006;21;345–351.

The Acute Respiratory Distress Syndrome Network. Ventilation with lower tidal volumes as compared with traditional tidal volumes for acute lung injury and the acute respiratory distress syndrome. N Engl J Med. 2000;342(18):1301–8.

Zaugg M, Lucchinetti E. Respiratory function in the elderly. Anesthesiol Clin North Am. 2000;18(1):47–58, vi.

Zeleznik J. Normative aging of the respiratory system. Clin Geriatr Med. 2003;19(1):1–18.

Chapter 16
Vascular Surgery: Endovascular and Major Vascular Surgery

Shamsuddin Akhtar

Introduction

Over a 100 million adults undergo noncardiac surgery worldwide, and a significant proportion of these patients are elderly patients with complex medical histories undergoing vascular surgery. The risk of adverse events, especially cardiac events, increases with age. Elderly patients with significant comorbidities who undergo high-risk procedures are more likely to sustain perioperative adverse events than their healthy counterparts in the same age cohort. Perioperative management of elderly patients scheduled for vascular surgery poses a unique challenge for the anesthesiologist. This chapter will focus on the demographics of an elderly patient presenting for vascular surgery, risks of commonly performed vascular procedures, preoperative evaluation, and perioperative management of elderly patients undergoing vascular surgery.

Demographics of a Vascular Surgery Patient

The probability of suffering from cardiovascular comorbidities increases dramatically with age. According to the latest American Heart Association (AHA) statistics, the prevalence of cardiovascular disease (CVD) in patients > 80 years is 78–85%. The incidence of hypertension is 65% (>75 years), CAD is 23–37% (>80 years), and congestive heart failure (CHF) is 13–15% (>80 years) (Fig. 16.1). Among Americans older than 60 years of age, 21% have diabetes (DM) and 38% have chronic kidney disease, and 10–15% of patients older than 70 years suffer from

S. Akhtar, MBBS (✉)
Department of Anesthesiologist, Yale University School of Medicine,
333 Cedar Street, TMP#3, New Haven, CT 06520, USA
e-mail: shamsuddin.akhtar@yale.edu

S.R. Barnett (ed.), *Manual of Geriatric Anesthesia*, DOI 10.1007/978-1-4614-3888-5_16,

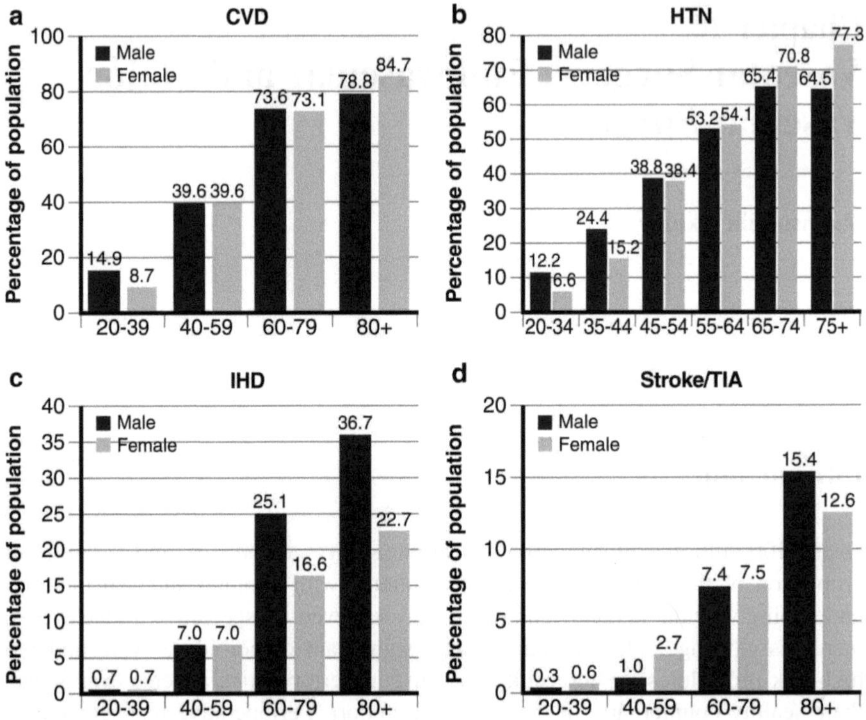

Fig. 16.1 The incidence of cardiovascular disease based on age and gender. (**a**) cardiovascular disease; (**b**) hypertension; (**c**) ischemic heart disease; and (**d**) stroke/transient ischemic attacks. Data from American Heart Association Statistics 2010

atrial fibrillation. The incidence of chronic obstructive pulmonary disease also increases significantly with age.

Approximately eight million Americans suffer from peripheral vascular or arterial disease (PAD). PAD affects 12–20% of Americans > 65 years of age and it disproportionately affects African-Americans. Prevalence of PAD increases dramatically with age, for example, the prevalence of abdominal aortic aneurysms (AAAs) 2.9–4.9 cm in diameter increases from 1.3% in men 45–54 years of age to 12.5% in men 75–84 years of age. For women, the prevalence ranges from zero in the youngest to 5.2% in the oldest age groups.

Typically, vascular disease is divided into three distinct categories: cerebrovascular disease (CVD) involving the carotid and intracranial vasculature, coronary artery disease (CAD) involving the vasculature of the heart, or peripheral vascular disease (PAD) involving aorta and its branches. At one extreme are individuals who have disease predominantly in one vascular bed, for example have only CAD or CVD. However, there are many patients who have disease in more than one vascular bed and some patients suffer from disease in all three vascular areas. By some estimates, only 10% of patients scheduled for vascular surgery have pristine coronary arteries and up to 60% have significant CAD. It is not unexpected that vascular patients are also on multiple medications. In a series of patients undergoing vascular surgery, the incidence of baseline medication was beta-blockers 80%, statins 72%, aspirin 58%, oral anticoagulants 19%, angiotensin-converting enzyme inhibitors (ACE-inhibitors) 35.5%, angiotensin-receptor blockers (ARBs) 17%, and diuretics 30%. Apart from the risk of unfavorable drug–drug interactions, many of these medications have perioperative implications and undesirable drug–anesthetic interactions.

Risk of Vascular Surgery

Vascular surgery inherently carries a significant risk of perioperative mortality [>5%], however, not all types of vascular surgeries are considered high risk. Based on the recent guidelines, open aortic surgery and lower extremity bypass surgery are associated with highest risk of perioperative morbidity and mortality and thus are considered high-risk surgeries. Mortality after elective open abdominal aortic aneurysm repair increases with advancing age, from 2.2% for patients in the sixth decade to 7.3% for octogenarians. Though the perioperative morbidity and mortality continues to improve overall, the risk of mortality following an emergent ruptured AAA repair is still significantly high at 20–40%.

With recent advancement in stent technology more than 60% of infrarenal AAA are now managed endovascularly (EVARs). More and more thoracic aneurysms (TAAA) are also being managed endovascularly or through a combination of open and endovascular procedure. This trend is likely to continue. Short-term morbidity and mortality seems to be lower for EVARs; however, long-term mortality is not much different from open AAAs. In contrast to an open AAA repair, an EVAR is considered intermediate risk surgery, with the risk of events to be <3%. EVARs are the preferred options in the elderly population especially patients older than 80 years.

All techniques for repairing AAA are associated with complications. Open AAA repairs are associated with higher surgical stress response, longer hospital stay and recovery times, and a high frequency of delayed interventions for incisional hernia and small bowel obstruction. On the other hand, EVARs are also associated with systemic complications. These range from cardiac, pulmonary, and renal dysfunction to embolic disease and spinal cord ischemic injury. In addition to endoleaks (which describes *incomplete* exclusion of blood flow from the aneurysm sac), EVARs also present with other unique access and endograft-related complications that are not encountered in open surgical repair. Early complications include: endograft limb thrombosis, unintentional occlusion of critical artery leading to organ ischemia (e.g., renal or mesenteric artery), or iatrogenic arterial injuries. Late complications include endoleaks, graft migration, late limb thrombosis or fractures, component separation, or fabric tears of the implant. Long-term surveillance is strongly recommended to ensure clinically efficacious results.

Though some studies report that older patients undergoing infrapopliteal bypass procedures for critical limb ischemia have a greater perioperative mortality rate than their matching younger cohort, other studies have failed to identify any difference in the perioperative mortality rates. However, all these types of vascular procedures are considered high risk for major adverse cardiac events (MACE).

The role of a carotid endarterectomy (CEA) in symptomatic and asymptomatic patients with internal carotid artery occlusive disease is well established. Though initial reports reported an increase in 30-day mortality in octogenarians, recent trials have not been able to support those results. By some estimates, almost 9% of patients undergoing CEA are older than 75 years, while octogenarians appear to make up 10% of CEA cases. It should be noted that CEA has been performed successfully, without additional morbidity and mortality even in nonagenarians. A review of contemporary results of CEA performed among 2,564 octogenarians showed a 30-day stroke/death rate of 3.5%. In one recent study, stroke/death rate was 2.3% in patients > 80 years and 2.1% in patients aged <80 years. The initial enthusiasm for treating carotid occlusive disease with stenting in the octogenarians has waned due to higher incidence of stroke in the carotid arterial stenting group (12.1 vs. 3.2%). Current evidence establishes CEA as a safer carotid intervention in the elderly and is considered intermediate risk surgery with the risk of events to be <5%.

Management of Elderly Patients Scheduled for Vascular Surgery

A typical approach and management of any patient (irrespective of age) is to identify patients at risk for perioperative events. The risk then may have to be quantified by further testing and the patient will be managed to improve outcomes if possible. This management can include specific monitoring techniques [for example, central venous pressure monitoring (CVP), pulmonary artery catheter monitoring (PAC), transesophageal echocardiography (TEE), continuous arterial blood pressure, or noninvasive cardiac output monitoring], perioperative adjustment of medications, or intensive postoperative care (Fig. 16.2). Postponing surgery, the adoption of specific anesthetic techniques or medications may also have an impact on improving outcomes. Due to high incidence of concomitant coronary artery disease (CAD), select (and rare) vascular surgery patients may even benefit from preoperative coronary revascularization.

Risk Assessment

A number of risk indices have been developed over the years to predict major adverse cardiac events (MACE) after noncardiac surgery. Currently, the most commonly used and recommended index in North America is the revised cardiac risk index (RCRI). The most recent AHA guidelines recommend use of RCRI for risk assessment. It is based on six factors: (1) history of ischemic heart disease,

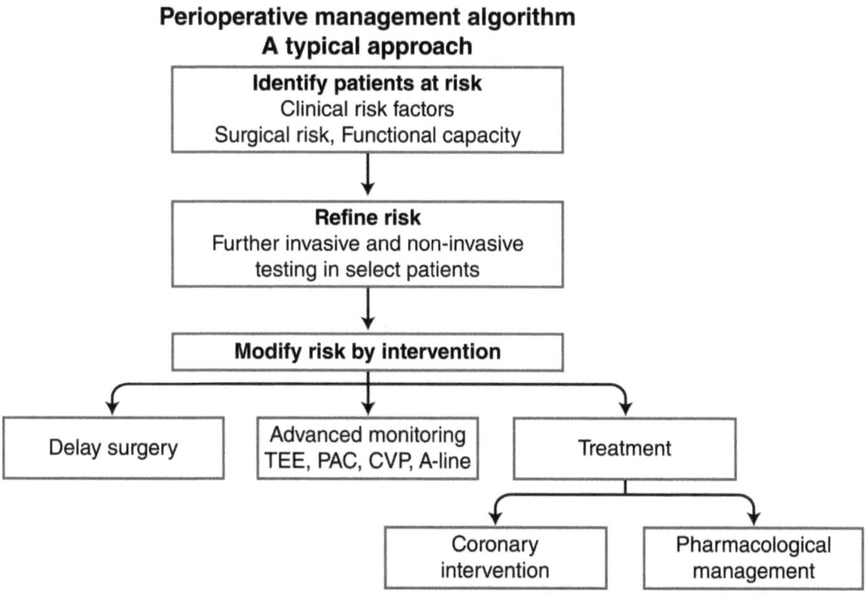

Fig. 16.2 Perioperative management algorithm for patient undergoing noncardiac surgery

(2) congestive heart failure, (3) diabetes, (4) cerebrovascular disease, (5) renal insufficiency, and (6) supra-inguinal aortic surgery. Each factor is allocated one point. Risk of MACE increases incrementally with increasing number of points. The predictive value of RCRI has been substantiated by many investigations; however, some modifications have also been suggested by the European group and include age as one of the factors (Table 16.1). The practitioner should keep in mind the following caveats regarding the RCRI:

(a) The index was developed based on patients who were recruited between 1991 and 1994. The medical management of patients, especially for cardiac ailments (e.g., use of statins, ACE inhibitors, ARBs, and anticoagulants) has changed radically in the past 15 years.
(b) The index is not developed selectively for elderly patients and age is not included as a factor for MACE, though post hoc analysis suggests that for each number of risk factors, increasing age confers incremental risk. A recent study suggested age > 80 years may be an independent risk factor for higher incidence of perioperative major adverse cardiac events.
(c) Though the patients who have CAD, CVD, DM, and renal insufficiency can be identified readily, a significant proportion of these patients have asymptomatic, systolic, and diastolic heart failure and may not be recognized. Up to 50% of patients presenting for vascular surgery may be suffering from echocardiographic-proven symptomatic or asymptomatic heart failure. Asymptomatic diastolic heart failure contributes to increased perioperative MACE.

Table 16.1 Clinical risk factors used for preoperative cardiac risk stratification: Lee index and European index (Erasmus model)

Clinical risk factor	Lee index	European index (Erasmus)
Ischemic heart disease	+	+
Surgical risk	+	+
Congestive heart failure	+	+
Stroke/transient ischemic attack	+	+
Diabetes requiring insulin	+	+
Renal dysfunction (Cr >2.0)	+	+
Age		+

Table 16.2 Frailty index

Shrinking (weight loss) was defined as unintentional weight loss >10 pounds in the last year
Decreased grip strength (weakness) as measured by a hand-held dynamometer. The strength measurement was adjusted by gender and body mass index
Exhaustion was measured by responses to questions about effort and motivation
Low physical activity was ascertained by inquiring about leisure time activities
Slowed walking speed was measured by the speed at which patient could walk 15 feet

It is well recognized that elderly patients have significantly decreased reserve and hence are more prone to major adverse events. Frailty index (Table 16.2) is able to predict outcomes in nonsurgical population and hence may have a role in perioperative risk assessment. In a recent study, adding frailty index to the established RCRI improved risk prediction by 8–10%. Though adding frailty index to establish the RCRI may be off incremental value, large control studies are required before it can be recommended as routine assessment tool in the elderly. Cost-effectiveness, logistics, time to conduct the test (~10 min per assessment), and its implications on the perioperative management of patient have to be considered.

Preoperative Assessment

An important goal of the history is to elicit from the patient or the caregivers the severity, progression, and functional limitations introduced by comorbidities. It should focus on determining the presence of major (unstable coronary syndrome, decompensated heart failure, significant arrhythmias, severe valvular disease), moderate (stable angina pectoris, previous MI by history or pathologic Q waves, compensated or prior heart failure, diabetes mellitus, renal insufficiency), and minor (uncontrolled hypertension, left bundle branch block, nonspecific ST-T wave changes, history of stroke) clinical risk factors in a particular patient. A history of CAD or an abnormal ECG suggestive of a prior myocardial infarction is associated with an increased incidence of silent myocardial ischemia. Myocardial ischemia, left ventricular dysfunction, and cardiac dysrhythmias are usually responsible for the symptoms of angina pectoris, dyspnea, limited exercise tolerance, and peripheral edema. Symptoms of CAD may be absent at rest, emphasizing the importance of evaluating the patient's responses to various physical activities such as walking or climbing stairs. Though limited exercise tolerance in the absence of significant lung disease is the most striking evidence of decreased cardiac reserve, many patients with significant vascular disease may also have limited exercise tolerance due to claudication. If a patient can climb two to three flights of stairs without symptoms, it is likely that cardiac reserve is adequate. It is important to recognize the presence of incipient congestive heart failure (CHF) preoperatively, as the added stress of anesthesia, surgery, fluid replacement, and postoperative pain may result in overt congestive heart failure.

A history of myocardial infarction is important information for the preoperative evaluation. It is common practice to delay elective operations for some time (up to 4–6 weeks) following an acute myocardial infarction. The incidence of myocardial reinfarction during the perioperative period is influenced by the time elapsed since the previous myocardial infarction. Acute (1–7 days) and recent myocardial infarction (8–30 days) and unstable angina would incur the highest risk of sustaining perioperative myocardial ischemia, infarction, and cardiac death.

It is also important to determine if the patient had an angioplasty with stent placement. Stent placement (drug eluting or bare metal) is routinely followed by postprocedure antiplatelet therapy to prevent acute coronary thrombosis and maintain long-term patency of the intervened vessel. Elective noncardiac procedure surgery should be delayed for 6 weeks after percutaneous intervention (PCI) with bare-metal stents and possibly 6–12 months in patients with drug-eluting stents, to allow for some re-endothelialization of the stent and completion of antiplatelet therapy with GIIb/IIIa inhibitors. The patient's cardiologist should be involved in any decisions surrounding cardiac stents and anticoagulation and antiplatelet therapies.

The history obtained from these patients should elicit symptoms and information relevant to co-existing noncardiac diseases. A history of syncope may reflect cerebrovascular disease, seizure disorders, or cardiac dysrhythmias. Cough is often pulmonary rather than cardiac in origin. It may be difficult to differentiate dyspnea due to cardiac dysfunction from that due to chronic lung disease, although patients with CAD often complain of associated orthopnea and paroxysmal nocturnal dyspnea. Chronic obstructive pulmonary disease is predictable in patients with a long history of cigarette smoking. The history of DM and renal insufficiency (creatinine >2.0 mg/dl) should be elicited.

Current Medications

Many patients with PVD who present for vascular surgery are on β-blockers, nitrates, calcium entry blockers, statins, antiplatelet agents, and ACE inhibitors. Except for withholding diuretics on the day of surgery or anticoagulants (per the patient's cardiologist or internist), most patients are usual advised to continue their antihypertensive and cardiac medications. In particular, beta-blockers, statins, and nitrates should be continued. There is continued controversy about withholding ACE inhibitors and ARBs 24 h prior to surgery. Prolonged hypotension has been observed in patients who are undergoing general anesthesia and who have chronically been treated with ACE inhibitors. Some recommend withholding ACE inhibitors for 24 h prior to surgical procedures involving major body fluid shifts on significant blood loss. Hypotension attributed to ACE inhibitors is frequently responsive to fluid and/or administration or sympathomimetic drugs. If hypotension is refractory to these measures treatment with vasopressin or its long-acting analogue terlipressin may be effective.

Antiplatelet agents are an essential component in the pharmacotherapy of acute coronary syndromes and long-term management of CAD and PAD. Aspirin irreversibly inhibits cyclo-oxygenase and prevents platelet activation and should be continued. Clopidogrel and ticlopidine bind irreversibly to ADP receptor on the platelets, thereby preventing transformation of platelet glycoprotein IIb/IIIa receptor and further platelet activation. These agents are strongly recommended after coronary stent insertion and early discontinuation in the perioperative period can lead to acute thrombosis and fatal myocardial infarction. However, dual antiplatelet therapy precludes neuroaxial anesthesia. Clopidogrel and ticlopidine can increase the risk of significant perioperative bleeding, which may require platelet transfusions in urgent clinical situations.

Physical Examination

In an elderly patient scheduled for vascular surgery, signs of left ventricular failure must be sought. A carotid bruit may indicate previously unrecognized CVD. Orthostatic hypotension may reflect an attenuated autonomic nervous system activity due to treatment with antihypertensive drugs. Peripheral edema is usually a late finding in patients with left ventricular failure and can also be due to venous insufficiency. Examination of the jugular venous pulse for abnormalities reflects right ventricular failure as does peripheral edema. Auscultation of the chest may reveal evidence of left ventricular dysfunction (S3 gallop) and incipient pulmonary edema. Evaluation of the patient's upper airway and the anticipated technical ease of laryngoscopy for tracheal intubation and determination of peripheral venous sites are useful. If regional anesthesia or neuroaxial block is contemplated, the respective areas should be examined for skin breakdown, active infection, and the ease of landmark identification. Significant osteoarthritis, kyphoscoliosis, or contractures may preclude a planned regional technique.

Preoperative electrocardiogram in elderly patients scheduled for vascular surgery is strongly recommended. Specialized preoperative testing such as echocardiography or thallium scintigraphy should be reserved for patients in whom the results are critical for guiding therapy.

Thallium Scintigraphy

Dipyridamole-thallium testing mimics the coronary vasodilator response associated with exercise, and similar to stress echocardiography is a useful test in patients with limited exercise capacity. Defects or "cold spots" on the nuclear scan denote areas of myocardial ischemia or infarction. This test is restricted to patients who cannot exercise and whose risk for perioperative cardiac complications cannot be estimated on the basis of clinical factors.

Echocardiography

Preoperative transthoracic or TEE is useful for diagnosing left ventricular dysfunction and for assessing the presence of cardiac valve disease. Echocardiographic wall motion analysis during the infusion of dipyridamole or dobutamine or atropine (pharmacologic stress) is an accurate technique for evaluating CAD, particularly in patients with no history of prior myocardial infarction. These tests have low false positive rates and high negative predictive values. Dobutamine stress echocardiography provides comparable (if not better) results to myocardial perfusion scintigraphy and provides additional information about valvular dysfunction.

Risk Stratification Algorithm

The AHA and the European Society of Cardiologist (ESC) guidelines provide a multistep algorithm for determining the need for preoperative cardiac evaluation and are very similar in their approach. The first step assesses the urgency of surgery: the need for emergency surgery takes precedence over the need for additional workup. The second step assesses whether the patient has undergone revascularization, i.e., coronary artery bypass grafting (CABG) or a percutaneous coronary intervention (PCI). The third step determines if and when the patient underwent invasive or noninvasive coronary evaluation. If the patient had revascularization within the last 5 years or had an appropriate coronary evaluation in the last 2 years—*with no subsequent deterioration of cardiac status*—then further cardiac evaluation is not warranted.

The next steps of the AHA Guidelines integrate risk stratification according to clinical risk factors, functional capacity, and surgery-specific risk factors. Clinical risk factors—obtained by history, physical examination, and review of EKG—are grouped into three categories, major, moderate, and minor risk factors. Next, functional capacity, also referred to as exercise tolerance, is evaluated. Many elderly patients with vascular disease may not be able to demonstrate good functional capacity.

Finally, surgery-specific risk of the vascular procedure is graded as high, intermediate, or low. High-risk surgeries include emergent major operations, aortic and

Clinical risk factors

Surgical risk factors	Major	Moderate				Minor
		Poor functional capacity			Good functional capacity	
		3 or more Risk factors	1-2 Risk factors	No Risk factors		
High risk surgery	E	Send for further testing	May send for further testing	No testing	No testing	No testing
Intermediate risk surgery	E	May send for further testing	May send for further testing	No testing	No testing	No testing
Low risk surgery	E	No testing	No testing	No testing	No testing	No testing

Fig. 16.3 Preoperative evaluation table to determine the need for further cardiac workup. Patients are divided based on clinical risk factors, surgical risk factors, and functional capacity. Patient with major risk factors should be sent for cardiology evaluation, further testing or surgery should be postponed unless it is emergent (E). Those with three or more risk factors scheduled for elective high-risk surgery should be referred for further testing. Others can be referred for testing or managed without testing based on the grid

other major vascular surgery, peripheral vascular surgery, anticipated prolonged surgical procedures associated with large fluid shift, and/or anticipated blood loss. Intermediate risk surgeries include CEA, EVARs, and lower limb amputations. Low-risk procedures are reported to have <1% risk of cardiac events. A-V fistula can be considered a low-risk procedure.

The presence of major clinical factors mandates possible delay of elective surgery, cardiology evaluation, and/or intensive perioperative management, if surgery is urgent or emergent and unavoidable. According to the ACC/AHA and ESC guidelines, patient scheduled for elective high-risk surgery, with low functional capacity and three or more RCRI factors should be considered for further cardiac evaluation or stress testing (Fig. 16.3). Patients that have 1–2 clinical risk factors with low functional capacity scheduled for high to intermediate risk surgery may be considered for further stress testing (Fig. 16.3). Patients who have low functional capacity, or in whom it is difficult to assess functional capacity, who are scheduled for high to intermediate risk surgery and have 1–2 moderate clinical risk factors may be considered for stress testing (Fig. 16.3). Though some patients may be candidates for exercise stress testing, many are likely to have poor functional capacity and are referred for pharmacological stress testing: stress echocardiography after dobutamine or atropine administration (DSE) or nuclear imaging with dipyridamole thallium (DTS). Both DSE and DTS have high negative predictive value (94 and 88%, respectively). The positive predictive value of DSE is better than DTS (67 vs. 37%) and DSE is more physiologically representative of the postoperative state.

Preoperative coronary angiography, at the discretion of cardiologist and possibly when there is significant variation of opinion, will be most suitable for patients with a positive stress test that suggests significant myocardium at risk. The aim of additional testing is to identify patients with significant CAD; left main or equivalent three-vessel CAD. Further management in patients with significant CAD would be dictated by patient's clinical condition, overall risk of an intervention, and resources available.

Management After Risk Stratification

The primary reason for risk stratification is to identify patients at increased risk so as to manage them with pharmacological and other perioperative interventions that can ameliorate perioperative cardiac events. Three therapeutic options are available prior to elective noncardiac surgery: (1) revascularization by surgery (CABG); (2) revascularization by percutaneous coronary intervention (PCI); (3) optimize medical management.

In nonoperative settings, treatment strategies like PCI with or without stenting, CABG in selected patients, and medical management with aspirin, statins, β-blockers, and anticoagulants, ACE inhibitors, ARBs have proven efficacy in improving long-term morbidity. Hence, patients with significant cardiovascular disease and symptoms who present for vascular surgery are likely to be candidates for one or more of the above-mentioned therapies regardless of whether they are scheduled for surgery. However, it may not be necessary to intervene preoperatively to improve perioperative outcomes. Coronary intervention should be guided by the patient's cardiac condition and by the potential consequences of delaying the noncardiac surgery for recovery after coronary revascularization.

Coronary Revascularization

Earlier studies had shown that patients who underwent coronary revascularization prior to major risk surgery had better outcomes postoperatively. However, for CABG surgery to be beneficial, the institutional risk for noncardiac surgery alone should be greater than the combined risk of coronary catheterization, coronary revascularization, and the subsequent vascular surgery. Benefit of preoperative coronary revascularization (CABG and/or PCI) has not been confirmed by more recent randomized studies in patients undergoing vascular surgery. In optimally treated patients (β-blockers, aspirin, statins, and ACE inhibitors), almost 3 years after randomization, there was no difference in mortality. This was attributed to better medical management in both the groups. Hence, the indications for coronary revascularization are the same as in the nonoperative setting (unstable angina, left main CAD or equivalent, 3-vessel disease, and decreased LV function). In general there seems to be no value of preoperative coronary intervention in patients with stable CAD.

Similarly, initial evaluations of PCI revealed that patients who underwent angioplasty prior to elective noncardiac surgery had better outcomes. However, angioplasty is now often accompanied by stenting, with postprocedure antiplatelet therapy, to prevent acute coronary thrombosis and maintain long-term patency of the intervened vessel. Though many factors influence the chance of stent thrombosis it is becoming clear that discontinuation of antiplatelet therapy, in the perioperative period, predisposes to stent thrombosis, with inherent high mortality. The following precautions can be adopted: (1) determine the date, kind of stent, and any history of complications in patients with history of PCI or coronary stent; (2) consider patients with recent stent placement (<6 weeks for bare mental stents and <1 year for drug-eluting stents) as high risk and consult an interventional cardiologist; and (3) review timing of proposed surgery. Discontinuing or modifying antiplatelet therapy should involve a multidisciplinary team which consists of cardiologist, surgeon, and anesthesiologist. Ideally, the procedure (especially emergent/urgent) should be performed in centers with interventional cardiologists, who can address the complication of stent thrombosis emergently.

Aortic stenosis is one of the most common valvular diseases in the elderly and predisposes to significant perioperative cardiac morbidity and mortality after noncardiac surgery. In symptomatic patients with critical aortic stenosis, aortic valve replacement or balloon angioplasty should be considered prior to elective surgery.

Pharmacological Management

In view of the serious limitations of current PCIs (and lack of utility of CABG and PCI in patients with stable CAD), very few patients with stable CAD will be revascularized prior to surgery. Most patients with stable CAD and or risk factors for CAD should be managed pharmacologically, although it should be recognized that most recommendations for pharmacological management are derived from studies performed in younger population (<80 years) and are extrapolated to an older age group.

Several pharmacological agents have been used to reduce perioperative injury, primarily because they have demonstrated pharmacological efficacy in the management of coronary ischemia in nonsurgical setting. Nitroglycerin may be helpful in the management of active perioperative ischemia. However, prophylactic use of nitroglycerin has not been shown to be efficacious in reducing perioperative morbidity and mortality.

Perioperative use of β-blockers has been shown to be efficacious in some studies in reducing perioperative cardiac morbidity and mortality in high-risk patients undergoing vascular surgery. However, results of recent trials have not shown efficacy of high-dose, acutely administered, perioperative beta-blockers to reduce overall mortality in patients undergoing noncardiac surgery. The largest of these trials, the POISE study, did show better perioperative *cardiac* outcomes with beta-blocker use; however, increased mortality and stroke rate were also noted in the beta-blocker group. Interestingly, subanalysis of vascular surgery patients in the study does demonstrate efficacy of perioperative beta-blockers. Currently, the only Class I recommendation for perioperative beta-blockers use is to continue their use in the patients who are already on beta-blockers. Patients undergoing vascular surgery who have multiple risk factors or have reversible ischemia on preoperative testing may benefit from perioperative beta-blockers (Class IIa). Though there are some differences between the ESC and the AHA Guidelines, they both agree that if beta-blockers are used for prophylactic purposes, they should be slowly titrated (at least a week prior to elective surgery) and acute administration of high-dose beta-blockers in high-risk population is not recommended (Table 16.3).

Patients with vascular disease should receive statin therapy for secondary prevention, independent of noncardiac surgery. Clinical trials have demonstrated a beneficial effect of perioperative statin use. European guidelines recommend starting therapy 7–30 days prior to high-risk surgery. Discontinuation of statins in the perioperative period may cause a rebound effect and may be harmful. Thus, it is recommended that statins be continued perioperatively (Table 16.4).

Alpha-2 agonists, by virtue of their central action, have analgesic, sedative, and sympatholytic effects. Perioperative use of alpha-2 agonists may be considered in patients scheduled for vascular surgery, to reduced MACE. However, their role in elderly vascular patients has not been specifically determined (Table 16.4).

Controlling hyperglycemia in patients undergoing cardiac surgery and in surgical intensive care patients has been associated with improved outcomes. To date appreciable decrease in morbidity and mortality with tight glucose control (120 mg/dl) has not been demonstrated in patients undergoing *major noncardiac surgery*. However, in light of recent discoveries of nonmetabolic effects of insulin and harmful effects of hyperglycemia, it is prudent to actively manage hyperglycemia with insulin, especially, in patients who are at high risk for cardiac injury and aim to keep perioperative glucose to <180 mg/dl.

Intraoperative and Postoperative Management

The basic challenge during induction and maintenance of anesthesia for patients with PVD is to prevent myocardial ischemia. The goals of intraoperative management in patients with vascular disease are: (1) prevent myocardial ischemia by optimizing myocardial oxygen supply and reduce oxygen demand; (2) monitor for ischemia and heart failure; (3) treat ischemia/infarction if it develops. These goals are logically achieved by maintaining the balance between myocardial oxygen delivery and myocardial oxygen requirements. Intraoperative events associated with persistent tachycardia, systolic hypertension, sympathetic nervous system stimulation, arterial hypoxemia, or diastolic hypotension can adversely influence this delicate balance. Perioperative myocardial injury is closely associated with perioperative heart rate in vascular surgery patients. Iatrogenic hyperventilation of the patient's

Table 16.3 Guidelines for perioperative beta-blocker use: American Heart Association (AHA) vs. European Society of Cardiology (ESC) recommendations

Recommendation class	Recommendation class	Recommendation class
Class I	Beta-blockers should be continued in patients undergoing surgery who are receiving beta-blockers for treatment of conditions with AHA Class I guideline indications for the drugs	Beta-blockers are recommended in patients who have known IHD or myocardial ischemia according to preoperative stress testing
		Beta-blockers are recommended in patients scheduled for high-risk surgery
		Continuation of beta-blockers is recommended in patients previously treated with beta-blockers because of IHD, arrhythmias, or hypertension
Class IIa	Beta-blockers titrated to heart rate and blood pressure are probably recommended for patients undergoing vascular surgery who are at high cardiac risk owing to coronary artery disease or the finding of cardiac ischemia on preoperative testing	Beta-blockers should be considered for patients scheduled for intermediate-risk surgery
	Beta-blockers titrated to heart rate and blood pressure are reasonable for patients in whom preoperative assessment for vascular surgery identifies high cardiac risk, as defined by the presence of more than 1 clinical risk factor	Continuation in patients previously treated with beta-blockers because of chronic heart failure with systolic dysfunction should be considered
	Beta-blockers titrated to heart rate and blood pressure are reasonable for patients in whom preoperative assessment identifies coronary artery disease or high cardiac risk, as defined by the presence of more than 1 clinical risk factor who are undergoing intermediate-risk surgery	
Class IIb	The usefulness of beta-blockers is uncertain for patients who are undergoing either intermediate-risk procedures or vascular surgery in whom preoperative assessment identifies a single clinical risk factor in the absence of coronary artery disease	Beta-blockers may be considered in patients scheduled for low-risk surgery with risk factor(s)
	The usefulness of beta-blockers is uncertain in patients undergoing vascular surgery with no clinical risk factors who are not currently taking beta-blockers	
Class III	Beta-blockers should not be given to patients undergoing surgery who have absolute contraindications to beta blockade	Perioperative high-dose beta-blockers without titration are not recommended
	Routine administration of high-dose beta-blockers in the absence of dose titration is not useful and may be harmful to patients not currently taking beta-blockers who are undergoing noncardiac surgery	Beta-blockers are not recommended in patients scheduled for low-risk surgery without risk factors

lungs, which greatly decreases the $PaCO_2$, should be avoided, as hypocapnia may evoke coronary artery vasoconstriction.

Open repair of AAA typically require general anesthesia, however, EVAR can be performed under general, regional, or local anesthesia. CEA can be performed either under general or regional anesthesia. Initial studies suggested that regional anesthesia for CEA may lead to better outcomes; however, subsequent larger trials (GALA trial) have not been able to show any clear difference between the techniques. Similarly, no significant difference in outcomes has been shown between neuroaxial and general anesthesia for lower extremity bypass surgery. Thus, maintenance of the balance between myocardial oxygen requirements and myocardial oxygen delivery is probably more important than the specific anesthetic technique or drugs selected to produce anesthesia (isoflurane, desflurane, sevoflurane, opioids) and skeletal muscle relaxation. Use of inhalational anesthetics is associated with preconditioning of the myocardium and their use, especially of sevoflurane, is recommended. The effect of prolonged nitrous oxide may predispose patients to perioperative myocardial ischemia; however, there is insufficient data at present to make firm recommendations about the use of nitrous. Most importantly, it is important to avoid persistent and excessive changes in heart rate and systemic blood pressure. A common recommendation is to strive to maintain the patient's heart rate and systemic blood pressure within 20% of the normal awake value. Nevertheless, most episodes of intraoperative myocardial ischemia seen on the ECG occur in the absence of hemodynamic changes. Furthermore, myocardial ischemia and dysfunction is not limited to the diseased vessels and does not correlate with the severity and distribution of CAD, suggesting that it is unlikely that this form of myocardial ischemia will be predictably preventable by the anesthesiologist. Vigilance, early detection, and treatment of myocardial dysfunction are of utmost importance.

No study to date has clearly demonstrated a difference in outcomes with advanced monitoring techniques. Right heart catheterization, which was in vogue 10 years ago, has not been shown to improve outcomes in large randomized studies. Intraoperative TEE may be considered in patients who develop significant and prolonged ST changes or who demonstrate sustained severe hemodynamic disturbances. The impact of noninvasive cardiac output monitors is yet to be defined in the elderly population.

Likewise, no definite recommendations can be made for transfusion triggers and fluid management for elderly patients undergoing vascular surgery. Due to advanced atherosclerosis, stiff ventricles, diastolic dysfunction, and occult coronary artery disease, elderly patients do not tolerate hypovolemia or hypervolemia. Hypovolemia leads to severe hypotension and organ hypoperfusion while over hydration can lead to congestive heart failure. Even in younger patients, liberal hydration is no longer considered innocuous and is associated with poor postoperative outcomes. Higher hemoglobin and hematocrit values may be more desirable in the elderly patients. It is appropriate to keep hematocrit levels above 22 and preferably around 27 mg/dl in the elderly.

Postoperative care of the elderly vascular patient is also governed by the same goals as intraoperative care. Presence of comorbidities and intraoperative course

Table 16.4 Guidelines for perioperative use of statins and alpha-2 agonists: American Heart Association (AHA) vs. European Society of Cardiology (ESC) recommendations

Recommendation class	AHA (2009)	ESC (2009)
Statins		
Class I	For patients currently taking statins and scheduled for noncardiac surgery, statins should be continued	It is recommended that statins be started in high-risk surgery patients, optimally between 30 days and at least 1 week before surgery It is recommended that statins be continued perioperatively
Class IIa	For patients undergoing vascular surgery with or without clinical risk factors, statin use is reasonable.	
Class IIb	For patients with at least one clinical risk factor who are undergoing intermediate-risk procedures, statins may be considered	
Alpha-2 agonists		
Class IIb	Alpha-2 agonists for perioperative control of hypertension may be considered for patients with known CAD or at least one clinical risk factor who are undergoing surgery	Alpha-2 receptor agonists may be considered to reduce the risk of perioperative cardiovascular complications in vascular surgery patients
Class III	Alpha-2 agonists should not be given to patients undergoing surgery who have contraindications to this medication	

determine the intensity of postoperative monitoring. It is not uncommon to expect elderly patients to be transferred to the intensive care unit on mechanical ventilation after open AAA. However, after an uncomplicated EVAR, it is very likely that the patient will be extubated in the operating room and discharged to a regular floor. For sedation in the critical units, dexmedetomidine may be a better drug than benzodiazepines, as it is associated with less delirium early recovery.

Summary

A large proportion of patients who undergo vascular surgery are elderly, with significant comorbidities. The risk of adverse events, especially cardiac events, is particularly increased in this patient population. Perioperative management of elderly patients scheduled for vascular surgery is geared towards clinical risk assessment based on AHA and ESC guidelines. Preoperative coronary revascularization prior to vascular surgery has not been shown to improve outcomes. Advanced monitoring techniques and intensive care may be required perioperatively to manage patient with severe comorbidities. Medical management of the patients with aspirin, beta-blockers, ACE inhibitors, statins, and glycemic control in the perioperative period are important interventions for improving outcomes.

Key Points

- Peripheral arterial disease (PAD) affects 12–20% of Americans >65 years of age and the prevalence of PAD increases dramatically with age.
- Vascular disease is divided into three distinct categories: cerebrovascular disease (CVD) involving the carotid and intracranial vasculature, coronary artery disease (CAD) involving the vasculature of the heart, or peripheral vascular disease (PAD) involving aorta and its branches.
- Vascular surgery carries a significant risk of perioperative mortality [>5%]. Open aortic surgery and lower extremity bypass surgery are associated with highest risk of perioperative morbidity and mortality.
- Short-term morbidity and mortality is lower for endovascular aortic aneurysm repair compared to open surgery and is the preferred option for patients over 80 years; however, long-term mortality is not much different from open aortic aneurysm repair.
- The most commonly used and recommended index is the revised cardiac risk index (RCRI). It is based on six factors: (1) history of ischemic heart disease, (2) congestive heart failure, (3) diabetes, (4) cerebrovascular disease, (5) renal insufficiency, and (6) supra-inguinal aortic surgery.
- Prolonged hypotension has been observed in patients who have chronically been treated with ACE inhibitors following the induction of general anesthesia.
- Perioperative beta-blockers should be continued in patients who are already on beta-blockers. Patients undergoing vascular surgery who have multiple risk factors or have reversible ischemia on preoperative testing may benefit from perioperative beta-blockers.
- Patients with vascular disease should receive statin therapy for secondary prevention of a cardiac event, independent of noncardiac surgery.
- Discontinuation of statins in the perioperative period may cause a rebound effect and may be harmful.

Suggested Reading

Akhtar S, Barash PG, Inzucchi SE. Scientific Principles and Clinical Implications of Perioperative Glucose Regulation and Control. Anesthesia & Analgesia. 2010.

Amato B, Markabaoui AK, Piscitelli V, Mastrobuoni G, Persico F, Iuliano G, Masone S, Persico G. Carotid endarterectomy under local anesthesia in elderly: is it worthwhile? Acta Biomed. 2005; 76 Suppl 1: 64–8.

Ballotta E, Da Giau G, Ermani M, Meneghetti G, Saladini M, Manara R, Baracchini C: Early and long-term outcomes of carotid endarterectomy in the very elderly: an 18-year single-center study. J Vasc Surg. 2009; 50: 518–25.

Barbosa FT, Cavalcante JC, Juca MJ, Castro AA. Neuraxial anaesthesia for lower-limb revascularization. Cochrane Database Syst Rev. 2010: CD007083.

Biccard BM, Rodseth RN. A meta-analysis of the prospective randomised trials of coronary revascularisation before noncardiac vascular surgery with attention to the type of coronary revascularisation performed. Anaesthesia. 2009; 64: 1105–13.

Bodenham AR, Howell SJ. General anaesthesia vs local anaesthesia: an ongoing story. Br J Anaesth. 2009; 103: 785–9.

Bundgaard-Nielsen M, Secher NH, Kehlet H. 'Liberal' vs. 'restrictive' perioperative fluid therapy--a critical assessment of the evidence. Acta Anaesthesiol Scand. 2009; 53: 843–51.

Fleisher LA, Beckman JA, Brown KA, Calkins H, Chaikof EL, Fleischmann KE, Freeman WK, Froehlich JB, Kasper EK, Kersten JR, Riegel B, Robb JF. 2009 ACCF/AHA focused update on perioperative beta blockade incorporated into the ACC/AHA 2007 guidelines on perioperative cardiovascular evaluation and care for noncardiac surgery: a report of the American college of cardiology foundation/American heart association task force on practice guidelines. Circulation. 2009; 120: e169–276.

Flu WJ, van Kuijk JP, Hoeks SE, Kuiper R, Schouten O, Goei D, Elhendy A, Verhagen HJ, Thomson IR, Bax JJ, Fleisher LA, Poldermans D. Prognostic implications of asymptomatic left ventricular dysfunction in patients undergoing vascular surgery. Anesthesiology. 2010; 112: 1316–24.

Galal W, Hoeks SE, Flu WJ, van Kuijk JP, Goei D, Galema T, den Uil C, van Gestel YR, Bax JJ, Verhagen HJ, Poldermans D. Relation between preoperative and intraoperative new wall motion abnormalities in vascular surgery patients: a transesophageal echocardiographic study. Anesthesiology. 2010; 112: 557–66.

Jim J, Sanchez LA. Abdominal aortic aneurysms: endovascular repair. Mt Sinai J Med. 2010; 77: 238–49.

Kang JL, Chung TK, Lancaster RT, Lamuraglia GM, Conrad MF, Cambria RP. Outcomes after carotid endarterectomy: is there a high-risk population? A National Surgical Quality Improvement Program report. J Vasc Surg. 2009; 49: 331-8, 339 e1; discussion 338-9.

Karkos CD, Harkin DW, Giannakou A, Gerassimidis TS. Mortality after endovascular repair of ruptured abdominal aortic aneurysms: a systematic review and meta-analysis. Arch Surg. 2009; 144: 770–8.

Lange C, Leurs LJ, Buth J, Myhre HO. Endovascular repair of abdominal aortic aneurysm in octogenarians: an analysis based on EUROSTAR data. J Vasc Surg. 2005; 42: 624-30; discussion 630.

Makary MA, Segev DL, Pronovost PJ, Syin D, Bandeen-Roche K, Patel P, Takenaga R, Devgan L, Holzmueller CG, Tian J, Fried LP. Frailty as a predictor of surgical outcomes in older patients. J Am Coll Surg. 2010; 210: 901–8.

Mayer D, Pfammatter T, Rancic Z, Hechelhammer L, Wilhelm M, Veith FJ, Lachat M. 10 years of emergency endovascular aneurysm repair for ruptured abdominal aortoiliac aneurysms: lessons learned. Ann Surg. 2009; 249: 510-5.

McArdle GT, McAuley DF, McKinley A, Blair P, Hoper M, Harkin DW. Preliminary results of a prospective randomized trial of restrictive versus standard fluid regime in elective open abdominal aortic aneurysm repair. Ann Surg. 2009; 250: 28–34.

Noordzij PG, Poldermans D, Schouten O, Bax JJ, Schreiner FA, Boersma E. Postoperative mortality in The Netherlands: a population-based analysis of surgery-specific risk in adults. Anesthesiology. 2010; 112: 1105–15.

Poldermans D, Bax JJ, Boersma E, De Hert S, Eeckhout E, Fowkes G, Gorenek B, Hennerici MG, Iung B, Kelm M, Kjeldsen KP, Kristensen SD, Lopez-Sendon J, Pelosi P, Philippe F, Pierard L, Ponikowski P, Schmid JP, Sellevold OF, Sicari R, Van den Berghe G, Vermassen F, Hoeks SE, Vanhorebeek I. Guidelines for pre-operative cardiac risk assessment and perioperative cardiac management in non-cardiac surgery: the Task Force for Preoperative Cardiac Risk Assessment and Perioperative Cardiac Management in Non-cardiac Surgery of the European Society of

Cardiology (ESC) and endorsed by the European Society of Anaesthesiology (ESA). Eur Heart J. 2009; 30: 2769–812.

Schouten O, Boersma E, Hoeks SE, Benner R, van Urk H, van Sambeek MR, Verhagen HJ, Khan NA, Dunkelgrun M, Bax JJ, Poldermans D, Dutch Echocardiographic Cardiac Risk Evaluation Applying Stress Echocardiography Study G. Fluvastatin and perioperative events in patients undergoing vascular surgery. N Engl J Med. 2009; 361: 980–9.

Trivedi RA, Weerakkody RA, Turner C, Kirkpatrick PJ. Carotid artery stenosis-an evidence-based review of surgical and non-surgical treatments. Br J Neurosurg. 2009; 23: 387–92.

Schermerhorn ML, O'Malley AJ, Jhaveri A, Cotterill P, Pomposelli F, Landon BE. Endovascular vs. open repair of abdominal aortic aneurysms in the Medicare population. N Engl J Med. 2008; 358: 464–74.

Chapter 17
Spine Surgery: Choosing the Patient and Handling the Surgery

Stacie Deiner

Background

Neck and back pain is one of our society's most common medical problems. According to the National Institute of Arthritis, Musculoskeletal, and Skin Diseases, about one-fourth of U.S. adults experience at least 1 day of back pain in a 3-month period. The first episode of low back pain typically occurs between the ages of 30 and 40 and becomes more common with age. As the number of elderly persons in the United States increases, so will the number of symptomatic age-related degenerative disorders of the spine. Back pain is a symptom of a medical condition, not a diagnosis itself. Common causes of back pain include mechanical problems such as degenerative disc, injuries, acquired conditions and diseases, and infections and tumors.

Initially, most spine practitioners utilize conservative modalities for patients suffering from degenerative disorders of the spine, in the absence of neurologic deficits and intractable pain. Conservative therapies include over-the-counter analgesics, anti-inflammatory medication like nonsteroidal anti-inflammatory drugs and oral steroids, muscle relaxants, physical therapy, exercise, and steroid injections. When conservative treatment fails or when neurologic deficits or cancer is present, surgery is often indicated. Osteoporotic compression fractures, which used to be repaired with extensive instrumentation and fusions can now often be fixed with minimally invasive techniques like kyphoplasty and vertebroplasty, resulting in a reduction in morbidity. Despite increases in noninvasive modalities, the mainstay of most spinal therapies remains traditional surgery. While spinal surgery in the general population comes with many risks, the geriatric population has many unique concerns such as chronic medical problems, polypharmacy, and limited cognitive

S. Deiner, MD (✉)
Department of Anesthesiology, Mount Sinai School of Medicine,
1 Gustave L. Levy Place, New York, NY 10029, USA
e-mail: Stacie.Deiner@mountsinai.org

S.R. Barnett (ed.), *Manual of Geriatric Anesthesia*, DOI 10.1007/978-1-4614-3888-5_17,

reserve. All of these factors may contribute to a decreased quality of life and an ability to live independently after major spine surgery.

In this chapter we will discuss the most common types of spine pathology affecting geriatric surgical patients, the surgical options available, and the evidence for their efficacy and safety. We will also discuss the anesthetic management of geriatric patients undergoing spine surgery that include preoperative evaluation of medical issues and polypharmacy, consideration of acute-on-chronic pain management for the elderly, and cognitive outcomes. Intraoperative anesthetic management of the geriatric spine patient also includes awareness of the potential for occult cervical spine pathology, such as unrecognized cervical stenosis and myelopathy that can complicate airway management, complications of prone positioning, issues related to neuromonitoring, and the pharmacokinetics and pharmacodynamics of total intravenous anesthesia (TIVA). During the postoperative period, the surgical and anesthesia team must remain vigilant for common postoperative medical problems seen in geriatric spine patients and recognize the potential for short- and long-term cognitive dysfunction.

Geriatric Spine Pathology

There are several categories of spinal pathology common to geriatric patients. The most common conditions include cervical stenosis causing myelopathy or radiculopathy, lumbar stenosis, lumbar spondylolisthesis, degenerative thoracolumbar scoliosis, osteoporotic burst/compression fractures, and spinal metastases.

Spondylolisthesis is any displacement of the cephalad vertebral body on the caudal vertebral body. The most common type of spondylolisthesis seen in the geriatric population is degenerative spondylolisthesis, which is due to osteoarthritis of the facet joints and disc degeneration. This occurs most often at the L4–L5 vertebrae and is usually accompanied by central spinal stenosis at the same vertebral level (see Fig. 17.1). Spondylolisthesis can also occur as a result of trauma or surgery (iatrogenic), spondylolysis (isthmic), tumor (pathologic), or may be congenital. The most widely accepted theory on its etiopathogenesis is that as the disc degenerates there is micromotion at the disc space level that evolves to macromotion, visible on imaging studies. The spinal structures around the degenerative and mobile segment often hypertrophy in response to this abnormal segmental motion, leading to spinal stenosis. Patients often complain of back pain, radiculopathy, and neurogenic claudication; however, neurologic deficits are uncommon in this population of patients. As mentioned previously, this subtype of spondylolisthesis is also associated with tandem stenosis (concomitant cervical stenosis) and should alert the practitioner to inquire about neck and arm symptoms, in addition to examining patient for spinal cord related problems, such as myelopathy.

Spinal stenosis is a narrowing of the spinal canal and a common cause of back and radicular pain in the geriatric population. Spinal stenosis can be congenital or acquired; factors that lead to acquired stenosis include degenerative conditions of

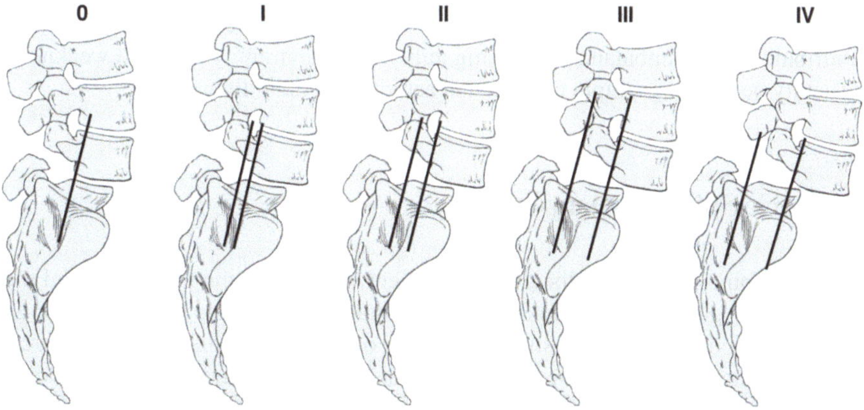

Fig. 17.1 Spondylolisthesis. Permission pending from Borenstein. Low Back Pain: Medical Diagnosis and Comprehensive Management. 1989

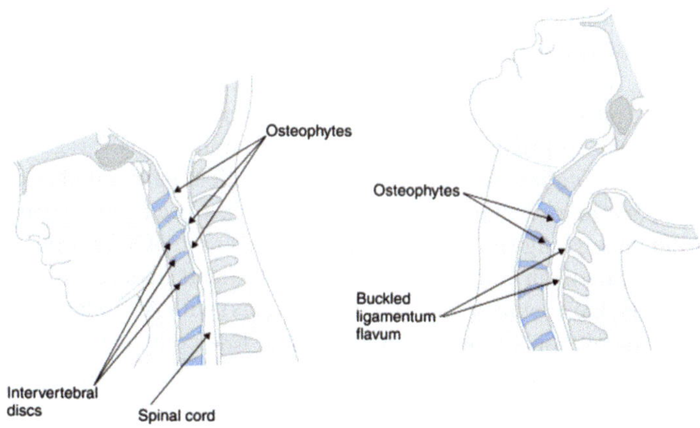

Fig. 17.2 Cervical stenosis (This article was published in Essentials of Physical Medicine and Rehabilitation. 2nd Ed, Frontera, Chapter 6, 6-1, Copyright Elsevier 2008)

the spine (e.g., spondylosis, degenerative disc disease), trauma, surgery (e.g., postlaminectomy), and metabolic or endocrine abnormalities (e.g., osteoporosis, hypoparathyroidism). Stenosis occurs most often in the cervical and lumbar regions and results from degeneration and bulging of the intervertebral disc anteriorly, with hypertrophy of the facet joints and ligamentum flavum posteriorly (see Fig. 17.2).

Although many of these degenerative changes occur normally with aging, in some instances may lead to a significant compression of the dural sac and nerve roots. When spinal stenosis affects the cervical canal it often leads to spinal cord compression with myelopathic and radicular features. In many patients, cervical and lumbar stenosis can co-exist, aptly named "tandem stenosis." Symptomatic cervical stenosis has been estimated to occur in 5% of patients with symptomatic degenerative spondylolisthesis. Lastly, cervical stenosis is often overlooked as a contributor to gait imbalance, easy fatigability, lower extremity pain and weakness, difficulty performing simple coordinated activities of daily living.

Geriatric Spine Surgery—Safety

Safety of spine surgery for the geriatric patient varies with the individual and the procedure. In general, spinal fusion, instrumentation, harvesting of autograft (e.g., iliac crest harvest), and increasing the number of involved spinal levels are associated with longer surgery, greater blood loss, and more postoperative pain. However quantification of outcomes has proved to be difficult. Although several studies have been published looking at the safety of spine surgery in older adults, the literature suffers from a lack of uniformity of basic definitions, including the definition of geriatric and what constitutes a complication. Complications are frequently defined as either minor or major; minor complications usually describe conditions that may recorded in patient's chart but do not affect long-term recovery (e.g., urinary retention), where as major complications describe conditions that affected recovery (e.g., pneumonia, new-onset atrial fibrillation). These definitions are broad, and it is not surprising the overall rate of complications varies from 2.5 to 80%. In general, more invasive surgeries in older patient have a higher complication rate. A 35% rate of major complications for has been reported in patients >85 years old undergoing spinal fusion, with an odds ratio of 9.2 for postoperative medical complications in comparison to younger patients undergoing similar surgery. Conversely, the "younger old" (age 65–75 years) with ASA status I–II having a simple decompression for spinal stenosis have low complication rates. There have been similar trends noted for lumbar stenosis and cervical myelopathy patients.

Few of the current studies take into account longer term outcomes. Poor bone quality predisposes older patients to vertebral fractures progression of spinal deformity after a spinal procedure. Thus, older patients often require more aggressive surgeries to prevent further injury, thereby exposing them to additional surgical risks and potentially repeat procedures.

Geriatric Spine Surgery Efficacy

There is considerable controversy regarding the benefits of surgery compared to conservative treatment for back pain and injures in the geriatric patient. The ongoing Spine Patient Outcomes Research Trial (SPORT) is a large, randomized multicenter trial which has examined conservative versus surgical therapy for lumbar herniated discs, spondylothesis, and spinal stenosis. This study found that for a mixed age group, surgical treatment was associated with better outcomes and patient satisfaction up to 2 years after surgery. This trial did not look specifically at geriatric patients and confounding factors include a high incidence of crossover from the conservative therapy to the surgical therapy group during the study period.

In general the quality of literature for geriatric-specific clinical outcomes for lumbar spine surgery is poor. Limitations include small sample sizes, frequent case series with sample sizes <100 patients, and a lack of appropriate control groups or standardized outcome measures. Studies reporting good or excellent outcomes in elderly patients range between 53 and 93%, varying with length of follow-up, patient population, surgical indication, and procedure.

Traditionally, the addition of fusion to decompression (arthrodesis) had been thought to be associated with better results for stenosis accompanied by spondylolisthesis. However this has been questioned and at least two studies suggest that fusion and decompression do not confer additional benefits in comparison to decompression alone.

With respect to long-term outcomes, little information is available regarding fusion rates in elderly patients. In one study of patients 70 years and above undergoing posterior lumbar interbody fusion, radiographic evaluation performed using CT found that the patients had higher rates of collapsed union and delayed union than younger patients. Additionally, a study of the effects of age on surgical outcomes for adult idiopathic scoliosis found that although pain relief was more consistently obtained in the older population, radiographic results were inferior when comparing the older population to their younger counterparts. This suggests good outcomes in geriatric patients undergoing fusion may not persist in the long term. However, the spine surgery literature has not shown a complete correlation with fusion and outcome; many spine surgery patients who are not fused often remain asymptomatic. A more recent study of patients treated with laminectomy and fusion for spondylolisthesis revealed that patients who were fused had better outcomes than those who were not fused; however, it took over 10 years to see this benefit as the differences were negligible early on. It is important to note that both of these groups were superior to laminectomy alone.

Preoperative Evaluation of the Geriatric Patient for Spine Surgery

Perhaps the most important consideration guiding appropriate preoperative evaluation of the geriatric patient for spine surgery is an understanding of the invasiveness of the surgical procedure. As discussed in the previous section, there are a wide range of surgical procedures performed on patients with neck and back pain. These procedures can vary in terms of operative time and estimated blood loss. Once the anesthesiologist understands the nature of the planned procedure, preoperative evaluation can be focused on patient risk factors. We will examine these in a geriatric specific systems focused manner.

Polypharmacy

Data from recent surveys reveal that more than 90% of people older than 65 years of age use at least one drug per week, 40% take five or more drugs, and 12–19% use ten or more medications. Polypharmacy is particularly relevant for patients undergoing spinal surgery as these patients frequently have chronic pain and may have attempted conservative treatment prior to choosing surgery which can include numerous medications. Acute-on-chronic pain complicates matters further in these vulnerable patients. It is important for the anesthesiologist to be aware of the patient's pain issues preoperatively especially the use of narcotic and multimodal pain medications, additionally, the patient should be informed which medications should be taken the morning of surgery. Ideally, the anesthesiologist will work with the patient's pain management physicians or anticipate difficult cases and consult pain medicine appropriately. With this information, the anesthesiologist can counsel the patient and family about what to expect in the postoperative period.

Cardiac Evaluation

The 2007 ACC/AHA guidelines have streamlined the process of cardiac evaluation of the patient for noncardiac surgery (see Fig. 17.3). Most geriatric spine surgery patients are in the intermediate risk procedure category for nonemergency surgery and will not require extensive cardiac evaluations (see Table 17.1). For patients with limited exercise tolerance, due most often to pain from their neck or back, the need for further evaluation will depend on the likelihood that any findings on cardiac testing will change management. After obtaining a full history, the anesthesiologist can use ACC/AHA guidelines to determine whether further evaluation is likely to be warranted, and then have a discussion with the patient, surgeon, and primary care doctor/cardiologist. Patients who have had cardiac stents placed present a particular challenge. It is important to ascertain when the stents were placed, what type of stents were used, and the location of the stents. The patient's cardiologist should be involved in the preoperative planning process to provide this information, including any recent studies documenting whether there is any residual myocardium at risk. If the need for spine surgery is anticipated in a patient who has a stent, a collaborative discussion should take place between the patient, surgeon, and cardiologist to determine appropriate timing and type of intervention. Patients who have had drug eluting stents placed <1 year prior to their procedure are not candidates for elective surgery because of the risk of thrombosis from the discontinuation of antiplatelet agents in the perioperative period (see Fig. 17.4). The management of antiplatelet drugs in the perioperative period can be extremely complex. In general it is recommended that based on current recommendations clopidogrel should be discontinued a minimum of 7 days and ticlopidine 14 days prior to

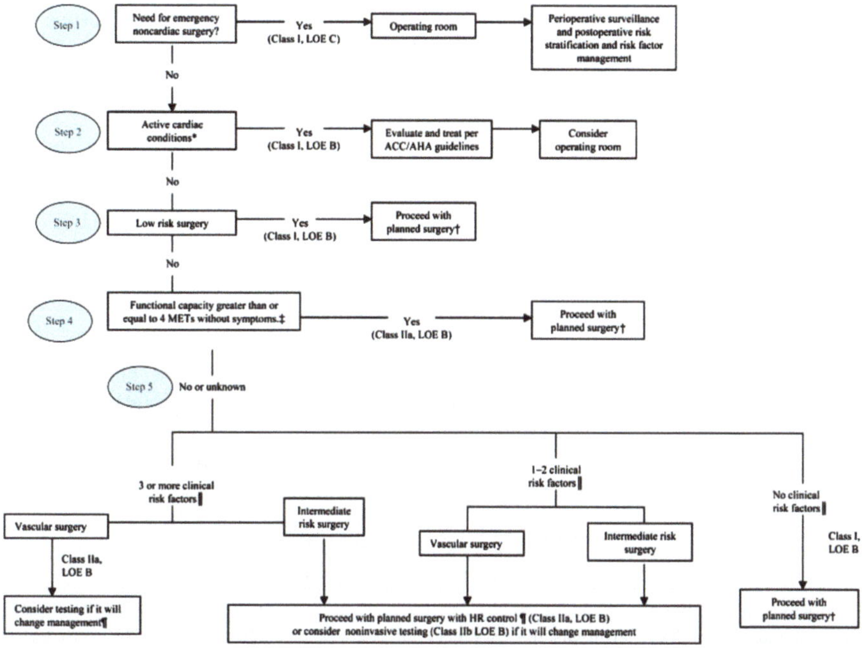

Fig. 17.3 ACC/AHA Algorithm for Perioperative Evaluation of the Patient for Noncardiac Surgery, from 2009 ACCF/AHA Focused Update on Perioperative Beta Blockade Incorporated Into the ACC/AHA 2007 Guidelines on Perioperative Cardiovascular Evaluation and Care for Noncardiac Surgery: A Report of the American College of Cardiology Foundation/American Heart Association Task Force on Practice Guidelines (Reprinted with Permission, Circulation.2009;120:e169–e276. ©2009 American Heart Association, Inc.)

surgery. However, since there is a large variation in response to clopidogrel, it is possible to use point-of-care testing of platelet function to discontinue agents for shorter periods of time. Unfortunately, due to the risk of epidural hematoma, most spine surgeons are wary to continue aspirin in the perioperative period, and many surgeons will not allow antiplatelet agents to be restarted for as long as 4 weeks postsurgery.

Airway/Respiratory Considerations

Managing the airway of geriatric patients undergoing spine surgery may be extremely challenging. These patients can have extensive arthritis beyond the surgical site and may manifest end stage effects of systemic diseases such as rheumatoid arthritis. The geriatric patient with cervical spine instability can represent the most challenging airway cases encountered. Fortunately the explosion in the airway

Table 17.1 Active cardiac conditions for which the patient should undergo evaluation and treatment before noncardiac surgery (Class I, Level of Evidence: B)

Condition	Examples
Unstable coronary syndromes	Unstable or severe angina[a] (CCS class III or IV)[b] Recent MI[c]
Decompensated HF (NYHA functional class IV; worsening or new-onset HF)	
Significant arrhythmias	High-grade atrioventricular block Mobitz II atrioventricular block Third-degree atrioventricular heart block Symptomatic ventricular arrhythmias Supraventricular arrhythmias (including atrial fibrillation) with uncontrolled ventricular rate (HR >100 bpm at rest) Symptomatic bradycardia Newly recognized ventricular tachycardia
Severe valvular disease	Severe aortic stenosis (mean pressure gradient >40 mm Hg, aortic valve area <1.0 cm^2, or symptomatic) Symptomatic mitral stenosis (progressive dyspnea on exertion, exertional presyncope, or HF)

Reprinted with Permission, Circulation 2009;120:e169–e276. ©2009 American Heart Association, Inc.
CCS indicates Canadian Cardiovascular Society; *HF* heart failure, *HR* heart rate, *MI* myocardial infarction, and *NYHA* New York Heart Association

[a]According to Campeau

[b]May include "stable" angina in patients who are unusually sedentary

[c]The American College of Cardiology National Database Library defines recent MI as >7 days but less than or equal to 1 month (within 30 days)

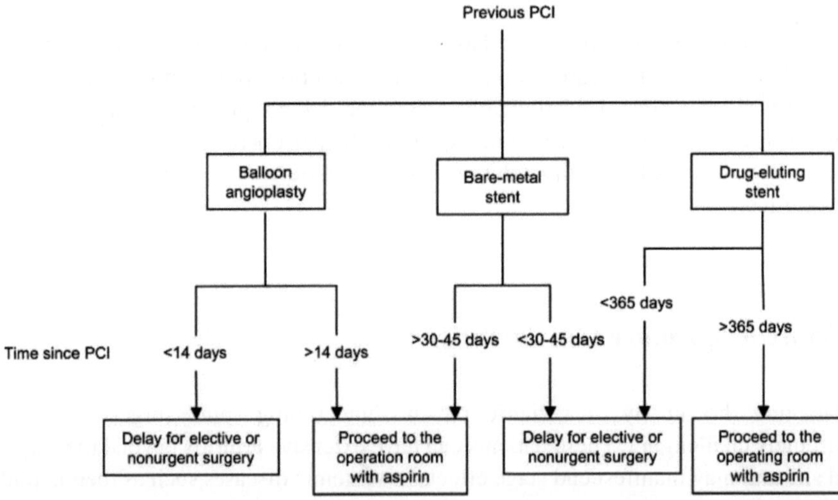

Fig. 17.4 AHA/ACC: Perioperative management of the patient with previous percutaneous cardiac intervention (PCI) (Reprinted with Permission, Circulation.2009;120:e169–e276. ©2009 American Heart Association, Inc.)

device industry has given anesthesia and emergency care practitioners a multitude of options for managing the patient with a pathologic or unstable cervical spine. Many of the new devices are extremely user friendly and are able to produce better laryngoscopic grade views in immobilized patients. However, the practitioner must understand how they perform with respect to efficacy and cervical motion. Because there is no evidence that a brief and successful laryngoscopy has resulted in quadriplegia, it is clear that patients with respiratory insufficiency should be ventilated and intubated. With knowledge of the patient's injury, clinical scenario and device capabilities, one can select the best technique.

Depending on the level of the surgery and planned the invasiveness of the surgery, patient risk varies with procedure and preexisting comorbidity. For example a single level laminectomy may involve only a 2 cm incision with minimal blood loss. In contrast a thoracic level spinal decompression can involve the lateral approach necessitating a thoracotomy and the opportunity for substantial blood loss. In the latter case, the anesthesiologist must be ready to perform one lung ventilation and arrange for appropriate preoperative and postoperative care. Postoperative intensive care and ventilation may need to be considered in these more complex and extensive cases.

An appreciation of renal function is especially important in patients undergoing more invasive procedures where large fluid shifts are anticipated and blood replacement is planned. Normal aging leads to a steady decline in baseline renal function and even normal or slightly elevated creatinine levels may signify significant renal dysfunction in an elderly patient with decreased muscle mass. Preoperative urinalysis to exclude UTI and the potential for bacteremia is especially important in patients who will undergo fusion.

Cognitive reserve and its impact on perioperative outcomes in geriatric patients has been an area of controversy. In the short term, geriatric patients undergoing major surgery are at risk for delirium, which is associated with an increased risk of mortality. Persistence of long-term postoperative cognitive decline is more nebulous. However, it is safe to say that in geriatric patients even relatively short periods of cognitive decline are likely to result in the need for discharge to skilled nursing facilities, with the associated financial and psychosocial costs. High-risk patients who have manifested mild cognitive impairment may warrant a preoperative geriatric consult, which is associated with improved outcomes. Delirium intervention programs which have focused on nonpharmacologic strategies (e.g., environmental cues, maintenance of sleep–wake cycles) have had significant success.

Finally, although postoperative blindness is not necessarily a complication specific for elderly spine patients, many elderly spine patients have risk factors for perioperative blindness and should be counseled. These risk factors include a prolonged procedure, the need for significant amounts of blood transfusion, and prolonged prone positioning. Concomitant vasculopathy and smoking history may further increase patients' risk. In high-risk patients, consideration should be given to performing a staged procedure to decrease operative time and blood loss. Staging a lengthy procedure also has the added advantage of reducing the risk for postoperative airway complications.

Intraoperative Considerations

Positioning

The majority of spine surgery is performed with the patient in the prone position. This is not necessarily a dangerous position, and with appropriate support and padding, being prone may actually lead to improved ventilation. However malpositioning in prone position can lead to significant morbidity. Furthermore in osteoporotic older people, the achievement of the prone position especially those with cervical instability can be a vulnerable period and attention should be given to the positioning process itself as well as the end position.

At the start, prior to induction, the patient should be allowed to position themselves comfortably in a supine position. After induction and intubation, it is important to recruit appropriate ancillary help to safely logroll the patient while maintaining in-line stabilization of the neck. There are many commercially available tables and frames, although it is also possible to use improvised bolsters and padding on a standard table to provide a safe position. Equipment and specialized tables will vary across institutions. For example the Jackson table is designed to allow the patient to be induced in the supine position and then secured to the table and rotated to the prone position. In all cases head and neck stability is of paramount importance and can be accomplished in multiple ways, and a few examples include the Mayfield headholder, Gardner-Wells tongs, or a specially molded foam (see Fig. 17.5a–c).

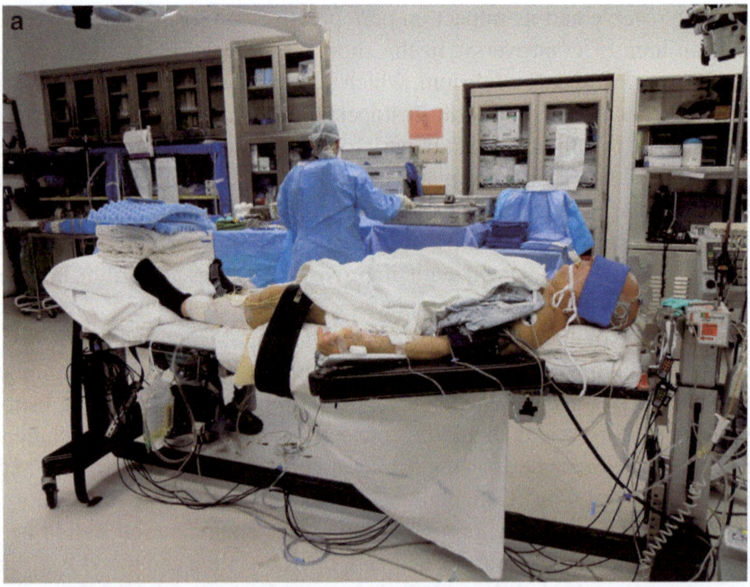

Fig. 17.5 (**a**) Jackson table—patient supine (S. Deiner) (**b**) Jackson table: preparing for prone positioning (S. Deiner) (**c**) Patient positioned in prone (S. Deiner)

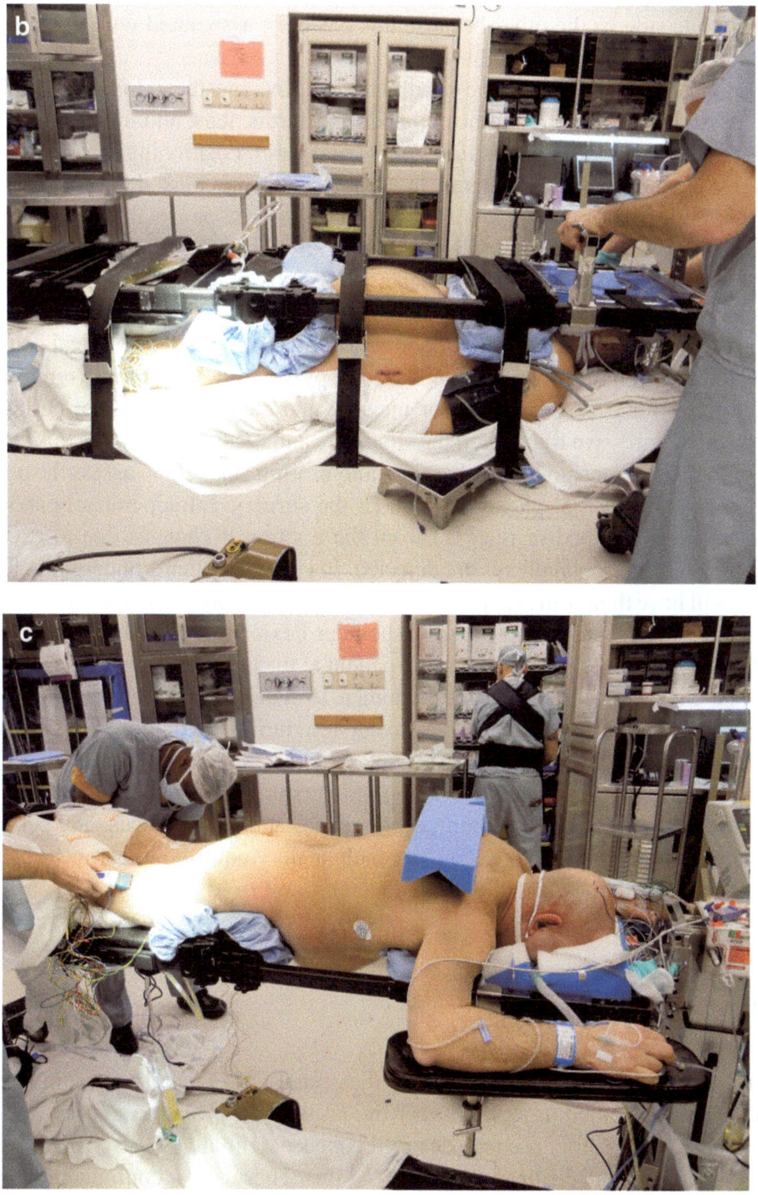

Fig. 17.5 (continued)

Regardless of specific equipment used, the overall goals in prone positioning are the same; the patient's neck should be maintained in a neutral position. Horseshoe head rests have fallen out of favor for prone positioning since they may impinge on the lateral canthus of the eye and this may be associated with postoperative blindness. Similarly the anesthesiologist should avoid positioning the patient with the face turned to one side or the other because this has been associated with postoperative blindness and stroke.

In addition to attending to the head and neck, the anesthesiologist must also be aware of positioning vulnerabilities related to the arms, legs, and torso of the geriatric patient. Next priority is the patients' arms and torso. Positioning an older person's arms can be especially challenging in patients with previous shoulder surgery or trauma. The intraoperative position of the patient's arms is usually dictated by the level of surgery and the need to use intraoperative imaging, either in the form of fluoroscopy (C-arm) or CT guided imaging. Usually, patients undergoing cervical spine surgery will have their arms secured at their sides. Surgeons occasionally tape the shoulders down to improve their ability to visualize the lower cervical spine and upper thoracic spine during routine fluoroscopy or to help contour (remove skin folds) a posterior cervical wound for incision and closure. Care must be taken to avoid overly aggressive traction on the shoulders and brachial plexus, as this can lead to neurologic issues postoperatively. Neuromonitoring can help to assess the position of the neck and brachial plexus throughout the surgery. Intraoperatively shoulders may need to be untaped or released from the traction if changes due to excessive stretching on the brachial plexus are detected. In general, patients undergoing lumbar surgery will have their arms supported by armboards and positioned at 90°. Typically, the shoulder is abducted, with minimal shoulder flexion and 5°–10° of internal rotation. Finally, bolsters should support the patient at the tips of the shoulders and upper chest and iliac crests allowing the abdomen to hang freely. This position favors venous return and adequate diaphragm excursion during ventilation. Legs should be bent at the knees, while the hips should be extended (to recreate lordosis of the lumbar spine) for fusion or flexed to widen the interspinous spaces for decompression procedures without fusion. All bony excrescences and prominences, and peripheral nerve areas subject to compression (e.g., ulnar nerve at elbow, peroneal nerve at fibular head) should be padded with foam.

Monitoring

The use of intraoperative monitoring of the spinal cord (IOM) is becoming more standard during spine surgery. Several modalities are available and can be used alone or in combination: somatosensory evoked potentials (SSEP), motor evoked potentials (MEP), and electromyography (EMG). These allow continual intraoperative assessment of the dorsal columns, anterior spinal cord, and nerve roots, respectively. The contraindications for evoked potential monitoring include implanted pacemaker, functioning implanted defibrillator (although in high-risk cases, the antitacharrythmia function can be disabled, making it possible to monitor evoked potentials), implanted metal in the cranial vault (aneurysm clips, etc.), epilepsy, increased intracranial pressure, and convexity defects of the skull. These are all relative contraindications, and the risk of the surgical procedure must be weighed against the risk of arrhythmia, seizure, or thermal injury.

The anesthesiologist must be aware of which modalities will be chosen, since each has anesthetic implications. SSEPs and MEPs are sensitive to inhalational agents, while MEPs and EMGs are sensitive to paralytic drugs. Although initial studies suggested that <0.5 MAC of inhalational agent still allowed for adequate monitoring of signals, a recent study suggests that this may not be the case for older patients with diabetes and/or hypertension. By establishing the association of clinical predictors and anesthetic technique on the baseline neuromonitoring signals, anesthesiologists can anticipate challenging patients and use this knowledge to choose the most appropriate anesthetic plan.

An anesthetic technique compatible with consistent IOM needs to be established well in advance to obtain monitoring signals. This is important because the transition from the relatively rapid dissipation of inhalational agents to the relatively slower onset of steady state blood levels of drug infusion may take significantly longer than several minutes when not temporally associated with an induction dose. When monitoring difficulties are anticipated, the anesthesiologist should select a combination of agents with a favorable effect profile and start their maintenance infusion around the time of induction. Examples include the addition of ketamine to a propofol infusion and the use of dexmedetomidine to decrease propofol and opioid requirements. If it is necessary to use inhalational agents (e.g., propofol shortage, patient history of adverse reaction, expense of TIVA), then there must be clear communication with the monitoring team. A single gas, either halogenated agent or nitrous oxide should be used. If baseline signals are not available, then a risk–benefit analysis should be discussed with the monitoring team and the surgeon. If the monitoring is compulsory, then the agent may need to be discontinued; if signals do not appear then the surgeon must decide whether to proceed without monitoring. In any case, whichever technique used to attain baseline signals must be continued throughout the case to avoid loss of signals at a critical portion of the procedure. For elderly patients with diabetes and/or hypertension, the increased cost of total intravenous anesthesia may be justified.

Management of TIVA during spine surgery and neuromonitoring for the geriatric patient has several goals, which may be challenging to achieve simultaneously. Often the patient needs to be immobile without the use of paralytic medication, have steady-state anesthesia compatible with neuromonitoring, and maintain adequate blood pressure to avoid blindness, loss of neuromonitoring signals, and perfusion pressure to the vital organs. Rapid awakening after surgery to facilitate a neurologic exam is also extremely important. In geriatric patients, this is complicated by the cardiodepressant effects of propofol and the age and disease altered pharmacokinetics and pharmacodynamics.

Normal aging results in a progressive decrease in muscle mass and an increase in body fat, leading to a decrease in total body water. The reduced volume of distribution for water-soluble drugs can lead to higher plasma concentrations; conversely, an increased volume of distribution for lipid-soluble drugs can lower their plasma concentration. These changes in volume of distribution may affect elimination half-life. If a drug's volume of distribution expands, its elimination half-life will be prolonged unless the rate of clearance is also increased. Additionally, because renal and

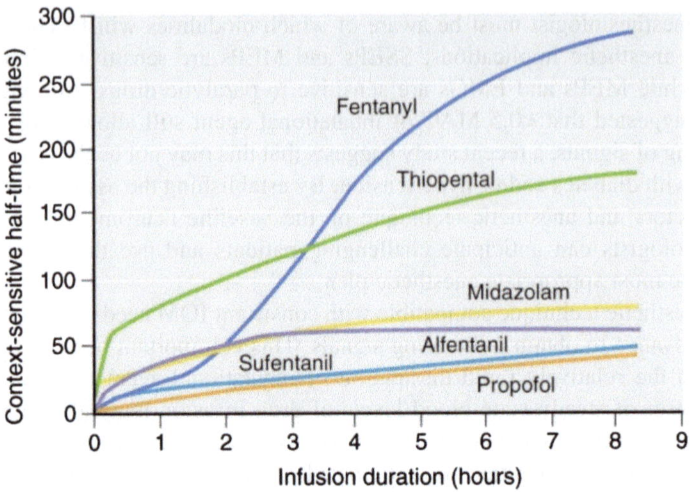

Fig. 17.6 Context sensitive half-life (This article was published in Miller's Anesthesia, 7th edition, Miller RD, Chapter 26, 26-3, Copyright Elsevier 2009.)

hepatic function normally declines with age, reductions in clearance further prolong the duration of action for many drugs. Distribution and elimination are also affected by altered plasma protein binding. Albumin tends to bind acidic drugs (e.g., barbiturates, benzodiazepines, upload agonists); its level typically decreases with age. Indeed, target concentration infusion pumps (TCI) use age as part of their algorithm. However, these pumps are not commonly used in the United States, so the anesthesiologist must use clinical judgment and titrate anesthetic infusions to clinical response throughout the case. The effects of age on drug metabolism may be further compounded by diseases related to renal or liver insufficiency and individual variation.

Processed EEG monitoring may be somewhat helpful to determine appropriate infusions required for amnesia, although not as an index of immobility. Studies have shown that sevoflurane and propofol effect movement to noxious stimuli differently. At an equivalent depression of BIS, sevoflurane suppresses the blink reflex more than propofol, indicating different pharmacodynamic properties of these anesthetics at brainstem level. The differential level of immobility at similar levels of hypnosis makes titration of TIVA during spine surgery, without use of paralytic drugs, somewhat complex.

If the patient is to awaken in a timely fashion at the end of the procedure, it is extremely important that the anesthesiologist is aware of the context sensitive half-life of the drugs they are using to maintain amnesia. Context sensitive half-life is the time for the plasma concentration to decrease by 50% from an infusion that maintains a constant concentration; context refers to the duration of the infusion. Time to 50% decrease in plasma concentration was chosen because a 50% reduction in drug concentration appears to be necessary for recovery after the administration of most intravenous hypnotics (see Fig. 17.6). During long spine surgery, this knowledge must be used to aggressively taper the intravenous anesthetic at the appropriate time, often 40 min prior to surgical finish. Often, during closure of the incision, the neuromonitoring team will stop monitoring and inhalational gas can be added if necessary.

Cardiodepressant effects of commonly used intravenous agents, namely propofol, may be particularly apparent in patients with decreased ejection fraction or certain valvular lesions. The normal increase in myocardial stiffness associated with aging makes geriatric patients somewhat more dependent on preload. Once the anesthesiologist has ascertained that the patient's intravascular volume status and blood volume are adequate, infusions of vasoactive agents may be necessary to ensure adequate perfusion to the vital organs and maintenance of neuromonitoring signals. Indeed, it may be more desirable to use a vasoactive agent and maintain a constant and deep level of anesthesia in a nonparalyzed patient, rather than to risk light anesthesia, movement, or the need to bolus an anesthetic at a critical time in the procedure (e.g., instrumentation).

"Adequate" intraoperative blood pressure during spine surgery may be a somewhat complicated issue. While both the brain and spinal cord are thought to autoregulate blood flow within a physiologic range of mean arterial pressures from 50 to 150 mm Hg, local factors (e.g., spinal stenosis) may contribute to acute or chronic decreases in blood flow. This may cause some individuals be more susceptible to regional ischemia even at "safe" systemic blood pressure. For example, during spinal surgery, the effects of hypotension may be aggravated by spinal distraction such that an acceptable limit of systemic hypotension cannot be determined without neuromonitoring.

Awareness of the patient's renal function and knowledge of the surgical procedure allows judicious titration of fluid. Goals include avoidance of anemia, because of its association with postoperative blindness in prone patients. Anemia can also affect neuromonitoring signals, but generally only below a hematocrit of 20%.

Postoperative Management

Postoperative care of the geriatric spine surgery patient has both similarities and differences when compared to younger spine patients. The choice of appropriate level of postoperative care (i.e., postsurgical floor versus intensive care unit) is heavily influenced by the geriatric patient's preoperative comorbidities and extent of surgery. Factors that have correlated significantly with the presence of postsurgical complications in geriatric postoperative spine patients are preexisting comorbidities, hospital stay, and the number of days in the ICU. Notably, there was no correlation between procedure type, surgery length, or transfusion requirement and inpatient complications. It makes sense that those geriatric patients who are sicker preoperatively may warrant higher levels of postoperative monitoring. Postoperative airway disasters are a particular risk following neck surgery. Multilevel anterior cervical fusion alone is a risk factor for postoperative airway swelling and reintubation; these patients may need to remain intubated or be observed closely in a monitored setting. Prolonged surgery in the prone position, fluid shifts, and multiple transfusions are all factors that may also necessitate a period of postoperative intubation and monitoring.

Conclusion

Care of the geriatric patient presenting for spine surgery has many specific considerations. Choosing the most appropriate procedure, timing, and patient selection may have a significant impact on outcomes. The literature, while still not well defined, can be used to facilitate a risk–benefit discussion with the patient and family prior to surgery. The anesthesiologist must understand the proposed procedure to perform an appropriate preoperative evaluation. Recommendations from the ACC/AHA for cardiac patients undergoing noncardiac surgery have made it clear that the anesthesiologist must collaborate with the surgeon, patient, and medical consultants to minimize patient risk. Airway management may prove challenging in some patients, especially when dealing with patients with limited cervical spine mobility. The anesthesiologist should strive to anticipate difficult airways and have significant knowledge and experience with a wide variety of devices for intubation. Intraoperatively, the geriatric spine patient must be positioned with care to avoid exacerbation of current pathology or creation of additional morbidity. Neuromonitoring has provided additional information in these cases, but has significant implications for anesthetic technique. Age- and disease-related changes to the pharmacokinetics and pharmacodynamics complicate the dosing of TIVA infusions. Maintenance of normotension and anesthetic technique are important for neuromonitoring and patient outcomes, especially with respect to postoperative blindness. Prevention, evaluation, and treatment of postoperative delirium can be accomplished by simple measures like appropriate pain control, but in some complicated cases may require a geriatric consult. With awareness of the specific issues of the geriatric patient undergoing spine surgery, the anesthesiologist can be poised to facilitate the best possible outcomes.

Key Points

- The most common conditions requiring spine surgery are cervical stenosis causing myelopathy or radiculopathy, lumbar stenosis, lumbar spondylolisthesis, degenerative thoracolumbar scoliosis, osteoporotic burst/compression fractures, and spinal metastases.
- *Spondylolisthesis* is any displacement of the cephalad vertebral body on the caudal vertebral body, in the geriatric population this is usually degenerative spondylolisthesis, due to osteoarthritis of the facet joints and disc degeneration.

This occurs most often at the L4–L5 vertebrae frequently accompanied by central spinal stenosis at the same vertebral level.

- Postoperative blindness is a potential complication for all spine patients; however, many elderly spine patients have risk factors that may increase their risk of perioperative blindness. These risk factors include a prolonged procedure, the need for significant amounts of blood transfusion, and prolonged prone positioning. Concomitant vasculopathy and smoking history may further increase patients' risk.
- Intraoperative monitoring of the spinal cord (IOM) can be used alone or in combination: somatosensory evoked potentials (SSEP), motor evoked potentials (MEP), and electromyography (EMG). These allow continual intraoperative assessment of the dorsal columns, anterior spinal cord, and nerve roots, respectively.
- Geriatric patients undergoing spine surgery often have extensive arthritis beyond the surgical site and may manifest end stage effects of systemic diseases such as rheumatoid arthritis resulting in extremely challenging airways.
- Correct positioning of the older patient in the prone position is an important step during spine surgery. Malpositioning can lead to increased morbidity and injury.
- Depending upon the surgery and monitoring TIVA (total intravenous anesthetic techniques) may offer significant advantages for the frail older patient.

Suggested Reading

American College of Cardiology Foundation/American Heart Association Task Force on Practice Guidelines; American Society of Echocardiography; American Society of Nuclear Cardiology; Heart Rhythm Society; Society of Cardiovascular Anesthesiologists; Society for Cardiovascular Angiography and Interventions; Society for Vascular Medicine; Society for Vascular Surgery, Fleischmann KE, Beckman JA, Buller CE, et al. 2009 ACCF/AHA focused update on perioperative beta blockade. J Am Coll Cardiol. 2009;54:e13-e118.

Back Pain. http://www.niams.nih.gov/Health_Info/Back_Pain/default.asp. Accessed March 28, 2010.

Barnett, SR. Polypharmacy and perioperative medications in the elderly. Anesthesiol Clin. 2009;27:377–389.

Cloyd JM, Acosta FL, Ames CP. Complications and outcomes of lumbar spine surgery in elderly people: a review of the literature. J Am Geriatr Soc. 2008;56:1318–1327.

Crosby ET. Airway management in adults after cervical spine trauma. Anesthesiology. 2006; 104:1293–318.

Deiner S, Kwatra S, Lin, Hung-Mo, Weisz, D. Patient characteristics and anesthetic technique are additive but not synergistic predictors of successful motor evoked potential monitoring. Anesth Analg (in press).

Deiner S, Silverstein JH. Postoperative delirium and cognitive dysfunction. Br J Anaesth. 2009; 103:i41–i46.

Deyo RA, Nachemson A, Mirza SK. Spinal fusion surgery- the case for restraint. N Engl J Med. 2004 Feb 12;350(7):722–6.

Epstein NE, Hollingsworth R, Nardi D, et al. Can airway complications following multilevel anterior cervical surgery be avoided? J Neurosurg. 2001;94:185–8.

Fine PG. Chronic pain management in older adults: special considerations. J Pain Symptom Manage. 2009;38:s4–s14.
Fredman B, Arinzon Z, Zohar E, et al. Observations on the safety and efficacy of surgical decompression for lumbar spinal stenosis in geriatric patients. Eur Spine J. 2002;11:571–574.
Glass PS, Shafer SL, Reves JG. Intravenous Drug Delivery Systems. In: Miller RD. Miller's Anesthesia. 7th ed. Philadelphia, PA: Elsevier Churchill Livingstone;2009.
Herkowitz HN, Kurz LT. Degenerative lumbar spondylolisthesis with spinal stenosis. A prospective study comparing decompression with decompression and intertransverse process arthrodesis. J Bone Joint Surg Am. 1991;73:802–8.
Hughes MA, Glass PS, Jacobs JR. Context-sensitive half-time in multicompartment pharmacokinetic models for intravenous anesthetic drugs. Anesthesiology. 1992;76:334–341.
Husebo BS, Strand LI, Moe-Nilssen R, et al. Who suffers most? dementia and pain in nursing home patients: a cross-sectional study. J Am Med Dir Assoc. 2008;9:427–433.
Kornblum MD, Fischgrund JS, Herkowitz HN et al. Degenerative lumbar spondylolisthesis with spinal stenosis: a prospective long-term study comparing fusion and pseudoarthrosis. Spine. 2004;29(7):726–33; discussion 733–4.
Okuda S, Oda T, Miyauchi A, et al. Surgical outcomes of posterior lumbar interbody fusion in elderly patients. J Bone Joint Surg Am. 2006;88:2714–2720.
MacDonald DB. Intraoperative motor evoked potential monitoring, overview and update. J Clin Monit Comput. 2006;20:347–77.
Marcantonio ER, Flacker JM, Wright RJ, et al. Reducing delirium after hip fracture: a randomized trial. J Am Geriatr Soc. 2001;49:516–522.
Mourisse J, Lerou J, Struys M, et al. Multi-level approach to anaesthetic effects produced by sevoflurane or propofol in humans: 1. BIS and blink reflex. Br J Anaesth 2007;98:737–745.
Mourisse J, Lerou J, Struys M, et al. Multi-level approach to anaesthetic effects produced by sevoflurane or propofol in humans: 2. BIS and tetanic stimulus induced withdrawal reflex. Br J Anaesth. 2007;98:746–755.
Practice advisory for perioperative visual loss associated with spine surgery: a report by the American Society of Anesthesiologists Task Force on Perioperative Blindness. Anesthesiology. 2006;104:1319–28.
Raffo CS, Lauerman WC. Predicting morbidity and mortality of lumbar spine arthrodesis in patients in their ninth decade. Spine. 2006;31:99–103.
Ragab AA, Fye MA, Bohlman HH. Surgery of the lumbar spine for spinal stenosis in 118 patients 70 years of age or older. Spine. 2003;28:348–353.
Razack N, Greenberg J, Green BA. Surgery for cervical myelopathy in geriatric patients. Spinal Cord. 1998;36:629–632.
Sadean MR, Glass PS. Pharmacokinetic–pharmacodynamic modeling in anesthesia, intensive care and pain medicine. Curr Opin Anaesthesiol. 2009;22:463–468.
Shore-Lesserson L. Evidence based coagulation monitors: heparin monitoring, thromboelastography, and platelet function. Semin Cardiothorac Vasc Anesth. 2005;9:41–52.
Sieber FE, Pauldine R. Geriatric Anesthesia. In: Miller RD. Miller's Anesthesia. 7th ed. Philadelphia, PA: Elsevier Churchill Livingstone; 2009.
Sloan TB, Heyer EJ. Anesthesia for intraoperative neurophysiologic monitoring of the spinal cord. J Clin Neurophys. 2002;19:430–443.
Weinstein JN, Tosteson TD, Lurie JD, et al. Surgical versus nonsurgical therapy for lumbar spinal stenosis. N Engl J Med. 2008;358:794–810.
Weinstein JN, Lurie JD, Tosteson TD, et al. Surgical versus nonsurgical treatment for lumbar degenerative spondylolisthesis. N Engl J Med. 2007;356:2257–2270.
Weinstein JN, Tosteson TD, Lurie JD, et al. Surgery vs. nonoperative treatment for lumbar disk herniation: the Spine Patient Outcomes Research Trial (SPORT): a randomized trial. JAMA. 2006;296:2441–2450.
Weinstein JN, Tosteson TD, Lurie JD, et al. Surgery vs. nonoperative treatment for lumbar disk herniation: the Spine Patient Outcomes Research Trial (SPORT) observational cohort. JAMA. 2006;296:2451–2459.

Chapter 18
Anesthesia for Genitourinary Surgery in the Elderly Patient

Christina M. Matadial and Jadelis Giquel

Introduction

Genitourinary surgery is a subspecialty of surgery which includes a wide spectrum of diseases involving the male and female urinary tract, the male reproductive system, and the female pelvic floor. Urological procedures account for 10–20% of most anesthetic practices, and many of these procedures are performed on elderly patients. This chapter reviews the anatomy and innervation of the genitourinary systems and anesthetic management of common urological procedures, highlighting special considerations for surgery in the elderly.

Innervation of the Genitourinary System

The intra-abdominal components of the genitourinary system receive their innervation from the autonomic nervous system. The pelvic urinary organs and genitalia are supplied by somatic and autonomic nerves. Figure 18.1 summarizes the neuronal conduction pathways and spinal levels of the nerves involved. Figure 18.2 shows diagrammatic representation of the anatomy of the genitourinary system.

Kidney and Abdominal Ureter

Sympathetic nerves to the kidney originate as preganglionic fibers from the eighth thoracic through the first lumbar segments and converge at the celiac plexus and

C.M. Matadial, MD (✉) • J. Giquel, MD
Department of Anesthesiology, University of Miami Miller School of Medicine,
1611 NW 12th Avenue, Room C300, Miami, FL 33136, USA
e-mail: CMatadial@med.miami.edu

S.R. Barnett (ed.), *Manual of Geriatric Anesthesia*, DOI 10.1007/978-1-4614-3888-5_18,

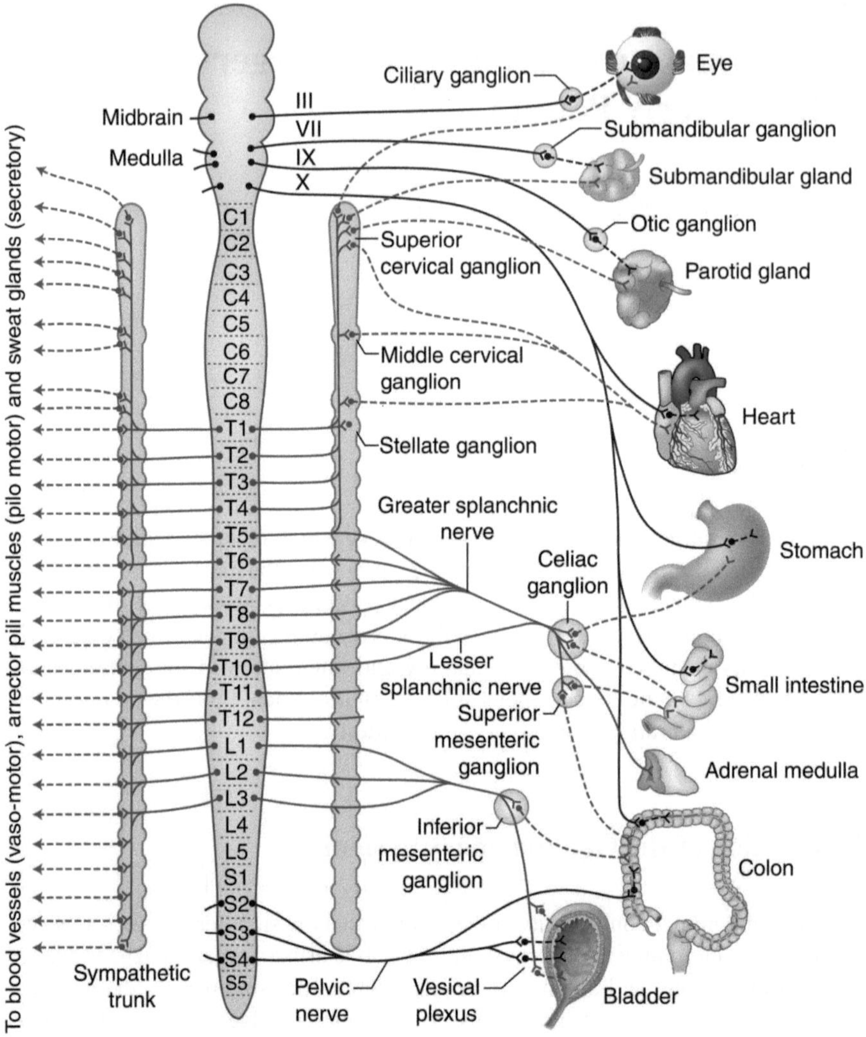

Fig. 18.1 Neuronal conduction pathways for genitourinary system

aorticorenal ganglia. Postganglionic fibers to the kidney arise mainly from the celiac and aorticorenal ganglia. Some sympathetic fibers may reach the kidney via the splanchnic nerves, and parasympathetic input is from the vagus nerve. Sympathetic fibers to the ureter originate from the tenth thoracic through the second lumbar segments and synapse with postganglionic fibers in the aorticorenal and superior and inferior hypogastric plexuses. Parasympathetic input is from the second through fourth sacral spinal segments. Nociceptive fibers travel along the sympathetic nerve roots to the corresponding spinal segments. Pain from the kidney and ureter is referred mainly to the somatic distribution of the tenth thoracic through the second lumbar segments—the lower part of the back, flank, ilioinguinal region. Effective

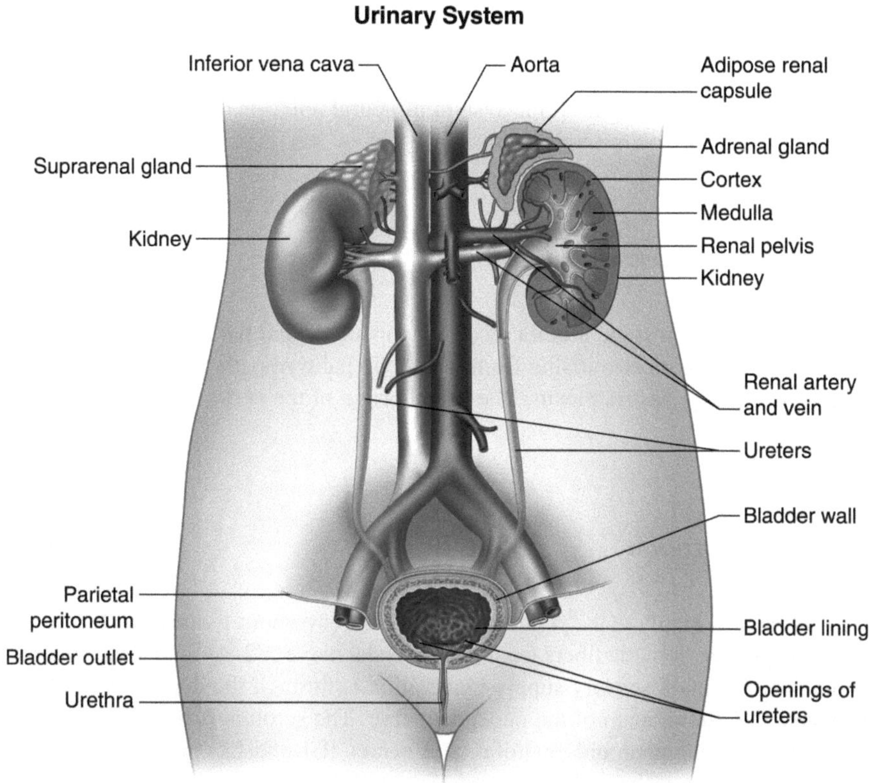

Fig. 18.2 Diagrammatic representation of the anatomy of the genitourinary system

neural block of these segments is necessary to provide adequate analgesia or anesthesia.

Bladder and Urethra

Sympathetic nerves to the bladder and urethra originate from the 11th thoracic to the 2nd lumbar segments, travel through the superior hypogastric plexus, and supply the bladder through the right and the left hypogastric nerves. Parasympathetic nerves arise from the second through the fourth sacral segments, forming the pelvic parasympathetic plexus, which is joined by fibers from the hypogastric plexus. Vesical branches proceed toward the bladder base, where they provide the nerve supply to the bladder and proximal part of the urethra. Parasympathetic fibers are the main motor supply to the bladder (with the exception of the trigone) and far outnumber sympathetic fibers in the bladder.

The afferents carrying sensations of stretch and fullness of the bladder are parasympathetic, whereas pain, touch, and temperature sensations are carried by sympathetic nerves. Sympathetic fibers are predominantly α-adrenergic in the bladder base and urethra, and β-adrenergic in the bladder dome and lateral wall. Knowledge of these aspects of neuroanatomy is important to appreciate the pharmacologic effects on the urologic system of neural ablation or regional block and drugs with adrenergic or cholinergic effects.

Prostate and Prostatic Urethra

The prostate and prostatic urethra receive sympathetic and parasympathetic supply from the prostatic plexus arising from the pelvic parasympathetic plexus, which is joined by the hypogastric plexus. The spinal origin of the nerve supply is primarily lumbosacral.

Penis and Scrotum

The autonomic supply to the penile urethra and the cavernous tissue comes from the prostatic plexus. Somatic fibers from the pudendal nerve (S2–4) supply the external sphincter. The main sensory supply innervation is through the dorsal nerve of the penis and the first branch of the pudendal nerve. The scrotum is innervated anteriorly by the ilioinguinal and genitofemoral nerves (L1 and L2) and posteriorly by perineal branches of the pudendal nerve (S2 and S4).

Testes

The testes descend from their intra-abdominal location to the scrotum during fetal development. Because they share their embryologic origin with the kidney, their nerve supply is similar to that of the kidney and upper part of the ureter and extends up to the T10 spinal segment.

Anesthetic Considerations

Radical Surgery for Urological Malignancies

Demographic changes resulting in an increasingly elderly population together with improved survival rates for patients with urological cancer following radical surgical resections have resulted in an increase in the number of procedures performed for prostatic, bladder, testicular, and renal cancer. Curative and palliative surgery plays an important role in treatment of these malignancies.

The desire for a quicker recovery with smaller, less painful incisions has prompted the successful development of laparoscopic operations for radical prostatectomy with pelvic lymph node dissection, nephrectomy, and laparoscopic retroperitoneal lymph node dissections for early malignancies. Robotic-assisted technology has also been applied to laparoscopic prostatectomy (da Vinci prostatectomy). The short-term results of these less invasive procedures appear to be comparable to standard open operations, at least for early malignancies. Whether long-term results are the same remains to be determined. A minimally invasive surgical approach in elderly patients can be particularly advantageous with more rapid return to baseline function.

Radical Nephrectomy

The operation may be carried out via an anterior subcostal, flank, midline, or thoracoabdominal incision. Smaller tumors may be resected with a hand-assisted laparoscopic technique. The kidney, adrenal gland, and perinephric fat are removed en bloc with the surrounding (Gerota's) fascia. The operation has the potential for extensive blood loss because these tumors are very vascular and often large at presentation. Retraction of the inferior vena cava may be associated with transient arterial hypotension. The surgery is performed under general endotracheal anesthesia, and invasive monitoring is frequently required, especially in very old patients who may not withstand swings in blood pressure and acute volume shifts as well as a younger patient. In addition to an arterial line and central venous access, a pulmonary artery catheter or cardiac output monitor may also be indicated for patients with impaired left ventricular function or significant cardiac disease.

Positioning Considerations for Nephrectomy

Many urological procedures are carried out in a hyperextended supine position to facilitate exposure of the pelvis during pelvic lymph node dissection, retropubic prostatectomy, or cystectomy. The patient is positioned supine with the iliac crest over the break in the operating table ("kidney rest"), and the table is extended such that distance between the iliac crest and the costal margin increases maximally. Care must be taken not to put excessive strain on the patient's back. The operating room table is also tilted head down to make the operative field horizontal. In the frog-leg position, a variation of the hyperextended supine position, the knees are also flexed and the hips are abducted and externally rotated. For thoracoabdominal surgery, the patient is placed in a hyperextended supine position close to the edge of the table on the operative side. The patient is tilted by flexing the leg on the nonoperative side 30° and the knee 90°, while the leg on the operative side remains straight. The shoulder on the ipsilateral side is elevated 30° with a roll to allow that arm to come across the chest into an adjustable arm rest ("airplane"), while the other arm is extended on an arm board. Although the adverse effects of the hyperextended supine position have not been studied, the physiological consequences of this position appear to be similar to the Trendelenburg position. Changes in pulmonary compliance and hemodynamic perturbation should be anticipated. The potential for neurological injuries and back injury exists because of the complex nature of the position. Careful positioning and generous padding of the arms and legs are therefore warranted. Positioning the pelvis above the heart may predispose patients to venous air embolism; however, this appears to be a rare complication.

Noncancer Surgery on the Upper Ureter and Kidney

Laparoscopic techniques are increasingly utilized in urology. Advantages for all patients, especially older ones, include shorter hospital stays, faster recovery, and less pain. Laparoscopic procedures include nephrectomy, partial nephrectomy, and pyeloplasty. Both transperitoneal and retroperitoneal approaches have been developed. A hand-assisted technique employs an additional larger incision that allows the surgeon to insert one hand for tactile sensation and dissection. Anesthetic management is similar to that for any laparoscopic procedure. Open procedures for kidney stones in the upper ureter and renal pelvis and nephrectomies for nonmalignant disease are often carried out in the "kidney rest position," also more accurately described as the lateral flexed position. With the patient in a full lateral position, the dependent leg is flexed and the other leg is extended. An axillary roll is placed underneath the dependent upper chest to prevent injury to the brachial plexus. The operating table is then extended to achieve maximal separation between the iliac crest and the costal margin on the operative side, and the kidney rest (a bar in the groove where the table bends) is elevated to raise the nondependent iliac crest higher and increase surgical exposure.

The lateral flexed position is associated with significant adverse respiratory and circulatory effects. Functional residual capacity is reduced in the dependent lung but may increase in the nondependent lung. In the anesthetized patient receiving controlled ventilation, ventilation/perfusion mismatching occurs because the dependent lung receives greater blood flow than the nondependent lung, whereas the nondependent lung receives greater ventilation, predisposing the patient to atelectasis in the dependent lung and hypoxemia. The arterial to end-tidal gradient for carbon dioxide progressively increases during general anesthesia in this position, indicating that dead space ventilation also increases in the nondependent lung. Moreover, elevation of the kidney rest can significantly decrease venous return to the heart in some patients by compressing the inferior vena cava. Venous pooling in the legs decreases venous return and aggravates any anesthesia-induced vasodilation.

Because of the potential for large blood loss and limited access to major vascular structures in the lateral flexed position, a large-bore intravenous catheter is advisable. Inadvertent entry into the pleural space can produce a pneumothorax, and diagnosis requires a high index of suspicion. The pneumothorax may be subclinical intraoperatively but can be diagnosed postoperatively with a chest radiograph.

Lower Genitourinary System

Cystoscopy

Cystoscopy is the most commonly performed urological procedure in older patients. Indications for cystoscopy include hematuria, recurrent urinary infections, renal calculi, and urinary obstruction. Bladder biopsies, retrograde pyelograms, resection of bladder tumors, extraction or laser lithotripsy of renal stones, and placement or manipulation of ureteral catheters (stents) can also be performed through the cystoscope.

Anesthetic management varies with the age and gender of the patient and the purpose of the procedure. Topical anesthesia in the form of viscous lidocaine with or without sedation may be used successfully for diagnostic studies in most women because of a short urethra. Operative cystoscopies involving biopsies, cauterization, or manipulation of ureteral catheters require regional or general anesthesia.

Lithotomy Position

The lithotomy position is most commonly used for patients undergoing endourological procedures. Failure to properly position patients can result in iatrogenic injuries. When moving the patient into the lithotomy position, two persons are required to safely move the patient's legs simultaneously up or down. Straps around the ankles or special holders support the legs in this position; these supports should be padded. Caution should be exercised to prevent the fingers from being caught between the mid and lower sections of the operating room table when the lower section is lowered and raised. Injury to the common peroneal nerve, resulting in loss of dorsiflexion of the foot, may result if the lateral aspect of the fibula rests on the strap support. If the legs are allowed to rest on medially placed strap supports, compression of the saphenous nerve can result in numbness along the medial calf. Excessive flexion of the thigh against the groin can injure the obturator nerve. Extreme flexion at the thigh can also stretch the sciatic nerve. A compartment syndrome of the lower extremities with rhabdomyolysis has been reported following a prolonged time in the lithotomy position.

The lithotomy position is associated with physiological alterations. Functional residual capacity decreases, predisposing patients to atelectasis and hypoxia. This effect is accentuated by the head-down (Trendelenburg) position (>30°). Elevation of the legs increases venous return acutely and may exacerbate congestive heart failure. Mean blood pressure often increases, but cardiac output does not change significantly. Conversely, rapid lowering of the legs acutely decreases venous return and can result in hypotension. Vasodilation from either general or regional anesthesia accentuates the hypotension. For this reason, blood pressure measurements should always be taken immediately after the legs are lowered, prior to transfer to a stretcher.

Choice of Anesthesia

General Anesthesia

Because of the short duration (15–20 min) and the outpatient setting of many cystoscopies, a deep sedation or general anesthesia is frequently used, and laryngeal mask airways (LMA) are common.

Regional Anesthesia

In the absence of contraindications such as anticoagulation, both epidural and spinal blocks can provide satisfactory anesthesia. Many clinicians prefer spinal over epidural anesthesia, which can have a more reliable and rapid onset particularly for procedures lasting more than 30 min.

Transurethral Surgery of the Prostate

Preoperative Considerations

Benign prostatic hypertrophy frequently leads to symptomatic bladder outlet obstruction in men older than 60 years. Indications of surgery include moderate to severe lower urinary tract symptoms in patients who do not respond to or decline medical therapy, persistent gross hematuria, recurrent urinary infections, renal insufficiency, or bladder stones. One of several operations may be selected to remove the hypertrophied and hyperplastic prostatic tissue: transurethral resection of the prostate (TURP), transurethral electrovaporization, transurethral incision, transurethral laser techniques, suprapubic (transvesical) prostatectomy, perineal prostatectomy, or retropubic prostatectomy. These surgeries require general or regional anesthesia. The transurethral approach for surgery is nearly always selected for patients with prostate gland volumes <40–50 g. Patients with advanced prostatic carcinoma may also present for transurethral resections to relieve symptomatic urinary obstruction. Regardless of its cause, long-standing obstruction can lead to impaired renal function.

Patients undergoing prostate surgery should be carefully evaluated for coexistent cardiac and pulmonary disease as well as renal dysfunction. Because of their age these patients have a relatively high (30–60%) prevalence of both cardiovascular and pulmonary disorders. TURP is reported to carry a 0.2–6% mortality rate, which correlates best with the American Society of Anesthesiologists' (ASA) physical status scale. Common causes of death include myocardial infarction, pulmonary edema, and renal failure.

Although a type and screen is adequate for most patients, blood should be available and crossmatched for anemic patients as well as patients with large glands (>40 g). Prostatic bleeding can be difficult to control through the cystoscope.

Intraoperative Considerations

TURP is performed by passing a loop through a special cystoscope (resectoscope). Using continuous irrigation and direct visualization, prostatic tissue is resected by applying a cutting current to the loop. Because of the characteristics of the prostate and the large amounts of irrigation fluid often used, TURP can be associated with a number of serious complications.

TURP Syndrome

Transurethral prostatic resection often opens the extensive network of venous sinuses in the prostate and potentially allows systemic absorption of the irrigating fluid. The absorption of large amounts of fluid (2 L or more) results in a constellation of symptoms and signs commonly referred to as the TURP syndrome. This syndrome presents intraoperatively or postoperatively as headache, restlessness, confusion, cyanosis, dyspnea, arrhythmias, hypotension, or seizures. Moreover, it can be rapidly fatal. The manifestations are primarily those of circulatory fluid overload, water intoxication, and, occasionally, toxicity from the solute in the irrigating fluid. Some maneuvers have been employed in an attempt to decrease the absorption of irrigant fluid during TURP. These include limiting the resection time to <1 h, limiting the height of the irrigation fluid to 60 cm above the resection level to prevent excessive rises in the hydrostatic pressure, maintaining a low intravesical pressure environment by suprapubic drainage or a continuous flow system, intraprostatic vasopressin injection, intraoperative monitoring of fluid absorption with markers such as ethanol-tagged irrigating solutions, and/or the use of diuretics during the procedure. The incidence of significant TURP syndrome approaches 2% despite these measures.

Irrigating Solutions

Saline solutions cannot be used for irrigation during TURP because they disperse the electrocautery current. Water provides excellent visibility; however, its hypotonicity lyses red blood cells, and significant absorption can readily result in acute water intoxication. For TURP, slightly hypotonic nonelectrolyte irrigating solutions such as glycine 1.5% (230 mOsm/L) or a mixture of sorbitol 2.7% and mannitol 0.54% (195 mOsm/L) are most commonly used. Less commonly used solutions include sorbitol 3.3%, mannitol 3%, dextrose 2.5–4%, and urea 1%. Absorption of irrigation fluid appears to be dependent on the duration of the resection as well as the height (pressure) of the irrigation fluid. Most resections last 45–60 min, and, on average, 20 ml of the irrigating fluid is absorbed into the patient's circulation per minute of operating time. Pulmonary congestion or florid pulmonary edema can readily result from the absorption of large amounts of irrigation fluid, particularly in patients with limited cardiac reserve. The hypotonicity of these fluids also results in acute hyponatremia and hypoosmolality, which can lead to serious neurological manifestations. Symptoms of hyponatremia usually do not develop until the serum sodium concentration decreases below 120 mEq/L. Marked hypotonicity in plasma ($[Na^+] < 100$ mEq/L) may also result in acute intravascular hemolysis.

Toxicity may also arise from absorption of the solutes in these fluids. Marked hyperglycinemia has been reported with glucose-containing solutions such as sorbitol and mannitol and is thought to contribute to circulatory depression and central nervous system toxicity. Glycine is known to be an inhibitory neurotransmitter in the central nervous system and has also been implicated in rare instances of transient blindness following TURP. Plasma glycine concentrations in excess of 1,000 mg/L have been recorded (normal is 13–17 mg/L). Hyperammonemia, presumably from the degradation of glycine, has also been documented in a few patients with marked central nervous system toxicity following TURP. Blood ammonia levels in some patients exceeded 500 μmol/L (normal is 5–50 μmol/L). Absorption of mannitol solutions causes intravascular volume expansion and exacerbates fluid overload.

Treatment of TURP syndrome depends on early recognition and should be based on the severity of the symptoms. The absorbed volume must be eliminated, and hypoxemia and hypoperfusion must be avoided. Most patients can be managed with fluid restriction and a loop diuretic. Symptomatic hyponatremia resulting in seizures or coma should be treated with hypertonic saline only in cases of extreme hyponatremia. Seizure activity can be managed with midazolam (2–4 mg), propofol (50–150 mg), or thiopental (50–100 mg). Phenytoin, 10–20 mg/kg intravenously (no faster than 50 mg/min), should also be considered to provide more sustained anticonvulsant activity. Endotracheal intubation is generally advisable to prevent aspiration until the patient's mental status normalizes. The amount and rate of hypertonic saline solution (3%) needed to correct the hyponatremia to a safe level should be based on the patient's serum sodium concentration. Hypertonic saline solution should not be given at a rate faster than 100 mL/h so as not to exacerbate circulatory fluid overload or induce cerebral pontine myelinolysis.

Recent technological and design advancements have led to the development of a bipolar resectoscope that allows resection using normal saline. The use of normal saline and bipolar electrocautery allows for excellent visualization, coagulation, and hemostasis, greatly reducing the risk of TURP syndrome by the use of isotonic irrigant.

Hypothermia

Large volumes of irrigating fluids at room temperature can be a major source of heat loss in patients. Irrigating solutions should be warmed to body temperature prior to use to prevent hypothermia. Postoperative shivering associated with hypothermia is particularly undesirable, as it can dislodge clots, contribute to postoperative bleeding, and, in extreme cases, induce cardiac dysrhythmias.

Bladder Perforation

The incidence of bladder perforation during TURP is estimated to be ~1%. Perforation may result from the resectoscope going through the bladder wall or from overdistention of the bladder with irrigation fluid. Most bladder perforations are extraperitoneal and are signaled by poor return of the irrigating fluid. Awake patients will typically complain of nausea, diaphoresis, and retropubic or lower abdominal pain and possibly shoulder pain secondary to referred pain from the diaphragmatic irritation. Large extraperitoneal and most intraperitoneal perforations are usually even more obvious, presenting as sudden unexplained hypotension (or hypertension) with generalized abdominal pain (in awake patients). Regardless of the anesthetic technique employed, perforation should be suspected in settings of sudden hypotension or hypertension, particularly with bradycardia (vagally mediated).

Coagulopathy

Disseminated intravascular coagulation (DIC) has on rare occasions been reported following TURP and is thought to result from the release of thromboplastins from the prostate into the circulation during surgery. Up to 6% of patients may have evidence of subclinical DIC. A dilutional thrombocytopenia can also develop during surgery as part of the TURP syndrome from absorption of irrigation fluids. Rarely, patients with metastatic carcinoma of the prostate develop a coagulopathy from primary fibrinolysis; the tumor is thought to secrete a fibrinolytic enzyme in such instances. The diagnosis of coagulopathy may be suspected from diffuse uncontrollable bleeding and should be confirmed by laboratory tests. Primary fibrinolysis should be treated with ε-aminocaproic acid (Amicar) 5 g followed by 1 g/h intravenously. The treatment of DIC in this setting may require heparin in addition to replacement of clotting factors and platelets.

Bacteremia

The prostate is often colonized with bacteria and may harbor chronic infection. Extensive surgical manipulation of the gland together with the opening of venous sinuses can allow entry of organisms into the bloodstream. Bacteremia following transurethral surgery is not uncommon and can lead to septicemia or septic shock. Prophylactic antibiotic therapy (most commonly gentamicin, levofloxacin, or cefazolin) prior to TURP may decrease the likelihood of bacteremic and septic episodes. Preoperative urinalysis and urine cultures should be evaluated prior to procedure, and treatment instituted prior to instrumentation.

Choice of Anesthesia

Either spinal or epidural anesthesia with a T10 sensory level provides excellent anesthesia and good operating conditions for TURP. When compared with general anesthesia, regional anesthesia appears to reduce the incidence of postoperative venous thrombosis; it is also less likely to mask symptoms and signs of the TURP syndrome or bladder perforation. Clinical studies have failed to show any differences in blood loss, postoperative cognitive function, and mortality between regional and general anesthesia. Regional anesthesia, however, does not abolish the obturator reflex (external rotation and adduction of the thigh secondary to stimulation of the obturator nerve by electrocautery current through the lateral bladder wall). The reflex (muscle contraction) is reliably blocked only by muscle paralysis during general anesthesia.

Monitoring

Evaluation of mental status in the awake patient is the best monitor for detection of early signs of the TURP syndrome and bladder perforation. A decrease in arterial oxygen saturation may be an early sign of fluid overload. Some studies have reported perioperative ischemic electrocardiographic changes in up to 18% of patients. Temperature monitoring should be used during long resections to detect hypothermia. Blood loss is particularly difficult to assess because of the use of irrigating solutions, so it is necessary to rely on clinical signs of hypovolemia. Blood loss can average 15 ml/g of resected tissue but is rarely life-threatening. Transient, postoperative decreases in hematocrit may simply reflect hemodilution from absorption of irrigation fluid. About 2.5% of patients require intraoperative transfusion; factors associated with transfusion include a procedure whose duration is longer than 90 min and resection of >45 g of prostate tissue.

Lithotripsy

The treatment of kidney stones has changed significantly over the past two decades from primarily open surgical procedures to less invasive or completely noninvasive techniques. Stones in the bladder and lower ureters are now usually treated with cystoscopic procedures, including flexible and rigid ureteroscopy, stone extraction, stent placement, and intracorporeal lithotripsy (laser or electrohydraulic). Laser lithotripsy typically utilizes a holmium: YAG laser. In contrast, stones in the upper two-thirds of the ureters or kidneys are treated with extracorporeal shock wave lithotripsy (ESWL) or percutaneous nephrolithotomy. The latter is reserved for large stones (>2 cm) and involves techniques similar to ureteroscopy; however, application is via a percutaneous sheath over the kidney in the prone position. Some stones (e.g., cystine, uric acid, and calcium oxalate monohydrate) are particularly hard and are more likely to require retreatment.

During ESWL, repetitive high-energy shocks (sound waves) are generated and focused on the stone, causing it to fragment as tensile and shear forces develop inside the stone and cavitation occurs outside on its surface.

Preoperative Considerations

Patients with a history of cardiac arrhythmias and those with a pacemaker or internal cardiac defibrillator (ICD) may be at risk for developing arrhythmias induced by shock waves during ESWL. Shock waves can rarely damage the internal components of pacemaker and ICD devices. Variability among devices may necessitate contacting the manufacturer for assistance in disabling and/or reprogramming the device. Synchronization of the shock waves to the R wave from the electrocardiogram (ECG) decreases the incidence of arrhythmias during ESWL. The shock waves are usually timed to be 20 ms after the R wave to correspond to the ventricular refractory period. Studies suggest that asynchronous delivery of shocks can be safe in patients without heart disease.

Intraoperative Considerations

Anesthetic considerations for ureteroscopy, stone manipulation, and laser lithotripsy are similar to those for cystoscopic procedures. ESWL requires special considerations, particularly when older lithotriptors, which require the patient to be immersed in water, are used.

Choice of Anesthesia

Pain during lithotripsy is from dissipation of a small amount of energy as shock waves enter the body through the skin. The pain is therefore localized to the skin and proportionate to the intensity of the shock waves. Older lithotripsy with units employing a water bath requires 1,000–2,400 relatively high-intensity shock waves (18–22 kV) that most patients do not tolerate without either regional or general anesthesia. In contrast, newer lithotripsy units that are coupled directly to the skin utilize 2,000–3,000 lower-intensity shock waves (10–18 kV) that usually require only light sedation.

Intravenous sedation is usually adequate for low-energy lithotripsy. Low-dose propofol infusions together with midazolam and opioid supplementation may be used.

Monitoring

Even with R wave-triggered shocks, supraventricular arrhythmias can still occur and may require treatment. Changes in functional residual capacity mandate close monitoring of oxygen saturation, particularly in patients at high risk for developing hypoxemia.

Prostate Cancer

Preoperative Considerations

Adenocarcinoma of the prostate is the most common cancer in men. It is the second most common cause of cancer deaths in men older than 55 years. The incidence of prostate cancer increases with age and is estimated to be 75% in patients over 75 years. Transrectal ultrasound is used to evaluate tumor size and the presence or absence of extracapsular extension. Clinical staging is based on the Gleason score of the biopsy, computed tomography (CT) scan or magnetic resonance imaging (MRI), and bone scan.

Intraoperative Considerations

Patients with prostate cancer may present to the operating room for a laparoscopic prostatectomy with pelvic lymph node dissection, radical prostatectomy, salvage prostatectomy (following failure of radiation therapy), or bilateral orchiectomy for hormonal therapy.

Laparoscopic Radical Prostatectomy

Laparoscopic radical prostatectomy with pelvic lymph node dissection differs from most other laparoscopic procedures in (1) the use of a steep (>30°) Trendelenburg position for surgical exposure and (2) the potential for greater carbon dioxide absorption from the retroperitoneum. The procedure is carried out under general endotracheal anesthesia because of the length of the procedure, steep Trendelenburg position, necessity for abdominal distention, and desirability of being able to increase the patient's minute ventilation. Most clinicians avoid nitrous oxide to prevent bowel distention and expansion of residual intra-abdominal gas.

Radical Retropubic Prostatectomy

Radical retropubic prostatectomy is usually performed together with a pelvic lymph node dissection through a lower, midline, abdominal position. It may be curative for localized prostatic cancer or occasionally used as a salvage procedure after failure of radiation. The prostate is removed en bloc with the seminal vesicles, ejaculatory ducts, and part of the bladder neck. A "nerve-sparing" technique may be used to help preserve sexual function. Following the prostatectomy, the remaining bladder neck is anastomosed directly to the urethra over an indwelling urinary catheter. The surgeon may ask for intravenous administration of indigo carmine for visualization of the ureters. This dye can be associated with transient blood pressure fluctuations and inaccurately low saturation levels on the pulse oximeter.

Radical retropubic prostatectomy is often associated with significant operative blood loss. Direct arterial pressure monitoring is generally advisable and allows controlled hypotension. Factors that may affect blood loss include positioning, pelvic anatomy, and size of the prostate; early ligation of the dorsal vein complex of the penis and temporary clamping of the hypogastric artery appear to reduce blood loss. Blood loss is similar in patients receiving general anesthesia and those receiving regional anesthesia; operative morbidity and mortality also appear to be similar. Neuraxial anesthesia requires a T6 sensory level, but awake patients typically do not tolerate regional anesthesia without heavy sedation because of the hyperextended supine position. Moreover, the combination of a prolonged Trendelenburg position together with administration of large amounts of intravenous fluids can produce edema of the upper airway.

Clinical studies have found no differences in pain relief or recovery between patients receiving epidural opioids and those receiving intravenous patient-controlled analgesia. The NSAID ketorolac can be used as an analgesic adjuvant and has been reported to decrease opioid requirements, improve analgesia, and promote earlier return of bowel function without increasing transfusion requirements. Extensive surgical dissection around the pelvic veins increases the risk of thromboembolic complications. Epidural anesthesia may reduce the incidence of postoperative deep venous thrombosis following prostatectomy, but the beneficial effect may be insignificant due to the perioperative use of low-molecular-weight heparin. Prophylactic use of unfractionated heparin has been reported to increase operative blood loss and transfusion requirements, whereas sequential pneumatic (leg) compression devices appear to delay but not reduce deep venous thrombosis. Other postoperative complications include hemorrhage; injuries to the obturator nerve, ureter, and rectum; as well as urinary incontinence and impotence.

Bladder Cancer

Preoperative Considerations

Bladder cancer occurs at an average patient age of 65 years with a 3:1 male to female ratio. Transitional cell carcinoma of the bladder is the second most common malignancy of the genitourinary tract. The association of cigarette smoking with bladder carcinoma results in coexistent coronary artery and chronic obstructive pulmonary disease in many of these patients. Moreover, underlying renal impairment may be age related or secondary to urinary tract obstruction. Staging includes cystoscopy and CT or MRI scans. Intravesical chemotherapy is used for superficial tumors, and transurethral resection is carried out for low-grade noninvasive bladder tumors. Some patients may receive preoperative radiation to shrink the tumor before radical cystectomy. Urinary diversion is usually performed immediately following the cystectomy.

Intraoperative Considerations

Radical Cystectomy

Radical cystectomy is a major operation that is often associated with significant blood loss. It is usually performed through a midline incision that extends from the pubis to the xiphoid process. All anterior pelvic organs including the bladder, prostate, and seminal vesicles are removed in males; the uterus, cervix, ovaries, and part of the anterior vaginal vault may also be removed in females. Pelvic node dissection and urinary diversion are also carried out.

These procedures typically require at least 4–6 h and frequently necessitate blood transfusion. General endotracheal anesthesia with a muscle relaxant provides optimal operating conditions. Controlled hypotensive anesthesia may reduce intraoperative blood loss and transfusion requirements; however, many elderly patients may not tolerate hypotension. Supplementation of general anesthesia with spinal or continuous epidural anesthesia can facilitate induced hypotension, decrease general anesthetic requirements, and provide postoperative analgesia. A major drawback of the use of neuraxial anesthesia is the hyperperistalsis that produces a very small contracted bowel, which complicates construction of a urinary reservoir.

Close monitoring of blood pressure, intravascular volume, and blood loss is essential. Direct intra-arterial pressure monitoring and central venous pressure monitoring are advisable in patients with limited cardiac reserve. Urinary output should be monitored continuously and correlated with the progress of the operation, as the urinary path is interrupted at an early point during most of these procedures. Scrupulous intraoperative active warming techniques are essential for prevention of hypothermia.

Urinary Diversion

Urinary diversion is usually performed immediately following radical cystectomy. The procedure entails implanting the ureters into a segment of bowel. The selected bowel segment is either left in situ, such as in ureterosigmoidostomy, or divided with its mesenteric blood supply intact and attached to a cutaneous stoma or urethra. The isolated bowel can either function as a conduit (e.g., ileal conduit) or be reconstructed to form a continent reservoir (neobladder). Conduits may be formed from ileum, jejunum, or colon.

Major anesthetic goals include keeping the patient well hydrated and maintaining a brisk urinary output once the ureters are opened. Central venous pressure monitoring is often employed to guide intravenous fluid administration. Neuraxial anesthesia may produce unopposed parasympathetic activity due to sympathetic blockade, which results in a markedly contracted, hyperactive bowel that makes construction of a continent ileal reservoir technically difficult; sometimes, glucagon (1 mg) may alleviate this problem.

Prolonged contact of urine with bowel mucosa (slow urine flow) may produce significant metabolic disturbances. Hyponatremia, hypochloremia, hyperkalemia, and metabolic acidosis can occur following jejunal conduits. In contrast, colonic and ileal conduits may be associated with hyperchloremic metabolic acidosis. The use of temporary ureteral stents and maintenance of high urinary flow help alleviate this problem in the early postoperative period.

Bilateral Orchiectomy

Bilateral orchiectomy is usually performed for local control of metastatic adenocarcinoma of the prostate. The procedure is relatively short (20–45 min) and is performed through a single midline scrotal incision. Although bilateral orchiectomy can be performed under local anesthesia, most patients and many clinicians prefer general anesthesia.

Genitourinary Surgery in the Elderly Female

Genitourinary disorders occur frequently among women ≥70 years old, and many of these disorders are best treated with surgery. The number of elderly women who seek surgical treatment of gynecologic disorders such as pelvic organ prolapse and stress urinary incontinence is expected to increase. There is limited data on perioperative morbidity and mortality rates of major genitourinary surgery in very elderly women, and the risks of such surgery have not been defined clearly in this population. Information about postoperative morbidity and mortality rates is essential for the assistance of elderly patients and their families in making decisions regarding elective surgery. There is often reluctance to perform major surgical procedures in elderly patients because of multiple comorbidities, presumed limited life expectancy, and the perception that elderly patients require prolonged and extensive hospital care.

Key Points

- Patient positioning is important in urologic surgery because of the variety and complexity of the positions used. Knowledge of the physiologic implications and the possible complications of these positions is critical to preventing untoward outcomes.
- For most endourologic procedures, rapid anesthetic onset and recovery are desired. These goals can be reached with either general or neuraxial anesthesia, provided appropriate pharmacologic choices are made.
- Use of neuraxial anesthesia for transurethral resection of the prostate (TURP) does not have proven outcome benefits over general anesthesia, but it may facilitate the detection of TURP syndrome. This is the most severe complication of TURP, although its frequency has decreased with the use of current irrigation fluids.
- TURP syndrome is a constellation of symptoms caused by the absorption of hypotonic bladder irrigants. Cardiovascular and neurologic changes are due to hypoosmolality, hyponatremia, hyperglycinemia, hyperammonemia, and hypervolemia. Newer techniques, such as laser prostatectomy, are making transurethral resection of the prostate (TURP) syndrome a rare event.
- Regional anesthesia offers several advantages over general anesthesia for standard, but not laser, TURP, although 30-day mortality rates remain unchanged at 0.2–0.8%.

- Radical prostatectomy is accompanied by significant blood loss. Intraoperative venous air embolism has been reported. Regional anesthesia with spontaneous ventilation is associated with less blood loss than general anesthesia and intermittent positive-pressure ventilation. Other advantages of epidural anesthesia include decreased deep vein thrombosis and preemptive analgesia.
- Robotic radical prostatectomy is associated with reduced blood loss and postoperative pain compared with open radical prostatectomy. Anesthetic concerns are related to steep head-down tilt and pneumoperitoneum and include hypercarbia, hypoxemia, increased intraocular and intracranial pressures, decreased perfusion pressure to lower extremity, and positional injuries.
- Due to increased longevity, more females are presenting with genitourinary conditions amenable to surgical repair. Ability to manage comorbidities of this anesthetic subset will be increasingly more important as the demand for surgery in females over 70 years increases.

Suggested Reading

Advances in Genitourinary Surgery. Highlights From the 114th Meeting of the American Association of Genitourinary Surgeons April 5–8, 2000, San Antonio, Tex Rev Urol. 2000 Fall; 2(4): 203–205, 210.-accessed online 07/23/2010.

The Bartleby.com edition of Gray's Anatomy of the Human Body-accessed 7/19/2010.

Chu J. Genitourinary Principles. Nelson LS, Lewin NA, Howland MA, Hoffman RS, Lewis R. Goldfrank, Flomenbaum NE, eds. In: Goldfrank's Toxicologic Emergencies, 9e: http://www.accesspharmacy.com/content.aspx?aID=6508360.

www.dkimages.com/discover/Home/Health-and-besuty/Human-Body/Reproductive-System/Female/Genitalia/Genitalia-04.html-accessed 7/21/2010.

www.dkimages.com/discover/Home/Health-and-besuty/Human-Body/Reproductive-System/Male/Genitalia/Genitalia-04.html-accessed 7/21/2010.

Durham D. Management of Status Epilepticus Critical Care and Resuscitation 1999; 1: 344–353.

Hsu GL, Hsieh CH, Chen HS, Ling PY, Wen HS, Liu LJ, Chen CW, Chua C. The advancement of pure local anesthesia for penile surgeries: Can an outpatient basis be sustainable? J Androl. 2007; 28:200–205.

www.ivy-rose.co.uk/HumanBody/Urinary/Urinary_System_Kidney_Diagram-accessed 7/28/2010.

Issa M, Young M, Bullock A, Bouet R, Petros J. Dilutional hyponatremia of TURP syndrome: A historical event in the 21st century. Urology - Volume 64, Issue 2 August 2004.

Longnecker DE, Brown DL, Newman MF, Zapol WM. Anesthesiology. McGraw-Hill; 2008; 194–215: 1450-1470.

Miller R, ed. Miller's Anesthesia, 7th ed. Churchill Livingstone; 2009: 2105–2134.

Morgan GE, Jr., Mikhail MS, Murray MJ. Clinical Anesthesiology. McGraw-Hill; 2002: 692–707.

The goal of the clinical evaluation of the genitourinary system is the diagnosis or abnormal innervation of the bladder and its sphincteric mechanism. www.ncbi.nlm.nih.gov ›accessed 07/27/2010.

Preston T, Fletcher R, Lucchesi B, Judge R. Changes in myocardial threshold. Physiologic and pharmacologic factors in patients with implanted pacemakers. American Heart Journal. August 1967; 74(2): 235–242.

pro2services.com/Lectures/Spring/RenalTests/renaltests-accessed 7/02/2010.

Sweitzer B. Handbook of Preoperative Assessment and Management. Philadelphia, Pa: Lippincott Williams & Wilkins; 2000: 196–212.

Toglia MR, Nolan TE. Morbidity and mortality rates of elective gynecologic surgery in the elderly woman. American Journal of Obstetrics and Gynecology. December 2003; 189, 6:1584–1587.

Chapter 19
Anesthetic Management for ECT

Punita Tripathi

Introduction

Depression in the elderly is a growing public health problem. Depression affects more than 6.5 million of the 35 million Americans aged 65 years or older. Depression in the older person can have significant impact including loss of function, social isolation, and even death; 20% of all suicides occur in individuals over the age of 65 years. Older patients with primary depression have frequently experienced episodes of the illness during much of their lives. However, late-life depressive syndromes also arise secondary to medical and neurological disorders common to elderly patients. Unfortunately depression in elderly people can go undiagnosed and untreated because it is thought to be a normal part of aging or an "accepted" sign of chronic illness.

Electroconvulsive therapy (ECT) in elderly patients is one of the most controversial treatments in all of medicine; however, old patients can do particularly well with ECT. When considering all patients receiving ECT, individuals over 65 years are more than twice as likely to receive ECT than those less than 65 years. Older women are overrepresented in the category of people treated with ECT; however, this may merely reflect the demographic shift with aging and the frequency of depression found in older women versus men. Later life depression is more likely to be resistant to drug therapy, and this partly explains the resurgence in the popularity of ECT for older individuals. Geriatric patients should not be denied treatment just based on their age.

P. Tripathi, MD (✉)
Department of Anesthesia and Critical Care Medicine, Johns Hopkins Medical Center,
4940 Eastern Avenue, Baltimore, MD 21224, USA
e-mail: Ptripat2@jhmi.edu

S.R. Barnett (ed.), *Manual of Geriatric Anesthesia*, DOI 10.1007/978-1-4614-3888-5_19,

Pharmacotherapy

When treating depression with pharmacotherapy, the drug of choice in the elderly are selective serotonin reuptake inhibitors (SSRIs), i.e., fluoxetine, nefazodone, sertraline, and paroxetine, have few adverse cardiovascular and anticholinergic effects. Agitation, a common adverse effect of SSRIs (e.g., fluoxetine), can be troublesome in elderly depressed patients. Although tricyclic antidepressants (e.g., nortriptyline, desipramine, amitriptyline) are used often, elderly patients may have difficulty tolerating the anticholinergic effects (especially those of amitriptyline) and the postural hypotension these drugs are likely to induce. Monoamine oxidase inhibitors (MAOIs) are less commonly used because of significant adverse effects. Low-dose lithium may augment the effect of tricyclic antidepressants and SSRIs. Carbamazepine may be added as it may reduce a patient's tendency to cycle in and out of depressive episodes. Methylphenidate has been used as an adjunct to antidepressants, especially in patients who are in long-term care facilities. It is generally reserved for patients who have stopped eating and have significant weight loss. It has a quick onset of action, stimulates appetite, is relatively safe, and rarely leads to dependence. Despite the vast array of pharmacologic agents for depression, a percentage of older patients either cannot tolerate the side effects of the medications or they do not respond to the therapy prescribed. ECT can provide a safe alternative for treatment in individuals who have failed or who cannot tolerate more conventional pharmacotherapy for their depression.

Electroconvulsive Therapy

Electroconvulsive therapy (ECT) consists of a course of treatments administered over weeks and months. During ECT treatment general anesthesia is induced and a small electrical stimulation is applied to the scalp to induce a generalized cerebral seizure. ECT can be effective in treating depression when all else has failed. ECT is used for severely depressed elderly patients who have responded to ECT in the past; have psychotic symptoms, catatonia, and self-destructive suicidal behavior; refuse to eat secondary to depression; and those who do not tolerate or respond to antidepressants.

Mechanism of Action

The exact mechanism of how ECT works is not known. There are several hypotheses. The most widely accepted hypothesis is that ECT reduces neuronal activity in some cortical regions, which have anticonvulsant and antidepressant effects. Another theory is that ECT works by raising levels of norepinephrine and serotonin while also enhancing the activity of the dopaminergic system in patients with depression. Depressed patients are known to be deficient in these neurotransmitters.

Frequency and Number of Treatments

During the initial treatment or acute phase, ECT is most commonly scheduled three times per week for a total of 6–12 treatments. Some initial clinical improvement is often seen after 3–5 treatments. Increased frequencies of ECT can be used in patients with severe symptoms, when a speedy recovery is deemed important, for example, with extreme malnutrition or catatonia. A reduction in the frequency of treatment is considered if severe cognitive dysfunction or delirium is present or develops. Maintenance ECT is often offered to prevent relapse. Generally these treatments are given at an interval of once a week to every 8 weeks for at least 6 months after remission. The frequency will depend on the patient and their response to treatment; it may continue indefinitely in selected circumstances.

Common Physiologic Responses and Side Effects Associated with ECT

Adverse Cognitive Effects

A successful ECT treatment results in a grand mal seizure with resultant increase in cerebral blood flow, cerebral metabolic rate, and intracranial pressure. The signs and symptoms following the induced seizure may include headache, dizziness, confusion, agitation, and amnesia which can be both retrograde and anterograde. Elderly patients may have a high seizure threshold, especially older men. This may increase the difficulty in eliciting an effective seizure in this subset of population. In patients with preexisting memory problems, cognitive adverse effects, especially impaired memory, are likely to be more common. ECT can be accompanied by a brief acute confusional state, generally only lasting 10–30 min after the seizure. Retrograde amnesia is one of the most disturbing side effects for older patients. This involves forgetting recent memories and can include the weeks preceding treatment as well as the treatment period. Retrograde amnesia is more common and may last longer with bilateral ECT compared with unilateral ECT treatment.

Cardiovascular Effects

Cardiovascular complications are rare with ECT; however, they are most common among patient with preexisting cardiac disease. The induced seizure stimulates the hypothalamo-pituitary axis resulting in the release of adrenocorticotropic hormone (ACTH). Cardiovascular responses are secondary to autonomic nervous system stimulation and release of catecholamines. There is an initial parasympathetic stimulation leading to bradycardia lasting 10–15 s. This can lead to varied arrhythmias including bradycardia, atrial arrhythmias, atrial and ventricular ectopy, and even asystole.

Table 19.1 Effects of IV anesthetic and cardiovascular drugs on the duration of ECT-induced seizure activity

Drugs	Increase in duration of seizure	Decrease in duration of seizure
Induction agents	Etomidate, methohexital	Thiopental, thiamylal, lorazepam, midazolam, ketamine, propofol
Narcotics	Alfentanil, remifentanil	Fentanyl
Cardiovascular drugs	Aminophylline	Diltiazem, lidocaine, labetalol, esmolol

The parasympathetic phase is followed by sympathetically mediated release of catecholamines leading to tachycardia and hypertension. The tachycardic interval usually correlates with the length of the seizure. These hemodynamic responses may last for 10–20 min following the seizure. The cardiovascular sympathetic stimulation can be intense and has been associated with serious cardiac arrhythmias such as asystole and ventricular tachycardia. It is not uncommon for patient to develop transient ECG changes during the ECT treatment. A transient decrease in left-ventricular systolic and diastolic function has been described after ECT treatments even in patients without cardiac diseases. It is not surprising that cardiopulmonary events are the most common cause of mortality following ECT. However overall mortality is rare with a mortality rate of 2–4 per 100,000 treatments (Table 19.1).

Musculoskeletal System

Myalgia may arise from the seizure itself and/or may be due to succinylcholine-induced fasciculations. Dislocation of joints and in extreme cases fracture of bones may occur secondary to seizures, although this has been largely eliminated through the coadministration of succinylcholine or other short-acting muscle relaxants.

Miscellaneous

Other side effects include dental and tongue injuries from biting, bladder rupture, raised intraocular pressure, and in rare case death.

Contraindication

Intracranial tumor with evidence of raised intracranial tension is the only absolute contraindication to ECT. Other relative contraindications include pheochromocytoma, unstable cardiovascular conditions such as a recent myocardial infarction, congestive heart failure, severe valvular heart disease, a recent stroke, and an intracranial aneurysm or vascular malformation that might be susceptible to rupture with increased blood pressure.

Anesthetic Management for ECT

ECT is performed under general anesthesia either as an outpatient or an inpatient. The goals for anesthetic management include premedication to attenuate unwanted cardiovascular physiological effects, a rapid induction and recovery, and protection of the patient from the effects of the tonic and clonic contractions due to the seizure itself. The minimal duration for a therapeutic seizure is 15 s; many seizures actually last between 15 and 70 s; continuous EEG monitoring is used to document the seizure occurrence and duration.

ECT is a low-risk procedure with a mortality rate similar to that of anesthesia for minor surgical procedure despite the fact that it is frequently used in the elderly with major medical problems. Responsibilities of the anesthesiologist include conducting an appropriate preprocedure assessment, managing the airway, administering a brief anesthetic including relaxant agents, monitoring cardiopulmonary functioning, and assisting in treating adverse events that may occur during or immediately following the seizure.

Preprocedure Evaluation

ECT is performed while the patient is under general anesthesia, and all patients must undergo a full preanesthetic evaluation to assess the risks. Informed consent is required for all patients. Since some of the patients may be delusional, paranoid, and uncommunicative, hospital policy should be followed regarding patients who are unable to give informed consents. Family members should be involved early in the decision-making process. Institutional operating room NPO guidelines should be followed:in general, patients should remain NPO after midnight. Benzodiazepines and anticonvulsant medications may need to be reduced or discontinued prior to treatment as they may interfere with the ability to generate a seizure in a patient. Most other psychotropic agents can be continued, and any changes in medications should be done only in consultation with the treating psychiatrist. All cardiac medications should be taken with a sip of water on the morning of procedure. A thorough preoperative evaluation should be conducted, and appropriate laboratory and diagnostic tests are recommended only if needed based on the preprocedure evaluation. An ECG is frequently required as a baseline test in adults over the age of 50 years and should be obtained in all patients with a cardiac history.

Special Considerations

Patients with pacemakers can receive ECT with full EKG monitoring. To avoid unnecessary triggering of the pacemaker, a demand pacemaker is converted to a fixed mode by application of a magnet. Patients with cardioverter-defibrillator should have defibrillator and antitachycardic function deactivated prior to ECT. This should be done in conjunction with the patient's cardiologist. Elderly patients with complete heart block may require pretreatment with atropine.

Diabetic patients should have blood sugar monitored before and after the treatment; some patients may experience a hyperglycemic effect secondary to the ECT. Dosing of insulin and oral hypoglycemic medications should follow standard preoperative recommendations for fasting patients.

Older individuals have a higher risk of aspiration and premedication with Bicitra, metoclopramide, and/or ranitidine should be considered in high-risk patients, for example, those with a hiatal hernia or documented reflux. Cricoid pressure can be applied during anesthesia, although the efficacy of this has been questioned by some anesthesiologists.

Premedications

The goal of premedication is to reduce the hemodynamic response to ECT and provide anxiolysis. The parasympathetic effects of ECT often result in increased salivation, transient bradycardia, and occasionally even asystole. An anticholinergic medication such as atropine or glycopyrrolate may be administered to prevent these adverse effects. Glycopyrrolate is preferred over atropine as it does not cross the blood–brain barrier and hence central anticholinergic side effects are avoided. Unfortunately the anticholinergic medications may themselves cause tachycardia. The sympathetic effects of ECT typically result in tachycardia, hypertension, and occasionally even myocardial ischemia and infarction. These hemodynamic effects can be decreased by use of beta-blocker agents. Short-acting agents like esmolol are preferred, but labetalol is often an acceptable longer-acting alternative. A vasodilator like nitroglycerine (NTG) in small doses may be given 1–2 min before ECT in high-risk patients.

Drug Interactions

All anesthesiologists must be aware of the drug interactions involved. Interaction of barbiturates and lithium leads to prolonged recovery. Benzodiazepines, valproate, carbamazepine, gabapentin, and topiramate may reduce seizure activity and hence the efficacy of ECT. Carbamazepine may prolong the action of succinylcholine. Patient on long-term carbamazepine therapy can develop resistance to nondepolarizing neuromuscular blocking agents except mivacurium. Increasing the dose may be required to achieve complete neuromuscular blockade in these patients. ECT in patients taking lithium increases the risk of delirium. ECT and calcium channel antagonists should be used with care to avoid cardiovascular depression. Barbiturates, propofol, or benzodiazepines in patients receiving MAOIs may result in hypotension and exaggeration of the CNS and respiratory depressant effects. MAOI also interacts with Demerol and ephedrine and can lead to a potentially fatal hypertensive crisis.

Intraprocedure

ECT may be bilateral, right unilateral, or bifrontal depending upon where the electrodes are placed. Bilateral or bitemporal ECT is the most common type administered in urgent situations. Right unilateral may be associated with less amnesia and may be selected in patients where this is of significant concern. If unilateral treatment is ineffective after 3–5 treatments, the treatment may be changed to bilateral ECT. The dose of electric stimulus can be variable but is usually administered as a pulse in the range of 0.5 to 2.0 ms. Most treatments will begin by establishing the lowest possible dose needed to induce a seizure; this is considered the seizure threshold. During ensuing treatments the dose is adjusted to deliver 1.5–2 times the seizure threshold for bilateral treatments. Up to six times the threshold dose may be needed for right unilateral treatments, and it is common in both types of treatment for the seizure threshold to go up during the course of ECT treatment. This may require an incremental upward adjustment of the dose. Older individuals and men, in particular, may have a higher seizure threshold requiring larger initial electrical pulses.

All patients receive a general anesthetic, and ASA standard monitoring of vital signs is required; invasive monitoring is rarely needed. The EEG (electroencephalogram) is monitored continuously during ECT to confirm seizure activity and to document the duration of seizure. The EEG is recorded on one or two channels, and a paper record of the seizure is frequently printed either during or following the treatment. The duration of the tonic-clonic portion of the seizure is noted. This may be done using EMG, but more commonly a tourniquet is placed around one of the patient's ankles before the administration of the succinylcholine or the chosen muscle relaxant to isolate the foot from the muscle relaxant. The duration of the tonic-clonic movements in the foot is generally recorded by nursing staff.

ECT requires a very brief general anesthetic, and a total intravenous anesthetic technique is preferred. Following preoxygenation and intravenous induction, bag-mask ventilation with supplemental oxygen is started. Hyperventilation is frequently performed to produce cerebral hypocarbia. The hypocarbia can increase the intensity of the ensuing seizure. Neuromuscular blocking agents are used to prevent skeletal muscle contraction and possible injury during seizures. A soft bite block is used to avoid tongue biting or dental injury; this should be placed just before the electrical stimulus is given.

Appropriate resuscitative equipment including a suction device must be available prior to induction of anesthesia. Although intubation is not generally required, a

Table 19.2 Dose of drugs recommended for ECT by the American Psychiatric Association

Drugs	Doses
Methohexital	0.75–1.0 mg/kg
Thiopental	1.5–2.5 mg/kg
Thiamylal	1.5–2.5 mg/kg
Etomidate	0.15–0.3 mg/kg
Propofol	0.75 mg/kg
Ketamine	0.5–2.0 mg/kg
Succinylcholine	0.75–1.0 mg/kg
Mivacurium	0.15–0.2 mg/kg

laryngoscope, endotracheal tube, and laryngeal mask airway should be available for management of an airway emergency. An oral airway may be needed in obese patients or those who are difficult to mask ventilate; this should be exchanged for the soft bite block prior to inducing a seizure to avoid injury to the teeth from the hard oral airway.

Induction Agents

Small to moderate doses of methohexital and propofol have been used for induction. Methohexital (0.75–1 mg/kg) remains the most widely used induction agent for ECT and is considered the "gold standard" against which all other anesthetics are compared. Propofol has anticonvulsant properties that may limit its effectiveness for ECT. Etomidate may be used in select patients, especially those with a significant cardiac history, and it has little effect on seizure duration. To optimize the seizure duration, the dose of the induction agent may need to be reduced or adjusted during the treatment course (Table 19.2).

Muscle Relaxant

Succinylcholine remains the most commonly used muscle relaxant to limit the motor seizure activity and reduce the potential for injury. This is most important in older patients with significant osteoporosis and arthritis. If succinylcholine is contraindicated, mivacurium or rocuronium may be substituted. A small single dose of vecuronium has been used for pretreatment in patients with severe succinylcholine-induced myalgias. In elderly patients it is very important to establish that the patient has completely recovered from the effects of the muscle relaxant. Weakness secondary to residual muscle relaxation in older patients can lead to hypoventilation and subsequent hypoxia and hypercarbia.

Seizure Duration

The goal of ECT treatment is to induce a grand mal type seizure that lasts 15–70 s on the EEG. Patients having a seizure duration of less than 15 s achieve a less favorable response to ECT. In some patients, it can be difficult to induce a seizure. A period of hyperventilation before treatment can lower the seizure threshold which can help these patients. Other strategies to obtain a seizure or lengthen the seizure include the preprocedure reduction of the dose of psychotropic medications and reduction of the induction dose of the anesthetic agent. Pretreatment with caffeine is no longer recommended.

Seizures that last longer than 120 s have been associated with serious injury including increased cognitive impairment. A prolonged seizure can generally be terminated with a small dose of propofol or a benzodiazepine.

Record Keeping

ECT treatment consists of a series of treatments, and the anesthetic chart can be used to communicate the success or limitations for the prior treatment. The dose of all the anesthetic drugs used, the patient's response, and seizure duration should be documented and signed. In the event of either a short or prolonged seizure, the remedy and recommendations for the next treatment should be documented for the next provider. Any other information pertinent to future treatment should also be noted such as the difficulty of the airway or the occurrence of post-ECT symptoms.

Adverse Effects

Fortunately, the most significant cardiovascular events such as asystole and ventricular tachycardia are usually transient. Other complications include prolonged seizures, prolonged apnea, emergent mania, and cognitive dysfunction. The most common adverse effect of ECT is a transient loss of memory. Older people treated with ECT have more severe memory deficits and cognitive dysfunction than younger individuals. Orientation and memory function should be assessed prior to each ECT and periodically during the course to monitor the presence of ECT-related memory issues.

Postanesthesia Recovery Period

Patients are usually monitored for 1–2 h by qualified nursing staff prior to discharge to their inpatient room or home. The most marked cognitive impairment in the elderly is characterized by periods of disorientation immediately postictally.

These effects are usually short lived and resolve over time. Rarely, patients develop postictal delirium which presents as agitation, aggression, and restlessness. This behavior usually responds to a low-dose benzodiazepine like midazolam (0.5–1 mg) intravenously. Increasing (or decreasing) the dose of the succinylcholine and adding a small bolus of methohexital (10 mg IV) at the end of the seizure may also be helpful in reducing the incidence of post-ECT agitation. Allowing the patient to rest in quiet surroundings in the immediate post-seizure period minimizes these episodes.

Headaches occur in up to 45% of patients receiving ECT. Patients in whom a post-ECT headache is significant may benefit from a single prophylactic dose of IV ketorolac 15 mg provided there is no contraindication to its use.

Summary

ECT provides a valuable method for the treatment of depression in the elderly population. The anesthesiologist's role is critical for the successful delivery of treatment.

Key Points

- Depression in the elderly is a growing public health problem and is frequently undiagnosed and untreated.
- ECT is a way of inducing grand mal type seizures by electrical stimulation applied to the scalp; the exact mechanism of how ECT works to reduce depressive symptoms is not fully understood.
- ECT in elderly patients is one of the most controversial treatments in all of medicine; however, age should not be considered a contraindication for ECT.
- ECT treatment in elderly patient can be very successful.
- ECT requires the administration of a general anesthesia, and coexisting medical or surgical conditions should be assessed and stabilized prior to treatment.
- Cardiovascular responses are secondary to autonomic nervous system stimulation and release of catecholamines.
- Intracranial tumor with evidence of raised intracranial tension is the only absolute contraindication to ECT.
- The goals for anesthetic management include premedication to attenuate the physiological effects of ECT, a rapid induction and recovery.
- The optimal EEG-documented seizure activity lasts between 20 and 70 s. The motor seizure is generally 30% shorter than the EEG seizure.
- Methohexital remains the most widely used induction agent for ECT and is considered the "gold standard." Succinylcholine is the most commonly used muscle relaxant for reduction of ECT-induced seizure.

Suggested Reading

Alexopoulos GS. Depression in the elderly. Lancet. 2005;365:1961–1970.
American Psychiatric Association Committee on Electroconvulsive Therapy. The practice of electroconvulsive therapy:recommendations for treatment, training, and privileging. 2nd ed. Washington, DC:American Psychiatric Association, 2001.
Boylan LS, Haskett RF, Mulsant BH, et al. Determinants of seizure threshold in ECT:benzodiazepine use, anesthetic dosage, and other factors. J ECT. 2000;16:3–18.
Dolenc TJ, Barnes RD, Hayes DL, Rasmussen KG. Electroconvulsive therapy in patients with cardiac pacemakers and implantable cardioverter defibrillators. Pacing ClinElectrophysiol. 2004;27:1257–1263.
Flint AJ, Rifat SL. The Treatment of Psychotic Depression in Later Life:A Comparison of Pharmacotherapy and ECT. Int J Geriatr Psychiatry. 1998;13:23–28.
Folk JW, Kellner CH, Beale MD, Conroy JM, Duc TA. Anesthesia for electroconvulsive therapy:a review. J ECT. 2000;16:157–170.
Kadoi Y, Saito S, Seki S, et al. Electroconvulsive therapy impairs systolic performance of the left ventricle. Can J Anaesth. 2001;48:405–8.
Larsen JR, Hein L, Stromgren LS. Ventricular tachycardia with ECT. J ECT. 1998;14:109–14.
McCall WV. Asystole in electroconvulsive therapy:report of four cases. J Clin Psychiatry. 1996;57:199–203.
Ng C, Schweitzer I, Alexopoulos P, et al. Efficacy and cognitive effects of right unilateral electroconvulsive therapy. J ECT. 2000;16:370–9.
Navines R, Bernardo M, Martinez-Palli G, et al. Optimization of electroconvulsive therapy:strategies for an adequate convulsion—role of caffeine. ActasEspPsiquiatr. 2000;28:194–201.
Saito S, Kadoi Y, Iriuchijima N, et al. Reduction of cerebral hyperemia with anti-hypertensive medication after electroconvulsive therapy. Can J Anaesth. 2000;47:767–74.
Swartz CM. Physiological response to ECT stimulus dose. Psychiatry Res. 2000;97:229–35.
Zielinski RJ, Roose SP, Devanand DP, Woodring S, Sackeim HA. Cardiovascular complications of ECT in depressed patients with cardiac disease. Am J Psychiatry. 1993;150:904–909.

Chapter 20
Ophthalmologic Surgery and the Management of Diabetes

Mary Ann Vann

Ophthalmologic procedures are the most common ambulatory surgeries for geriatric patients. In developed countries throughout the world, cataract surgery is the most frequently performed surgical procedure. As the incidence of diabetes increases in the population, retina surgery is also becoming more common.

Modern Cataract and Retina Surgery: General Information

In many ways ophthalmologic surgery is different than most other procedures. While the surgery is limited anatomically, manipulation of the eye can have systemic effects. A unique situation exists for the patient: they need to be cooperative yet remain still while the eye remains immobile during these delicate procedures. Even miniscule movements are noticeable as the surgery is done under a microscope. Although rare, the consequences of surgical misadventure are great, potentially leading to blindness.

Cataract surgery has undergone significant advances in recent years. Phacoemulsification cataract removal and foldable intraocular lenses have altered the procedure dramatically. Extracapsular cataract extractions are done only rarely now. During phacoemulsification the lens is broken up with ultrasound waves and the fragments are suctioned out. The surgeon utilizes two tiny incisions on opposite sides of the pupil, and when the instruments are in place, the surgeon can manually restrict eye movements. Often these incisions do not require suture closure. There is lesser need for lowered intraocular pressure (IOP) and akinesia of the eye during phacoemulsification procedures as opposed to other eye surgeries. As for most eye

M.A. Vann, MD (✉)
Department of Anesthesia, Pain, and Critical Care, Harvard Medical School, Beth Israel Deaconess Medical Center, 330 Brookline Ave, Boston, MA 02215, USA
e-mail: mvann@bidmc.harvard.edu

S.R. Barnett (ed.), *Manual of Geriatric Anesthesia*, DOI 10.1007/978-1-4614-3888-5_20,

surgeries, dilation of the pupil is necessary for this procedure. Phenylephrine is the most frequently utilized drug for this purpose and is administered in the holding area prior to surgery.

During ophthalmologic surgery there is always the possibility that patients may notice the bright light of the microscope. In addition, the ultrasound waves of the phacoemulsification may themselves create visual images for the patient. Several articles have displayed colorful artistic renderings produced by patients to illustrate their visual experiences during cataract extraction by phacoemulsification. Phenomena perceived by patients include lights, colors, shapes, and even operating instruments. These visual experiences occur more frequently during topical anesthesia as compared to peribulbar block anesthesia for the eye. Up to 16% of patients have described their visual experiences during ophthalmologic surgery as frightening. Preoperative education on what to expect during this surgery can allay these patient fears.

Retinal procedures include vitrectomies, scleral buckle, and laser treatments of the retina. These are most often performed for diabetic retinal disease and detached retinas. Complications of cataract surgery such as retained lens fragments may also require vitrectomy. Posterior chamber surgeries usually require block anesthesia.

Scleral buckle, a procedure for detached retina, is done on the surface of the globe, altering the shape of the eye to allow the detached retina to adhere. Occasionally a gas or oil bubble is introduced into the posterior chamber to compress the repaired retina against the back of the eye as an aid to healing. Once a patient receives such an injection, they need to keep their head in a certain position to maintain the proper location of the bubble in the eye. Often this is a face-down position. Gas injection into the eye places the patient at risk in situations where changes in pressure may occur such as during air travel or after administration of nitrous oxide. The patient wears a warning bracelet while the gas bubble is present in the eye.

During eye surgery, increased IOP may need to be reduced acutely. Intravenous Acetazolamide is often utilized for this purpose. This drug has a potential risk of expansion of intravascular volume and may precipitate pulmonary vascular congestion in susceptible patients. Rarely allergic reactions to Acetazolamide may occur.

After surgery, a protective shield usually covers the operative eye. This is to prevent injury such as corneal abrasion to the anesthetized eye and minimize possibility of disruption of incisions or introduction of infection. After topical anesthesia, this is often a clear shield, as the patient can see immediately after surgery. However, after an eye block, the patient is unable to focus. Usually the ophthalmologist examines the patient in the office on the day following surgery and removes the shield.

Preoperative Considerations

The preoperative evaluation of patients undergoing cataract surgery was revolutionized by a single study published by Schein in 2000. This Study of Medical Testing for Cataract Surgery (SMTCS) enrolled almost 20,000 patients. They concluded that as long as a patient undergoes routine medical care, they do not need any additional medical testing prior to cataract surgery. These findings were confirmed by the Cochrane Collaboration in 2009. A main point of emphasis about the STMCS is that all these patients received adequate care for their preexisting conditions and underwent medical testing when indicated. The Cochrane findings were dominated by the SMTCS as the two other comparable studies on preoperative evaluation only involved 2,300 patients. The Cochrane publication examined major outcomes and determined that there was no ability of the preoperative evaluation to predict perioperative events. They also determined that the majority of events occurred intraoperatively and were minor, such as hypertension and arrhythmias. The three studies covered by the Cochrane publication only considered patients undergoing local or regional anesthesia for the eye with or without sedation. Patients undergoing general anesthesia for cataract or retina surgery have been found to be more likely to have ischemic events. While most ischemia occurred during the intraoperative period, it was detected on Holter monitor for up to 24 h following surgery. Ischemic events were more common in diabetic patients undergoing retina surgery regardless of type of anesthesia.

Patients often present for ophthalmologic surgery with elevated blood pressures. A recent study found that patients presenting with elevated blood pressures, even without known hypertension, did not suffer any higher incidence of perioperative events up to 1 h postoperatively.

When any patient is not required to have a preoperative visit, as is true for many cataract surgery cases, there must be an adequate way to assure that the patient receives the proper instructions for fasting and medications preoperatively. This is especially important for the elderly patient with some cognitive impairment.

Preoperative Medications

Usually all preoperative prescription medications are continued up to and including the day of surgery. Oftentimes diuretics are held for patient comfort. There is general agreement that cataract patients on anticoagulants, such as aspirin or Coumadin, can continue them in the perioperative period. While topical anesthesia may be preferable for these patients, they can nonetheless undergo blocks without higher risk of retrobulbar hematoma, which is more attributable to vascular fragility rather than anticoagulant use. Stronger antiplatelet agents such as clopidogrel may require special considerations.

NPO

A practice of allowing relaxed fasting requirements prior to cataract surgery has crept into the ophthalmologic community over the last 10 years. In 2009 a study on the practice of suspending NPO requirements for cataract surgery was published.

This was a retrospective review of a single anesthesiologist's experience with 5,125 cases done under topical anesthesia. Fifty percent of these patients received IV sedation. The absence of events of aspiration was ascertained by review of the anesthesiologist's and surgeons' recollections and hospital admissions for pneumonia. However, aspiration is a rare occurrence even in general anesthesia patients, so a much larger population would be required to detect the true incidence of this event.

In general, cataract patients receiving anesthesia care should follow the ASA published guidelines for NPO and fasting until further data is available.

Perioperative Management of Diabetes for Patients Undergoing Ambulatory Surgery

While the incidence of diabetes is rising in the general population, the increase is even more substantial in the geriatric population. The presence of diabetes makes it more likely that the geriatric patient will require some type of surgery. This fact is especially true for cataract and retina procedures.

Diabetic patients benefit from scheduling as first case of the day. This allows a patient to experience minimal disruptions of their usual food and insulin schedules. In the case of early morning surgeries, usual insulin doses may be delayed and administered at normal levels prior to or immediately after surgery depending on the patient's blood sugar and anticipated length of the case. Normal meals are usually resumed promptly after ophthalmologic surgery.

Glucose Management

The perioperative management of blood glucose is controversial in general, but the management of diabetes and glucose has not been studied specifically in ambulatory patients. Management strategies instead must be gleaned from knowledge of routine treatments for diabetes as well as studies concerning glucose control for the critically ill. There are specific considerations for ambulatory surgery to be considered in the geriatric patients. For example the elderly diabetic patient has an exaggerated risk of hypoglycemia due to fewer symptoms. The psychosocial situations of elderly diabetic patients can be very challenging, and the delivery of clear instructions on perioperative medications and food intake for these patients is vital. There should also be an assessment of the patient's ability to understand the instructions, test their own blood glucose, and act in case of hypoglycemia. Additional comorbid conditions in older diabetic patients place them at higher risk for complications especially in light of the perioperative prothrombotic state that is worsened by hyperglycemia. Fortunately most ophthalmologic surgery is relatively low stress for patients, resulting in lower incidence of hyperglycemia and cardiac events than more invasive procedures.

Point-of-care glucometers are adequate for testing of perioperative blood sugars. All patients requiring medications for treatment of diabetes should have preoperative and postoperative glucose measurements. It is useful to know the patient's HbA1c value as this value can help guide decisions, for example, regarding case cancelation on the day of surgery for hyperglycemia or perioperative correction of blood glucose with insulin. Acute reductions of a patient's usual blood sugar can be harmful by causing systemic oxidative stress. Also some chronically hyperglycemic patients may experience hypoglycemic symptoms at normal blood glucose values.

All diabetic patients should be encouraged to bring their medications with them on the day of surgery to facilitate proper identification and administration of these agents. Also, diabetic patients should travel with their glucometers and receive instructions regarding suitable treatments for hypoglycemia, such as clear juices. Glucose tablets are particulate and should be avoided in the fasting patient.

Oral Agents

Type 2 diabetic patients on oral hypoglycemics are relatively easy to manage during ambulatory surgery. Oral hypoglycemics are held on the day of surgery only and may be restarted once the patient is able to eat. Even metformin does not pose any special risks for the patient undergoing ophthalmologic surgery, so it can be taken up to the day of surgery. Most oral medications have a low risk of causing hypoglycemic reactions, as noted in Table 20.1. Non-insulin injectable hypoglycemics such as exenatide and pramlintide are also held on the day of surgery until food intake resumes.

Insulin

Both type 1 and type 2 diabetic patients taking insulin pose a greater challenge. One must be clear of the exact type of insulin these geriatric patients are taking. Often, older patients use prefilled insulin pens. These relatively easy-to-use pens look alike, and their contents may sound alike, e.g., Humalog and Humalog Mix.

Patients taking insulin usually follow one of two modes of treatment. Basal–bolus regimens attempt to duplicate the body's normal insulin release and provide better glucose control. The basal component mimics the background or non-nutritional insulin needs while the patient administers the bolus component as required to cover food intake. The basal component should constitute approximately one-half of the total daily dose of insulin. Long-acting peakless insulins such as glargine or detemir, when comprising 50% of the total daily insulin, should not cause hypoglycemia even during fasting. Thus they can often be maintained at normal doses on the day of surgery, or reduced to 75% of usual amounts (see Table 20.2). Rapid-acting insulins, such as lispro or aspart, utilized for nutritional insulin boluses, are

Table 20.1 Oral and injectable hypoglycemics

Drug class examples	Action	Adverse effects	Risk of hypoglycemia
Oral medications			
Biguanide Metformin	Antihyperglycemic, decreases glucose production, increases insulin action	Lactic acidosis in susceptible patients (renal failure), certain cases (radiologic)	No
Meglitinides Repaglinide, nateglinide	Stimulate insulin release from beta cells	Hypoglycemia	Yes—moderate risk
Sulfonylureas First generation: chlorpropamide, tolbutamide Second generation: glyburide, glipizide, glimepiride	Stimulate insulin release from beta cells	Hypoglycemic effects for 12–24 h: Glimepiride more likely than glyburide	Yes—highest risk
Thiazolidinediones Pioglitazone, rosiglitazone	Decreases insulin resistance, glucose production	Hepatotoxicity, fluid retention, cardiac events	No
Alpha-glucosidase inhibitors Acarbose, miglitol	Reduces intestinal absorption of starch, disaccharides	Gastrointestinal symptoms	No
Dipeptidyl peptidase-4 (DPP-4) inhibitors Sitagliptin, saxagliptin, linagliptin	An incretin drug: increases insulin production, decreases glucose production	Respiratory tract infection	No
Injectable medications (not insulin)			
Exenatide	An incretin drug: increases insulin production, decreases glucose production	Gastrointestinal symptoms	Yes, when combined with sulfonylureas
Pramlintide	An incretin drug, analog of amylin: increases insulin production, decreases glucose production	Gastrointestinal symptoms	Yes

less likely to cause unexpected hypoglycemia due to the short time (30 min) to peak effect. Another basal–bolus regimen is continuous subcutaneous insulin infusion delivered by an insulin pump. These pumps are the most physiologic way to administer insulin as they may be programmed to deliver various basal rates as well as boluses of rapid-acting insulin on demand when the patient eats. Surgical patients can maintain their pumps on a "sick day" basal rate while fasting, and the pump can remain on throughout the procedure. This is especially true for eye surgery, as customary pump placement sites are far away from the surgical field.

Many type 2 diabetic patients today utilize insulin as part of a less rigorous regimen such as basal insulins only (no nutritional insulin) or scheduled doses of fixed combination insulins (such as NPH and regular insulin) as a supplement to oral hypoglycemics. These insulin regimens place a patient at risk of hypoglycemia perioperatively if maintained at usual doses. Basal (peakless) insulins taken alone or peaked insulins, such as NPH, should be reduced on the day of surgery to approximately 50% to simulate basal activity only. Fixed combination insulins such as 75/25 NPH/Regular or Humalog Mix (75% lispro protamine, 25% lispro) need to be reduced as well. Ideally the patient should receive a partial dose of only the longer-acting component, e.g., NPH or lispro protamine. However, this may not be easily accomplished outside of the hospital or surgery center. Patients utilizing the fixed combination insulins often do not possess NPH insulin alone, and lispro protamine is not available outside the mix. On the day of surgery, NPH may be substituted for the lispro protamine component. Usually NPH is dosed at 50% of its usual amount (i.e., 50% of 75% of the units of 75/25 mix insulin administered). These changes in insulin dosage are best administered to the patient once they reach the facility.

Correction of hyperglycemia on the day of surgery should be done with subcutaneous doses of rapid-acting insulin (lispro or aspart) which act reliably and are easily administered by patients, nurses, or physicians. Patients should not be discharged home from the facility until the peak effect for correction doses of insulin has passed. For rapid-acting insulins, this is less than 1 h.

Methods of Local/Regional Anesthesia for the Eye

Risks

In almost all ophthalmologic surgery cases, the patient receives local or regional anesthesia for the eye. The patient's experience during eye surgery varies with the type of local or regional used.

Objectives for the local or regional anesthesia for ophthalmologic surgery include anesthesia of the conjunctiva and globe, elimination of intraoperative and postoperative pain, akinesia of the globe and orbicularis oculi, and reduction in IOP. Typical injection blocks include retrobulbar and peribulbar blocks, where

Table 20.2 Insulin preparations and day of surgery management recommendations

Type of insulin	Onset (O) and duration(D) of action	Day before surgery dosing	Day of surgery dosing
Basal insulin (part of basal–bolus regimen)			
Glargine	O: 2–5 h D: 5–24 h	Basal insulin should be maintained, if history of hypoglycemia, can reduce to 75%. Pump at sick day basal rate	Basal insulin should be maintained, pump at sick day basal rate Check BS frequently (every 1–2 h)
Detemir	O: 3–4 h D: 5–25 h		
CSII (insulin pump)	Continuous, usually rapid-acting insulin		
Nutritional insulin			
Lispro	O: 15 min D: 30–90 min	No change	Restart nutritional insulin when food intake resumes, can also be given to correct hyperglycemia
Aspart	Same as above		
Glulisine	Same as above		
Regular (subq dosing)	O: 30 min D: 90 min–4 h		
Intermediate or fixed combination insulin			
NPH	O: 2–4 h D: 6–12 h	Nighttime doses can be given as usual or reduced by up to 50%, dependent on whether patient experiences hypoglycemia during sleep or when morning meal omitted	Morning doses of intermediate insulins can be given in full for early case when food intake expected at normal time, can be reduced by up to 50% for later cases. For fixed combinations, only intermediate insulin portion should usually be given and reduced as above
70/30 NPH/Regular	O: 30–90 min D: 6–12 h		
70/30 Lispro/Lispro Protamine (or Aspart Mix)	O: 15 min D: 14–20 h		
50/50 NPH/Regular	O: 30–90 min D: 6–12 h		
Basal insulin solely (Pt takes NO other insulin)			
Glargine	O: 2–5 h D: 5–24 h	Usual nighttime doses can be given or reduced by up to 50%, dependent on whether patient experiences hypoglycemia when morning meal missed	Morning doses can be given in full for early case when food intake expected at normal time, can be reduced by up to 50% for later cases
Detemir	O: 3–4 h D: 5–24 h		

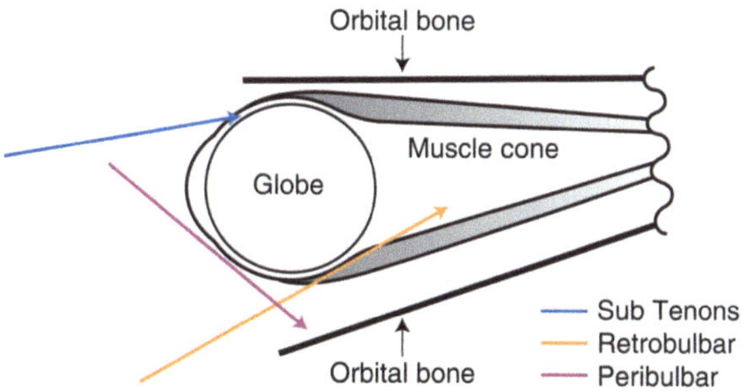

Fig. 20.1 Schematic of various eye blocks

local anesthetic is injected within the muscle cone or into the peribulbar space, respectively (Fig. 20.1). Sometimes these blocks are done in combination as well. Anesthesia personnel often perform these blocks in the holding area prior to entering the OR. Once the eye is blocked, the oculocardiac reflex will not occur. Some practitioners choose to place pressure on the eye immediately after injection either manually or with a Honan device to enhance spread of the block. If the block is not yet established, however, this pressure can cause bradycardia. The placement of injection blocks is painful, but they provide good analgesia and akinesia during the procedure. Occasionally a separate facial nerve block is administered to limit eyelid function. This injection is often more uncomfortable for the patient than block placement.

Risks of injection blocks are dependent on the skill and experience of the person performing them. Globe perforation and/or rupture is related to operator inexperience and also the axial length of the eye. The block needle can injure extraocular muscles. Seizures or brainstem anesthesia can occur if local anesthesia travels to the brain along the optic nerve or retrograde within the vascular system. The risk of retrobulbar hemorrhage is low. It has been reported as approximately 1/1,000. The main risk for hemorrhage is arterial fragility, which is increased in the elderly and in diabetic patients. If retrobulbar hemorrhage is suspected, the first response is placement of pressure on the globe.

A sub-Tenon's block is usually done on the surgical field by the surgeon. Tenon's capsule is a fascial sheath surrounding the globe. Beneath the episcleral region is a potential space called sub-Tenon's space. After local anesthesia is applied to the surface of the eye, the surgeon raises a flap and enters the sub-Tenon's space with a blunt cannula and administers the local anesthesia. Injection techniques for this block have also been described. In some centers the anesthesiologists may perform a sub-Tenon's block by injection. A sub-Tenon's block delivers good analgesia to the globe due to circumferential spread. Akinesia of the globe can be achieved with larger volumes of local anesthesia. Patients may feel an uncomfortable pressure sensation during injection in the sub-Tenon's space, especially when large volumes are given.

The local anesthetics utilized for eye blocks most often are lidocaine, bupivacaine, or a mix of the two. Hyaluronidase is often added to hasten onset and to improve quality of the block. With this additive, a good efficacy can be achieved utilizing lower volumes of local anesthesia. There is a small risk of allergic reactions to hyaluronidase.

As many as 60% of cataract surgeries are currently performed under topical anesthesia. Topical anesthesia involves application of local anesthesia as drops or gels to the surface of the eye. This technique does not limit the patient's extraocular movements. Some operators have reported improved pain control after supplemental intracameral injection of local anesthesia. Reports of transient vision loss after intracameral injection have been attributed to retinal dysfunction caused by the local anesthetic. During topical anesthesia, patients may feel pain during iris manipulation, globe expansion, and lens implantation. Lowering the microscope's light intensity may decrease patient complaints of light sensitivity during topical anesthesia. Increased sensations during topical anesthesia often translate into increased sedation requirements. Patients undergoing topical anesthesia may encounter additional surgical risks due to lack of akinesia, including an increased need for anterior vitrectomy due to posterior capsule rupture during cataract surgery. Cases of endophthalmitis have been attributed to local anesthetics applied to the eye, especially in gel form. The surgeon can identify patients who will not likely tolerate the increased sensations during topical anesthesia prior to surgery. Those unable to cooperate with eye measurements done in the office which require local anesthesia and contact with the eye will not endure surgery under topical anesthesia.

Several direct comparisons of patient experiences during injection blocks and topical anesthesia have been published. In one of the most interesting, 98 patients underwent bilateral cataract surgeries 1 week apart. They were randomized to receive topical anesthesia for one surgery and a combined peribulbar and retrobulbar block for the other. Seventy patients preferred the block, while 18 patients had no preference. Only ten patients preferred topical anesthesia, and all had topical anesthesia for their first cataract procedure. A recent study compared retrobulbar block, sub-Tenon's block, and topical anesthesia. All patients received patient-controlled sedation with propofol and remifentanil. Patients who had a retrobulbar block utilized the least amount of sedation, but they reported the most pain during block placement and experienced elevations in blood pressure and heart rate during the injection. Patients who had topical anesthesia reported the most intraoperative and postoperative pain and had the highest usage of patient-controlled sedation. Sub-Tenon's block provided the highest patient satisfaction scores. Another study compared the light sensitivity and pain perceptions during cataract surgery under sub-Tenon's block as compared to topical anesthesia with intracameral injection. Forty-four percent of patients with topical anesthesia reported light sensitivity, while 78% of patients with sub-Tenon's blocks reported no light sensitivity. Pain was minimal under sub-Tenon's block: 89% of patients reported no pain, and 11% reported only minimal pain. For patients under topical anesthesia, 33% had no pain, 33% reported minimal pain, 20% had mild pain, and 7% described moderate pain. Interestingly in this study, the surgical procedures done under sub-Tenon's block took longer than those under topical. Surgeons have previously reported

Table 20.3 Comparison of topical and blocks for cataract surgery

Type of block	Discomfort during placement	Intraoperative pain/ sensations	Eye movement capability	Postoperative pain
Topical	Minimal	++	+++	+
Sub-Tenon's	+	Minimal	Minimal	Minimal
Peribulbar	++	Minimal	None	Minimal
Retrobulbar	++	Minimal	None	Minimal

Range of comparative values: none to +++
Note: This table is based on a summary of findings from multiple publications; there is no single comparison of all four modalities

better operating conditions under blocks as compared to topical anesthesia, probably due to the akinesia and reduced IOP with blocks (Table 20.3).

Sedation for Ophthalmologic Surgery

The need for sedation during ophthalmologic surgery varies with the type of local or regional anesthesia utilized. Pain on injection of a block, light sensitivity, intraoperative and postoperative discomfort, and duration of surgery all influence a patient's need for sedation during ophthalmologic surgery.

Administration of sedation to geriatric patients is significantly more complicated than for younger patients. There are special risks to older patients not only during the procedure but also upon returning home from ambulatory surgery, such as the ability to conduct their activities of daily living.

The geriatric patient's risks for sedation must be considered. A review of Monitored Anesthesia Care (MAC) cases in the ASA Closed Claim Database showed that elderly patients were more likely to be harmed by sedation than younger patients. A fifth of these MAC claims occurred during ophthalmologic surgery. MAC claims had a higher percentage of patients with higher ASA physical status, 3 or 4, than general anesthesia claims. Events in geriatric patients were also more likely to occur when two or more classes of drugs were utilized for sedation. Elevated risks were ascribed to head and neck procedures during which the surgical draping can decrease the ability to detect hypoventilation and also allow carbon dioxide to accumulate. The use of ETCO2 monitoring can alleviate these risks.

Levels of sedation for ophthalmologic surgery range from none to minimal to temporarily deep. While anxiolysis is the main goal, some patients also desire amnesia or somnolence. The anesthesiologist, however, must maintain verbal communication with the patient in most cases. A patient who is oversedated or confused may move unexpectedly, leading to eye injury and usually blindness. Success with any type of anxiolysis or sedation is always partially dependent on patient expectations.

The ideal sedative for ophthalmologic surgery has rapid onset and short duration. Additional desirable characteristics for the geriatric patient include the lack of accumulation and predictability. All sedation regimens must be individualized to the patient, and even minimal sedation of a patient with dementia may lead to loss of cooperation. Even with sedation, certain patients may be unable to remain still during ophthalmologic surgery due to tremors, arthritis, or even dysuria. Fortunately, most eye procedures are relatively brief, so positioning issues are less significant. Some centers provide cataract surgery patients with music, utilize relaxation techniques, verbal reassurances, distraction methods, and/or handholding.

Benzodiazepines, usually midazolam, are frequently employed as first-line sedative drugs for eye surgery. Midazolam acts rapidly and is short acting, and pharmacological reversal is possible with flumazenil. There are no reports of cognitive dysfunction due to benzodiazepines in cataract surgery patients, probably due to a combination of a brief procedure, low doses, the patient's prompt return to home, and familiar surroundings after eye surgery.

Propofol is the most commonly employed hypnotic drug for ophthalmologic surgery. It is particularly useful for patients who want to be completely unaware of injection of the block. Onset of a bolus injection is 30 s, while its duration is 3–10 min. For eye surgery, propofol has the advantages of decreasing IOP and preventing nausea and vomiting. Disadvantages include patient movement during the block injection, which is not indicative of patient recall, and sneezing. Doses range from 0.5 to 1 mg/kg to an elaborate formula by Hocking and Balmer based on patient age and weight.

Ketamine is still occasionally used for sedation during eye cases. The peak effect is 2–4 min after a bolus of 10–50 mg. However, ketamine increases IOP and can have lasting effects including delirium.

A popular newer agent used for sedation during eye surgery is the opioid remifentanil. This drug has extremely rapid onset and a short duration due to plasma elimination. Remifentanil delivers intense analgesia resulting in minimal patient movement during block placement, but it does not eliminate patient recall. When administered solely at a dose of 0.3 mcg/kg, respiratory depression does not occur. However, at higher doses, or when combined with other drugs, profound respiratory depression, bradycardia, and hypotension have been reported. Occasionally, opioids, including remifentanil, cause nausea and vomiting. This is a serious concern in the eye surgery patient, as vomiting elevates IOP.

Dexmedetomidine, a selective alpha-2 agonist, has been studied for use during eye surgery. Advantages of dexmedetomidine include anxiolytic, sedative, and analgesic effects while the patient remains cooperative. It also reduces IOP. However, the long half-life and sympatholytic effects, causing significant drops in heart rate and blood pressure, are distinct disadvantages to use during eye surgery. If used at all, it should be reserved for difficult to sedate patients, or those unable to tolerate traditional agents.

The use of patient-controlled sedation for eye surgery has been described in the literature. Single agents such as midazolam, fentanyl, and propofol have been utilized, as well as drug combinations such as propofol and remifentanil. Today it is a costly and uncommon means of sedation for ophthalmologic surgery.

Occasionally a patient requires general anesthesia for eye surgery; often this is done for a movement disorder or cognitive impairment that does not allow the patient to lie still and remain cooperative during surgery. While the patient may be unconscious, unexpected movements such as coughing and bucking may occur, which could cause eye injury. If the eye is blocked in addition to the general anesthesia, it is less likely that the patient would move due to manipulations of the eye, or experience the oculocardiac reflex.

Outcomes After Ophthalmologic Surgery

Few studies have addressed whether there are measurable differences in outcomes such as pain, adverse events, and surgical complications that make one sedation regimen or regional anesthesia technique superior to the others. Adverse events due to sedation were examined for the patients in the SMTCS. The odds ratio for an adverse event rose sharply when more than one class of sedation drugs were used. However the majority of these events were minor, and there was not an increased risk of death or hospitalization for these patients. The Agency for Healthcare Research and Quality (AHRQ) found only weak evidence that sedation during eye surgery improved anxiety control, pain relief, or patient satisfaction. They found no evidence that any sedation technique resulted in a better outcome than any other.

Patient satisfaction scores for patients undergoing cataract surgery in a Canadian community hospital were published by Fung et al. Surgeries were performed under topical anesthesia, and most patients received bolus sedation with midazolam, 70% received fentanyl, 24% propofol, and less than 5% had remifentanil. The main finding of the study concerned the patients' regard for the role of the anesthesiologist, which was higher in the postoperative interview. In addition, 92% of patients indicated that there was nothing about their care that they would have changed. These authors felt their data supported the need for sedation during cataract surgery to relieve perioperative pain and to meet the needs of patients.

Overall patient satisfaction is high for eye surgery. Predictors of lower satisfaction scores in eye surgery patients include postoperative pain, preoperative anxiety, and the surgeon.

Future Trends for Anesthesia for Ophthalmologic Surgery

Sedation and regional anesthesia protocols for ophthalmologic surgery vary according to location in this country and worldwide. It is anticipated that the new surgical techniques in cataract surgery will result in expansion into developing countries where cataracts are a major cause of blindness. Some of the major stimulants for this growth include the use of minimal incision phacoemulsification techniques and topical anesthesia. It is anticipated that these new techniques will reduce costs.

Anesthesiologist's Role

The need for an anesthesiologist during a cataract procedure has been questioned. The presence or absence of anesthesia personnel during cataract surgery varied geographically in developed countries prior to the use of phacoemulsification. For example, in a study during the last decade, anesthesia presence during cataract surgery was common in the USA and Australia but rare in Scandinavia. However before eliminating the presence of the anesthesiologist for sedation, one must consider that current evidence actually suggests that patients undergoing topical anesthesia have more pain and sensation and thus may require more sedation as compared to those under injection blocks.

Other health care providers, including nurses and respiratory therapists, administer sedation for cataract surgery in the USA and Canada. In a Veterans Administration hospital in Iowa, the ophthalmologist directed the administration of sedation by registered nurses. An "available" anesthesiologist was called in for consultation in less than 9% of cases. The main reasons for anesthesiologist assistance were ECG interpretation and IV placement. Only one case required transfer of care to the anesthesiologist. ASA physical status III patients required consultation more often than ASA II patients. This VA system had utilized nurses as sedation providers for eye surgery due to a lack of anesthesia personnel and limited financial resources.

Investigators in Canada have published a large series of over 15,000 cases where Registered Respiratory Therapists (RRTs) provided sedation during eye surgery. These RRTs were required to have 2 years of critical care experience, a 30-day anesthesia training program, and ACLS certification. All patients were seen preoperatively by general practitioners, and the ASA physical status was ascertained. Certain patients were selected to have care by an anesthesiologist based on their visit to the preadmission clinic. Most surgeries were performed under topical anesthesia, and the majority of patients received IV sedation with midazolam and fentanyl, and only occasionally propofol, up to a predetermined level established by the anesthesiologist. Consultations with the anesthesiologist were mandated for specified perioperative events. Only 2.6% of cases required intervention by the anesthesiologist. Patients older than 75 years of age and those with higher ASA physical status were more likely to require anesthesiologist intervention. Most of these interventions occurred preoperatively. A significant component of this protocol is the fact that all patients were evaluated in a preoperative clinic, and some were selected to have care by an anesthesiologist at that time. It may be more difficult to identify those patients requiring anesthesia care among those not seen preoperatively, as is customary in many eye centers. It can also be challenging to provide an anesthesiologist if needed at the last minute. An older study found that the patients who required anesthesia interventions most frequently during cataract surgery suffered from hypertension, pulmonary disease, renal disease, or past or current cancers. Interestingly, older patients in this study required interventions less often than patients less than 60 years of age. All these patients had injection blocks for their surgeries, which in several studies has been shown to reduce the need for sedation.

Multiple factors will influence the need for anesthesia providers during ophthalmologic surgery in the future. These include surgical techniques and risks, patient expectations, anesthesiologist availability, and financial resources.

Summary

Ophthalmologic surgery is very common in geriatric patients. While it is focused on a small region of the body, the surgery has systemic effects. Local or regional anesthesia for the eye can be done in various ways. Retina or posterior chamber surgeries usually require injection blocks. The choice of anesthesia for the eye influences the need for sedation. The need for a cooperative but immobile patient creates a unique situation for sedating these elderly patients. Risks of sedation during ophthalmologic surgery are not serious and are more common when multiple categories of drugs are employed. More anesthesia interventions are required for those who are older and have higher ASA physical status. Overall, patients are satisfied with their experiences during cataract surgery.

Key Points

- There is no need for preoperative testing prior to ophthalmologic surgery under local or regional anesthesia if a patient has routine medical care and their preexisting conditions are managed.
- Ensure that elderly patients receive understandable preoperative instructions. Most medications, including anticoagulants, can be continued preoperatively.
- Knowledge of diabetic patients HbA1c can facilitate their perioperative management. Maintain a patient's blood glucose near their usual values.
- Oral hypoglycemic medications can be held on the day of surgery until oral intake resumes. Management of insulin depends on the patient's regimen.
- The patient experience during ophthalmologic surgery varies with type of local or regional anesthesia for the eye. This influences the level of pain and light sensitivity as well as the duration of surgery.
- The need for sedation varies with the type of regional or local anesthesia used for the eye.
- Risks of sedation for elderly patients undergoing eye surgery include the draping around the head and the use of more than one class of sedative.
- Overall, geriatric patients are usually satisfied with their anesthesia care during eye surgery.
- In the future, RNs and respiratory therapists, instead of anesthesia providers, may provide sedation during cataract surgery.

Suggested Reading

Agency for Healthcare Research and Quality Evidence Report Number 16: Anesthesia Management during Cataract Surgery. Washington, D.C. AHRQ Publication No. 00-E015, 2000. Accessed at: www.ahrq.gov.

Alhassan MB, Kyari F, Ejere HO. Peribulbar versus retrobulbar anaesthesia for cataract surgery. Cochrane Database Syst Rev. 2008 Jul 16;(3):CD004083.

Alhashemi JA. Dexmedetomidine versus Midazolam for Monitored Anesthesia Care during Cataract Surgery. Br J Anaesth. 2006;96:722–6.

Bhananker SM, Posner KL, Cheney FW, Caplar RA, Lee LA, Domino KB. Injury and Liability Associated with Monitored Anesthesia Care: A Closed Claim Analysis. Anesthesiology. 2006;104:228–34.

Boezaart A, Berry RA, Nell M. Topical Anesthesia versus Retrobulbar Block for Cataract Surgery: The Patient's Perspective. J Clin Anesth. 2000;12:58–60.

Boezaart AP, Berry RA, Nell ML, van Dyk AL. A comparison of propofol and remifentanil for sedation and limitation of movement during periretrobulbar block. J Clin Anesth. 2001;13:422–6.

Friedman DS, Bass EB, Lubomski LH, Fleisher LA, Kampen JH et al. Synthesis of the literature on the effectiveness of regional anesthesia for cataract surgery. Ophthalmology. 2001;108: 519–29.

Fung D, Cohen MM, Stewart S, Davies A. What determines patient satisfaction with cataract care under topical local anesthesia and monitored sedation in a community hospital setting? Anesth Analg. 2005;100:1644–50.

Hu K, Scotcher S. Seen from the other side: visual experiences during cataract surgery under topical anaesthesia. BMJ. 2005 Dec 24;331(7531):1511.

Ioannidis AS, Papageorgiou K, Alexandraki KI, Massaoutis P, Sinha AJ, Andreou PS. Light sensitivity and pain sensation during cataract surgery. A comparative study of two modes of anaesthesia. Int Ophthalmol. January 2010 published online.

Katz J, Feldman MA, Bass EB, Lubomski LH, et al. Adverse Intraoperative Medical Events and Their Association with Anesthesia Management Strategies in Cataract Surgery. Ophthalmology. 2001;108:1721–6.

Keay L, Lindsley K, Tielsch J, Katz J, Schein O. Routine preoperative medical testing for cataract surgery. Cochrane Database of Systematic Reviews. 2009; Issue 2. Ar. No.:CD007293.

Mathew MR, Williams A, Esakowitz L, Webb LA, Murray SB, Bennett HG. Patient comfort during clear corneal phacoemulsification with sub-Tenons local anesthesia. J Cataract Refract Surg. 2003;29:1132–6.

Maynard G, O'Malley CW, Kirsh SR. Perioperative Care of the Geriatric Patient with Diabetes or Hyperglycemia. Clin Geriatr Med. 2008;24:849–665.

Nouvellon E, Cuvillon P, Ripart J, Viel EJ. Anaesthesia for cataract surgery. Drugs Aging. 2010;27(1):21–38.

O'Brien PD, Fulcher T, Wallace D, Power W. Patient pain during different stages of phacoemulsification using topical anesthesia. J Cataract Refract Surg. 2001;27:880–3.

Rengaraj V, Radhakrishnan M, AuEong KG, Saw SM, Srinivasan A, Mathew J, Ramasamy K, Prajna NV. Visual experience during phacoemulsification under topical versus retrobulbar anesthesia: results of a prospective, randomized, controlled trial. Am J Ophthalmol. 2004;138: 782–7.

Ryu JH, Kim M, Bahk JH, Do SH, Cheong IY, Kim YC. A comparison of retrobulbar block, sub-Tenon block, and topical anesthesia during cataract surgery. Eur J Ophthalmol. 2009 Mar-Apr;19(2):240–6.

Sanmugasunderam S, Khalfan A. Is fasting required before cataract surgery? A retrospective review. Can J Ophthalmol. 2009 Dec;44(6):655–6. Review.

Schein OD, Katz J, Bass EB, et al. The Value of Routine Preoperative Medical Testing Before Cataract Surgery. NEJM. 2000;342:168–75.

Tantri A, Clark C, Huber P, Stark C, et al. Anesthesia monitoring by registered nurses during cataract surgery: Assessment of need for intraoperative anesthesia consultation. J Cataract Refract Surg. 2006;32:1115–8.

Vann MA, Ogunnaike BO, Joshi GP. Sedation and anesthesia care for ophthalmologic surgery during local/regional anesthesia. Anesthesiology. 2007;107:502–508.

Vann MA. Perioperative management of ambulatory surgical patients with diabetes mellitus. Curr Opin Anesthesiol. 2009;22:718–24.

Woo JH, Au Eong KG, Kumar CM. Conscious sedation during ophthalmic surgery under local anesthesia. Minerva Anesthesiol. 2009;75:211–9.

Zakrzewski PA, Banashkevich AV, Friel T, Braga-Mele R. Monitored Anesthesia Care by Registered Respiratory Therapists during Cataract Surgery: An Update. Ophthalmology. 2010;117(5):897–902.

Part V
Common Geriatric Issues

Chapter 21
Postoperative Central Nervous System Changes in Elderly Surgical Patients

Jeffrey H. Silverstein

Introduction

It has been clear since early in the history of modern anesthesia, and for some time in the much longer history of surgery, that patients have cognitive and behavioral changes following surgery. With the advent of ever safer anesthesia care, mortality has declined. In this milieu, two major trends are notable. The first is that increasing numbers of elderly patients are undergoing both elective and emergent surgery. While elective surgery for patients over 50 was considered risky 70 years ago, patients over 100 are routinely electing to have surgical treatments. This trend is clearly supported by the demographics of western societies, where the average longevity has exceeded 75 years of age and the elderly are the fastest growing demographic. Surgical techniques have evolved significantly, providing less invasive means of performing surgical procedures. The second major trend is an evolving sense in the anesthesia community that outcomes other than mortality are important end points. Some of the newest frontiers in the effort to improve anesthesia care include prevention of postoperative neurological complications.

In this chapter, the basis upon which CNS changes occur is first considered. These are the alterations in brain anatomy, physiology, and function that occur in a normal individual experiencing aging in the absence of any neurological disease. Specific diseases of the neurological system including dementia and Parkinson's disease are considered separately in Chap. 17. With this information as a background, the specific syndromes of postoperative delirium and postoperative cognitive dysfunction are considered.

J.H. Silverstein, MD (✉)
Department of Anesthesiology, Mount Sinai School of Medicine,
Box 1010, 1 Gustave L. Levy Place, New York, NY 10029, USA
e-mail: Jeff.Silverstein@mountsinai.org

S.R. Barnett (ed.), *Manual of Geriatric Anesthesia*, DOI 10.1007/978-1-4614-3888-5_21,

Changes in the Elderly Brain

For centuries, the aging brain was considered one of persistent deterioration and diminishment. Mammals in general, and humans in particular, were conceived as having been born with a fixed number of brain cells from which only a downhill course was possible. In 1913, Santiago Ramón y Cajal, the Nobel laureate Spanish neuroanatomist, wrote that the adult human brain was "fixed, ended, immutable." Evolving from that concept, it has been a commonly held notion that widespread neuron death in the neocortex and hippocampus is the substrate of brain aging. However, a number of lines of evidence now suggest that neuron death is relatively limited in normal aging and unlikely to account for age-related impairment of neocortical and hippocampal functions. Importantly, it appears that the primary neurobiological substrates for functional impairments that are found in normal aging differ in important ways from those in neurodegenerative disorders such as Alzheimer's disease. The most exciting of developments relative to brain aging is the evolving status of neurogenesis. Once thought impossible, the development of new neurons has been demonstrated in most subhuman mammals, and there is every reason to believe that neurogenesis occurs in humans. The nature of neurogenesis, what happens to new neurons and their role in processes such as learning and memory or the potential for neurogenesis to be controlled for therapeutic purposes such as recovery from stroke, remains to be understood.

Advances in histologic technique and, most importantly, imaging technology have revolutionized the conception of normal brain aging. It remains true that overall brain size tends to decrease with aging, although the number of neurons is not the primary alteration. The metabolic requirement of brain decreases but remains tightly coupled to brain mass such that aging is clearly not a failure or decrement in metabolic capacity.

For the practicing anesthesiologist, the clinical behavior of the aging patient is important to understand. There is an unfortunate tendency to ascribe a variety of deficits to the aging process, but all anesthesiologists have encountered patients of extreme age who are essentially intact from a mental and neurological perspective. As with all aspects of aging, variability is immensely important. The average function of any organ or system for a population of elderly individuals will have more variability than a sample of younger patients. This phenomenon is particularly notable in cognitive processes. The average decline for a population of elderly patients might not reflect the circumstance of any individual patient that presents for surgery and anesthesia.

On average, elderly humans retain fairly normal simple reaction time to stimuli, but when a choice is involved, that is, selecting from among different options or systems, reaction time tends to be diminished slightly. Time is an important variable. When elderly individuals are given as much time as they like to complete a test, they may do as well as younger patients. It is the speed of processing rather the ability to process that is altered. Intelligence, frequently divided into fluid intelligence and crystallized intelligence, has been thought to be differentially affected.

Fluid intelligence, associated with adaptability, has been thought to decline with aging, while crystallized intelligence, perhaps associated with accumulated wisdom, is thought to be maintained or even increase with age.

Memory is a complex function that may be affected by age in different ways. Researchers have delineated memory through many different systems, making the comparison between studies difficult. Most researchers believe that one type of memory, called working memory or short-term memory, is most affected by age. Working memory is the retention of information that must be manipulated or transformed in some way. Long-term memory of events long ago tends to be maintained, even in patients with dementing illness.

Auditory and visual capacity is diminished in many elderly patients. Auditory acuity, particularly as the higher range (particularly above 8,000 Hz), is frequently diminished. Slow and deliberate speech, particularly in direct sight of the patient, may improve perception during preoperative evaluations. There is no good evidence that elderly patients do not feel or have less pain than younger patients, although the speed at which a full painful reaction occurs may diminish.

Delirium

Delirium is a behavioral syndrome that was described in some detail in the 3rd edition of the American Psychiatric Associations Diagnostic and Statistical Manual. This was an important milestone in that this definition formed the basis for the formulation of the Confusion Assessment Method or CAM which will be described below. In a general sense, delirium refers to confusion and lack of orientation. Anesthesiologists have used this phrase for two fairly distinct syndromes. Emergence delirium or agitation occurs, as stated, during the emergence from anesthesia. Postoperative delirium occurs primarily in elderly patients at some distance from emergence, usually following an extended lucid interval of 24–48 h

Emergence Delirium

Some clinicians have postulated that emergence delirium is analogous to stage 2 excitement described by Snow as part of the induction phenomenon seen with slow-acting anesthetics of days past. Given recent evidence suggesting that orexigenic pathways are responsible for emergence though a different pathway than induction would occur, there is a fair likelihood that emergence delirium is not simply the converse of stage 2 excitement. Further, the idea that emergence delirium is stage 2 in reverse does not help to understand or treat the phenomena. Emergence delirium is not a uniquely geriatric syndrome. The agitated form of emergence delirium is the most well noted and occurs among all age groups. These are patients who emerge from anesthesia in a wild and uncontrollable state, failing to respond to commands and frequently exhibiting extreme behaviors such as self-removing intravenous lines or endotracheal tubes. These patients are not coherent and cannot follow commands. Extraordinary efforts may be necessary to keep the patient on the operating room table. For large, strong patients, this can be a challenge. There is little reason to believe that stating commands in ever louder voices is likely to be successful, although this is a common reaction among anesthesia personnel and other staff in the operating room. Children are particularly prone to emergence delirium;however, small children can usually be restrained without injury during emergence excitation or delirium. Adults can be difficult to manage and almost impossible to physically restrain. Such patients usually require some additional sedation with either a benzodiazepine or propofol to prevent them from injuring themselves or operating room staff. Care should be given to providing only enough sedation to control the behavior rather than re-inducing general anesthesia. In postoperative delirium, there is a form referred to as hypoactive, which is not associated with excitation and uncontrolled behavior. There has been very little exploration of emergence phenomenon to know whether such a form of emergence delirium exists. Clearly some patients emerge from anesthesia extremely coherent and following commands. Elderly patients frequently emerge but remain sedated and poorly responsive—this state has never been described as delirium but may be a hypoactive form of emergence delirium. Therefore, emergence delirium has not been considered a particular problem for the elderly, but that may be because we have not looked for it.

There is some thought that certain agents, most recently sevoflurane, are conducive to the presence of emergence delirium and that propofol or dexmedetomidine is associated with a lower incidence and less aggressive forms of emergence delirium. There is little concern that emergence delirium has long-lasting consequences in young patients, but there is some evolving concern that emergence delirium in the elderly can progress to more long-lasting delirium.

Postoperative Delirium

After a lucid period of 24–72 h, elderly patients may develop a form of delirium referred to as interval delirium or postoperative delirium. The principle instrument for the diagnosis of delirium is the CAM (see box). The CAM is designed to be used by individuals who are not trained psychiatrists or psychologists and thus can be effectively used by nursing staff. A key feature of delirium is the fluctuating nature, so a patient who is delirious at one point might appear normal sometime later. Postoperative delirium is classified as hypoactive, hyperactive, or mixed. The hyperactive type is easy to recognize as these patients are actively behaving in a confused manner, trying to get out of bed or verbalizing their confusion. Unfortunately, a larger majority of patients manifest the hypoactive form and will not be diagnosed in the absence of an active effort to do so. These patients are quiet, remaining in bed, and not acting out. Hypoactive delirium is frequently missed or passed over as minor dementia or what you would expect of an old patient who had surgery. This is unfortunate as the prognosis for hypoactive delirium is also poor.

The incidence of delirium appears to vary with surgical type. For general surgery patients, the incidence is reported between 5 and 15%. For patients who have suffered from hip fractures, the incidence is higher, being reported between 16 and 62% with an average estimated at 35% of patients. Cardiac surgical patients and ICU patients are thought to have much higher incidences of delirium, in the vicinity of 50–80%. The figures for ICU include medical patients as well as postoperative patients.

The impact of postoperative delirium is important. One major study indicated that patients with delirium increased the average hospital stay from 4.6 to 6.0 days at an average cost of $2,947 additional per patient. The overall cost of postoperative delirium has been estimated at $2 billion.

The etiology of delirium in general and postoperative delirium in particular remains essentially unknown. Associations with various inflammatory markers have been described; however, these associations tend to be nonspecific and are extremely difficult to distinguish from general inflammatory phenomena associated with surgical procedures. It is unlikely that any of the inflammatory mediators will be found to be specific to delirium. Some researchers have proposed a relationship to sleep disruption, which is extremely common in all hospitalized patients. There are some neuroendocrine patterns seen with patients with delirium that are similar to those noted in sleep disruption, and the time frame of postoperative delirium is also consistent. A major limitation to this area of research is the need to do polysomnography which requires extensive equipment that is not easily tolerated by postoperative patients. The work to date, accomplished using motion monitors referred to as actigraphs, is not well accepted by more traditional sleep researchers.

Among the most interesting recent findings in relationship to the etiology of postoperative delirium is the apparent importance of anesthesia depth. In a recent study by Seiber et al., patients under spinal anesthesia were randomized to either lighter or deeper sedation; the authors found a markedly different incidence of delirium in the groups. Approximately 19% of patients with a light level of sedation as determined by an observer's assessment of alertness/sedation scale score (OAA/S) of 4–5 and bispectral index (BIS) >80 were found to have delirium. In contrast patients with heavy sedation as defined by an OAA/S score of 0 and BIS < 50 had an incidence of over 40%. Although this is a small study that requires repetition, it is the first major study to suggest that the intraoperative management of elderly patients has a significant impact on the subsequent development of delirium. This result also has important implications for one of the most heavily speculated aspects of delirium (as well of POCD), which is the relationship to the choice of anesthetic. For years it has been suggested that regional anesthesia should be associated with a lower incidence of postoperative delirium. However, multiple studies and a subsequent major meta-analysis failed to show a significant difference in the incidence of delirium. The inability to find a difference between regional and general anesthesia might be attributable to the sedation that is frequently administered with regional anesthesia.

There have been a number of efforts to prevent delirium in postoperative patients with variable success. In general, a comprehensive geriatric assessment has been shown to be effective in improving the outcomes of geriatric surgical patients with two main caveats. First, this service is only effective if there is a system to implement the suggestions. A second possibly larger issue is that these consultations are not easily compensated by current reimbursement formulas. Given these caveats it is not surprising that they have failed to attain a significant level of acceptance. Other approaches to reducing postoperative delirium include using drug prophylaxis with a variety of medications, usually haloperidol or newer forms thereof;this approach has been only minorly effective. Although larger trials are currently under way, the side effect profile of these medications is uncomfortable, if not intolerable. For elective general surgery patients, this type of prophylaxis is unlikely to become popular.

Postoperative Cognitive Dysfunction

There is an extensive literature extending from the 1950s suggesting that patients are somehow cognitively impaired after undergoing surgery and anesthesia. This is sometimes described as "not being the same after surgery." Larry McMurtry, a well-known author and book enthusiast, related his experience following cardiac surgery as follows: "From being a living person with a distinct personality I began to feel more or less like an outline of that person—and then even the outline began to fade, erase by what had happened inside. I felt as if I was vanishing—or more accurately, had vanished." In McMurtry's case, the principal problem was that he no longer had any enthusiasm and capacity for reading. Other individuals will describe inability to manipulate numbers or difficulty in completing crossword puzzles that were easy immediately prior to surgery. Categorizing these complaints involves neurocognitive testing that must be done at baseline prior to surgery. The deficits that have been elucidated using this approach are referred to as postoperative cognitive dysfunction or POCD. Unlike delirium, which is defined in the American Psychiatric Associations Diagnostic and Statistical Manual, POCD has not been defined as a clear clinical entity. As preoperative cognitive testing is not a standard procedure, this finding only occurs in research settings. A number of controversies exist regarding POCD. First, POCD is defined by the tests incorporated into a battery of neuropsychological tests used to evaluate the patient. Most tests are focused on memory and executive function, so a phenomenon such as that described by Larry McMurtry would be hard to detect. Next the timing of testing is extremely varied between studies. For instance the literature to date indicates a fairly high degree of POCD immediately (1–3 days) following surgery with a decreasing incidence as time progresses afterwards. However an important and as yet unanswered question addresses distinguishing when the effects of anesthetic drugs and the response to surgery have dissipated, so that one can assume the cognitive alterations being discerned are no longer part of a transitory state. Finally, the degree of change that is used to define dysfunction has varied across studies, making comparison extremely difficult. The lack of consensus on these issues results in a situation where it is not possible to define a clear definition of POCD as either present or absent, particularly in an individual patient. Other caveats relate to the population groups represented in the reports. For example studies of POCD have included either general surgical patients or cardiac surgical patients; both populations are rarely, if ever, considered together. Patients with underlying dementia have not been studied to date, and patients undergoing neurosurgery have been routinely excluded from studies of POCD and delirium.

Because of these concerns, the clinical relevance of POCD has been questioned. For general surgery, the incidence (see below) seems to become hard to distinguish from the general decrease in cognitive function seen in the elderly population. This has also been questioned in the cardiac surgical population, where a few recent studies have suggested that patients with coronary artery disease managed via nonsurgical procedures have similar problems with cognitive decline. For noncardiac surgery, a recent retrospective review found, as have previous studies, that the trajectory of decline for patients with Alzheimer's disease and other forms of dementia is not influenced by surgery and anesthesia.

Testing

Most neurocognitive batteries include tests of memory and executive function. Memory includes short- and long-term memory and can be tested in different ways, including the recall of words, phrases, or numbers. Executive function is that aspect of cognition involved in the manipulation of information and includes psychomotor skills. Tests have not been created specifically to study POCD but rather have been adapted from other areas of neuropsychology. This has the distinct advantage of using tests with a proven record of repeatability and validity. However, returning to the story of Mr. McMurtry at the outset of this section, there are few tests that would clearly define the alterations he described. It is not clear that current batteries used to study POCD would have detected significant change in the author. Changes in personality, motivation, and drive are not well assessed by the batteries that have been used to date. The second aspect of understanding POCD is the timing of the tests. The literature contains reports of cognitive testing extending from the day of surgery to many years following surgery. As one might expect, patients tend to test poorly on the day or first few days after surgery. This type of deterioration is attributable to the anesthetic drugs, pain, analgesics, and the stress response of surgery. These types of studies seek to define the early recovery trajectory following an operation. Many studies have focused on an intermediate term of weeks to months following a procedure. One of the largest series of studies in the area, those conducted by the International Study of Postoperative Cognitive Dysfunction (ISPOCD), as well as some follow-up studies using the same battery and timing focused on a period from 1 week to 3 months following surgery. These studies sought to determine whether cognitive change occurred in a period after the initial trauma of surgery and the effect of anesthetic drugs has presumably dissipated. The incidence of POCD decreases as the time from surgery increases. By 1 year it is difficult to find a clear impact following noncardiac surgery. Studies that follow patients out to many years following surgery can be hard to understand in that intervening events that may have effected cognitive change are usually not well defined. A third and highly controversial question in the definition of POCD is how much change is considered deterioration. As an analogy, if a patient scored 100% on a test before surgery and 95% a month after surgery, would that difference be particularly meaningful? How about an 85%? In the realm of cognitive testing, the definitions vary as to how much change on how many tests is considered significant. Some investigators have used one or two standard deviations from baseline on one or more tests. Other investigators have used specifically defined clinically important differences defined by focus groups for a specific study. This variability has led to tremendous criticism of the entire field and calls for some attempt to develop a consensus definition. In this context, it is important to understand that the definition of dementia as defined by scales, such as the clinical dementia rating (CDR) scale, include not only cognitive testing but also extensive interviews and assessment of activities in addition to pure mental function. Therefore, the relationship of POCD to dementia is yet to be clearly defined. Finally, there is the question of control groups and their relevance to the types of changes being sought. Given that there is an underlying level of dementia in the elderly population, the question arises as to how to distinguish a specific effect of surgery or anesthesia from evolving dementia. Another aspect of this same problem is that individuals tend to improve with repeat testing, so it would be valuable to be able to remove that learning effect. The ISPOCD studies attempted to do this by recruiting a control group of similarly aged patients that were not undergoing surgery. Some investigators have argued that, if the point is to define the role of surgery and anesthesia, the comparison needs to be made to individuals with medical illness rather than to healthy patients. Of course, trying to define a group of patients before a medical illness ensues is essentially impossible. A second criticism of the control groups and the surgical patients included in these studies is that there was at most a single test performed preoperatively. Therefore, if patients were experiencing cognitive decline in the months leading up to surgery, this would not be captured. The relevance of this issue remains theoretical.

Every so often, a patient is found to have severe deterioration following surgery. These catastrophic cases are rare and are only reported as anecdotes—there is very little literature regarding such cases. The typical story is that an elderly patient is severely impaired, i.e., delirious immediately following surgery and goes on to have multiple complications, usually pneumonia and decubitus ulcers associated with a significant deterioration of mental function, leading to nursing home placement or death. The number of such cases is completely unknown. They are almost never captured in studies of POCD as the number of studies in progress is relatively small and perioperative cognitive testing is not common. Furthermore, such deterioration would usually preclude the completion of postoperative tests, so even if such a patient were in a study, the testing paradigms would not define their deterioration particularly well. This represents a systematic problem for studies of POCD. Some authors have recently argued that this type of catastrophic deterioration is a real, if poorly defined, phenomena, while the type of minor alterations defined by most studies of POCD is trivial or clinically irrelevant.

Given all of these limitations, what is the incidence of POCD? The first large ISPOCD study included 1,218 patients, aged 60 and older who underwent surgery under general anesthesia. At 1 week, 25.8% of patients showed deterioration of two standard deviations on one or more of five tests. At 3 months following the surgery, 9.9% of patients tested showed this level of deterioration. In another study that used a different battery and different end points, deterioration was noted in 5% of patients at 6 months following surgery. A long-term follow-up at 1 year of some of the patients in the original ISPOCD study showed about a 1% difference from similarly matched control patients. A review and meta-analysis of POCD studies, focusing to some extent on cardiac surgery, concluded that POCD appears to be primarily a transient phenomenon that resolves of a period of months. The clinical importance of such finding has been highlighted by the Copenhagen group who showed that there are both influences on activities of daily living as well as employability among patients with POCD. Therefore, it is difficult to advise patients who ask that anesthesia and surgery have no impact on cognition, although it is reassuring that these might be transient.

The etiology of POCD has not been determined. One of the prime candidates is cerebral ischemia. Unlike embolic stroke, in which specific area of the brain is impacted, a more global form of ischemia might cause the types of deterioration noted on neurocognitive tests. The ISPOCD study postulated that ischemia, as measured by hypotension (using continuous noninvasive blood pressure measurement) and hypoxemia (using pulse oximetry) would be associated with POCD. However, in this large study (1,218 patients), there were many instances of hypotension and hypoxemia but no relationship to POCD. Recent studies using cerebral oximetry have suggested that there may be regional ischemia, but these results need to be confirmed.

The potential for direct anesthetic toxicity is intriguing. There have been a number of recent animal and cell culture studies that suggest that some anesthetic agents, particularly isoflurane, have specific effects on the biochemistry associated with Alzheimer's dementia. There is also an evolving literature on the impact of anesthetics on neurocognitive performance in neonatal animals exposed to anesthesia. Arguing against an impact of anesthesia is the repeated failure to demonstrate a difference in either POCD or postoperative delirium in patients who are randomized to either regional or general anesthesia. If the anesthetic agents were the cause of either syndrome, they should be much less common in patients receiving regional anesthesia, even if the regional patients received sedation. This has not been the case in either individual studies or in a significant meta-analysis.

There is speculation regarding the role of inflammation and genetic markers in the development of POCD. To date, nothing specific has been shown to predict or be significantly associated with POCD.

The relationship between POCD and either dementing illness or delirium remains unclear. Attempts to find an impact of surgery and anesthesia on the incidence or trajectory of dementia have not proven fruitful. There is mixed evidence as to whether patients who develop postoperative delirium go on to have POCD.

There is no preventive measure that has even the suggestion of diminishing the incidence of POCD, and there are no treatments available to alter POCD.

Conclusions

Elderly patients seem particularly prone to specific neurological complications following anesthesia and surgery. Postoperative delirium occurs at 24–48 h following surgery. It is frequently missed by the anesthesia team but has important implications for patient outcomes and healthcare expenditures. Postoperative cognitive dysfunction is an evolving research area that requires extensive additional work to be able to define a present/absent syndromal definition of this entity. Important considerations include the areas to test, the timing of testing, and the amount of change that is considered clinically important. As the changes found to date tend to diminish over time, it is extremely difficult to counsel a particular patient given our current level of knowledge.

Key Points

- Our understanding of brain aging is evolving;modern histology indicates that we do not loose many neurons as part of the aging process.
- The primary neurobiological substrates for functional impairments that are found in normal aging differ in important ways from those in neurodegenerative disorders.
- While there is some decrease in function with aging, a successfully aging individual will have most of their faculties intact for their entire life span.
- The anesthesiologist should understand normal brain aging, as well as the aging of sensory function, to help them in their approach to these patients.
- Delirium is a behavioral syndrome. Emergence delirium or agitation occurs in all age groups. Postoperative delirium occurs mostly in elderly patients after a period of lucidity, usually 24–48 h postoperative.
- Delirium is best diagnosed using the confusion assessment method (CAM)
- Hypoactive delirium is frequently missed or misdiagnosed.
- Delirium is associated with increased medical complications and increased medical expenditures.
- The etiology of delirium is unknown, but early evidence suggests that the depth of sedation accompanying a spinal anesthetic can affect the incidence of delirium.
- Postoperative cognitive dysfunction (POCD) requires preoperative cognitive testing.
- The degree of dysfunction in POCD is dependent on the choice of tests, and the timing of the tests and the decision as to how much deterioration is significant.

The current state of information makes it difficult to properly counsel an individual patient as to their risk of deterioration following anesthesia and surgery.

Suggested Reading

Abildstrom H, Christiansen M, Siersma VD, Rasmussen LS. Apolipoprotein E genotype and cognitive dysfunction after noncardiac surgery. Anesthesiology. 2004;101:855–861.

Abildstrom H, Rasmussen LS, Rentowl P, Hanning CD, Rasmussen H, Kristensen PA, Moller JT. Cognitive dysfunction 1-2 years after non-cardiac surgery in the elderly. ISPOCD group. International Study of Post-Operative Cognitive Dysfunction. Acta Anaesthesiol Scand. 2000;44:1246–1251.

Avidan MS, Searleman AC, Storandt M, Barnett K, Vannucci A, Saager L, Xiong C, Grant EA, Kaiser D, Morris JC, Evers AS.:Long-term cognitive decline in older subjects was not attributable to noncardiac surgery or major illness. Anesthesiology. 2009 Nov;111(5):964–70. Also see correspondence in Anesthesiology. 2010 May;112(5):1280-1;author reply 1283–5.

Battaglia J. Pharmacologic management of acute agitation. Drugs. 2005;65:1207–1222.

Bekkar AY, Weeks EJ. Cognitive function after anaesthesia in the elderly. Best Pract Res Clin Anaesthesiol. 2003;17:259–272.

Beloosesky Y, Hendel D, Weiss A, Hershkovitz A, Grinblat J, Pirotsky A, Barak V. Cytokines and c-reactive protein production in hip-fracture-operated elderly patients. J of Gerontology. 2007;62A:420–426.

Bickel H, Gradinger R, Kochs E, Forstl H. High Risk of Cognitive and Functional Decline after Postoperative Delirium. Dement Geriatr Cogn Disord. 2008;26:26–31.

Bitsch M, Foss N, Kristensen B, Kehlet H. Pathogenesis of and management strategies for postoperative delirium after hip fracture. Acta Orthop Scand. 2004;75:378–389

Brauer C, Morrsion R, S Silberzweig SB, Siu AL. The cause of delirium in patients with hip fracture. Arch Intern Med. 2000;160:1856–1860.

Cole MG. Delirium in elderly patients. Am J Geriatr Psychiatry. 2004;12:7–21.

Culley DJ, Baxter MG, Crosby CA, Yukhananov R, Crosby G. Impaired acquisition of spatial memory 2 weeks after isoflurane and isoflurane-nitrous oxide anaesthesia in aged rats. Anesth Analg. 2004;99:1393–1397.

Deiner S, Silverstein JH. Postoperative delirium and cognitive dysfunction. Br J Anaesth. 2009 Dec;103 Suppl 1:i41–46.

Eckenhoff MF. Inhaled anesthetic enhancement of amyloid-beta oligomerization and cytotoxicity. Anesthesiology. 2004;101:703–709.

Etzioni DA, Liu JH, Maggard MA, Ko CY. The aging population and its impact on the surgery workforce. Ann Surg. 2003;238:170–177.

Fong HK, Sands LP, Leung JM. The role of postoperative analgesia in delirium and cognitive decline in elderly patients. Anesth Analg. 2006;102:1255–1266.

Franco K, Litaker D, Locala J, Bronson D. The cost of delirium in the surgical patient. Psychosomatics. 2001;42:68–77.

Gottesman RF, Grega MA, Bailey MM, Pham LD, Zeger SL, Baumgartner WA, Selnes OA, McKhann GM. Delirium after coronary artery bypass graft surgery and late mortality. Ann Neurol. 2010 Mar;67(3):338–344.

Green N, Attix DK, Weldon C, Smith PJ, McDonagh DL, Monk TG. Measures of Executive Function and Depression Identify Patients at Risk for Postoperative Delirium. Anesthesiology. 2009;110:788–795.

Gruber-Baldini AL, Zimmerman S, Morrison RS, Grattan LM, Hebel JR, Dolan MM, Hawkes W, Magaziner J. Cognitive impairment in hip fracture patients:timing of detection and longitudinal follow up. J Am Geriatr Soc. 2003;51:1227–1236.

Hattori H, Kamiya J, Shimada H, Akiyama H, Yasui A, Kuroiwa K, Oda K, Ando M, Kawamura T, Harada A, Kitagawa Y, Fukata S. Assessment of the risk of postoperative delirium in elderly patients using E-PASS and the NEECHAM Confusion Scale. Int J Geriatr Psychiatry. 2009;24(11):1304–10.

Hudetz J, Patterson KM, Iqbal Z, Gandhi SD, Byrne AJ, Hudetz AG, Warltier DC, Pagel PS. Ketamine attenuates delirium after cardiac surgery with cardiopulmonary bypass. J Cardthorac Vasc Anes. 2009;53(7):864–72.

Inouye S. Delirium in older persons. N Engl J Med. 2006;354:1157–1165.

Johnson T, Monk T, Rasmussen LS, Abildstrom H, Houx P, Korttila K, Kuipers HM, Hanning CD, Siersma VD, Kristensen D, Canet J, Ibanaz MT, Moller JT. Postoperative cognitive dysfunction in middle-aged patients. Anesthesiology. 2002;96:1351–1357.

Kain ZN, Caldwell-Andrews AA, Mayes LC, Weinberg ME, Wang SM, MacLaren JE, Blount RL. Family-centered preparation for surgery improves perioperative outcomes in children:a randomized controlled trial. Anesthesiology. 2007;106:65–74.

Kain ZN, Caldwell-Andrews AA. Maranets I, Gaal D, Mayes LC, Feng R, Zhang H. Preoperative anxiety and emergence delirium and postoperative maladaptive behaviors. Anesth Analg. 2004;99:1648–1654.

Kat MG, Vreeswijk R, de Jonghe JFM, van der Ploeg T, van Gool WA, Eikelenboom P, Kalisvaart KJ. Long-Term Cognitive Outcome of Delirium in Elderly Hip Surgery Patients. Dement Geriatr Cogn Disord. 2008;26:1–8.

Lemstra A, Kalisvaart KJ, Vreeswijk R, van Gool WA, Eikenlenboom P. Preoperative inflammatory markers and the risk of postoperative delirium in elderly patients. Int J Geriatr Psychiatry. 2008;23:943–948.

Litaker D, Locala J, Franco K, Bronson DL, Tannous Z. Preoperative risk factors for postoperative delirium. Gen Hosp Psychiatry. 2001;23:84–89.

Lowery DP, Wesnes K, Ballard CG. Subtle attentional deficits in the absence of dementia are associated with an increased risk of postoperative delirium. Dement Geriatr Cogn Disord. 2007;23:390–394.

Marcantonio ER, Flacker JM, Wright RJ, Resnick NM. Reducing delirium after hip fracture:a randomized trial. J Am Geriatr Soc. 2001;49:516–522.

McGory ML, Shekelle PG, Rubenstein LZ, Fink A, Ko CY. Developing quality indicators for elderly patients undergoing abdominal operations. J Am Coll Surg. 2005;201:870–883.

Moller JT, Cluitmans P, Rasmussen LS, Houx P, Rasmussen H, Canet J, Rabbitt P, Joles J, Larsen K, Hanning CD, Langeron O, Johnson T, Lauven PM, Kristensen PA, Bieldler A, van Beem H, Fraidakis O, Silverstein JH, Beneken JE, Gravenstein JS. Long-term postoperative cognitive dysfunction in the elderly ISPOCD1 study. ISPOCD investigators. International Study of Post-Operative Cognitive Dysfunction. Lancet. 1998;351:857–861.

Morimoto Y, Yoshimura M, Utada K, Setoyama K, Matsumoto M, Sakabe T. Prediction of postoperative delirium after abdominal surgery in the elderly. J Anesth. 2009;23:51–56.

Newman S, Stygall J, Hirani S, Shaefi S, Maze M. Postoperative cognitive dysfunction after noncardiac surgery:a systematic review. Anesthesiology. 2007;106:572–590.

Price RB, Nock MK, Charney DS, Mathew SJ. Effects of intravenous ketamine on explicit and implicit measures of suicidality in treatment-resistant depression. Biol Psychiatry. 2009;66:522–6.

Rasmussen LS, Larsen K, Houx P, Skovgaard LT, Hanning CD, Moller JT;ISPOCD group. The assessment of postoperative cognitive function. Acta Anaesthesiol Scand. 2001;45:275–289.

Rasmussen LS, Siersma VD;ISPOCD group. Postoperative cognitive dysfunction:true deterioration versus random variation. Acta Anaesthesiol Scand. 2004;48:1137–1143.

Rudolph JL, Jones RN, Rasmussen LS, Silverstein JH, Inouye SK, Marcantonio ER. Independent Vascular and Cognitive Risk Factors for Postoperative Delirium. Am J of Med. 2007;120:807–813.

Rudolph JL, Marcantonio ER, Culley DJ, Silverstein JH, Rasmussen LS. Delirium is associated with early postoperative cognitive dysfunction. Anaesthesia. 2008;63:941–947.

Rudolph JL, Ramlawi B, Kuchel GA, McElhaney JE, Xie D, Selke FW, Khabbaz K, Levkoff SE, Marcantonio E. Chemokines are associated with delirium after cardiac surgery. J of Gerontology. 2008;63A:184–189.

Schrader SL, Wellik KE, Demaerschalk BM, Caselli RJ, Woodruff BK, Wingerchuk DM. Adjunctive haloperidol prophylaxis reduces postoperative delirium severity and duration in at-risk elderly patients. The Neurologist. 2008;14:134–137.

Sieber FE, Zakriya KJ, Gottschalk A, Blute MR, Lee HB, Rosenberg PB, Mears SC. Sedation depth during spinal anesthesia and the development of postoperative delirium in elderly patients undergoing hip fracture repair. Mayo Clin Proc. 2010;85(1):18–26. Erratum in:Mayo Clin Proc. 2010;85(4):400.

Siddiqi N, Holt R, Britton AM, Holmes J. Interventions for preventing delirium in hospitalised patients (review). The Cochrane Collaboration. 2009.

Sidlecki KL, Stern Y, Reuben A, Sacco RL, Elkind MS, Wright CB. Construct validity of cognitive reserve in a multiethnic cohort:The Northern Manhattan Study. J Int Neuropsychol Soc. 2009;15:558–569.

Silverstein JH, Timberger M, Reich DL, Uysal S Central Nervous System Dysfunction following Noncardiac Surgery and Anesthesia in the Elderly. Anesthesiology. 2007;106(3):622–8.

Smith PJ, Attix DK, Weldon BC, Greene NH, Monk TG. Executive function and depression as independent risk factors for postoperative delirium. Anesthesiology. 2009;110:781–787.

Steinmetz J, Christensen KB, Lund T, Lohse N, Rasmussen LS, ISPOCD Group. Long-term consequences of postoperative cognitive dysfunction. Anesthesiology. 2009;110:548–555.

Tune L. Serum anticholinergic activity levels and delirium in the elderly. Semin Clin Neuropsychiatry. 2000;5:149–153.

Wacker P, Nunes PV, Cabrita H, Forlenza OV. Postoperative delirium is associated with poor cognitive outcome and dementia. Dement Geriatr Cogn Disord. 2006;21:221–227.

Williams-Russo P, Sharrock NE, Mattis S, Szatrowski TP, Charlson ME. Cognitive effects after epidural versus general anaesthesia in older adults:A randomized trial. JAMA. 1995;274:44–50.

Wu CL, Hsu W, Richman JM, Raja SN. Postoperative cognitive function as an outcome of regional and general anaesthesia. Reg Anesth Pain Med. 2004;29:257–268.

Yang FM, Marcantonio ER, Inouye SK, Kiely DK, Rudolph JL, Fearing MA, Jones RN. Phenomenological subtypes of delirium in older persons:patterns, prevalence, and prognosis. Psychosomatics. 2009;50:248–254.

[illegible]

Chapter 22
Management of the Hip Fracture Patient

Mark D. Neuman and Samir Mehta

Introduction

Hip fracture is a frequent and disabling injury among older adults, defining a distinctly vulnerable subset of the orthopedic trauma population. Hip fractures are associated with profound consequences, including an associated mortality of approximately 20% at 1 year, and high rates of morbidity and loss of function among survivors. Occurring approximately 340,000 times annually in the United States, the number of hip fractures is expected to rise to 500,000 per year by the year 2040 due to the aging of the American population. As these frequent adverse events are due both to a high burden of preexisting comorbidities among hip fracture patients and to the combined effects of immobilization, surgical stress, and pain, anesthesia providers play a potentially critical role in optimizing outcomes after hip fracture. This chapter is divided into two sections; the first provides background regarding hip fracture as a clinical syndrome, outlining the anatomy, epidemiology, risk factors for hip fracture, and data on outcomes following hip fracture. The second discusses the management of hip fracture patients in the perioperative period from the perspective of anesthesia care, highlighting recent evidence identifying opportunities for anesthesia providers to contribute to improved outcomes among hip fracture patients.

M.D. Neuman, MD, MS (✉)
Department of Anesthesiology, Hospital of the University of Pennsylvania,
423 Guardian Drive, 11th Floor Blockley Hall, Philadelphia, PA 19104, USA
e-mail: neumanm@mail.med.upenn.edu

S. Mehta, MD
Department of Orthopedic Surgery, University of Pennsylvania,
2 Silverstein, 3400 Spruce Street, Philadelphia, PA 19104, USA

S.R. Barnett (ed.), *Manual of Geriatric Anesthesia*, DOI 10.1007/978-1-4614-3888-5_22,

Background

Anatomy

The adult hip is a ball–and–socket joint formed by the femoral neck and the acetabulum of the pelvis; key landmarks relevant to the classification of hip fractures appear in Fig. 22.1. Extending distally from the femoral head, the neck of the femur includes the region between the base of the femoral head and a line between the greater and lesser trochanters of the femur. The intertrochanteric portion of the femur represents the segment between the greater and lesser trochanters and serves as a zone of transition to the femoral shaft. Lastly, the subtrochanteric portion of the femur extends from the lesser trochanter to a point 5 cm distal. As the hip capsule extends from the acetabulum to cover the full anterior aspect of the femoral neck and the proximal half of its posterior portion, fractures of the femoral neck are termed *intracapsular,*

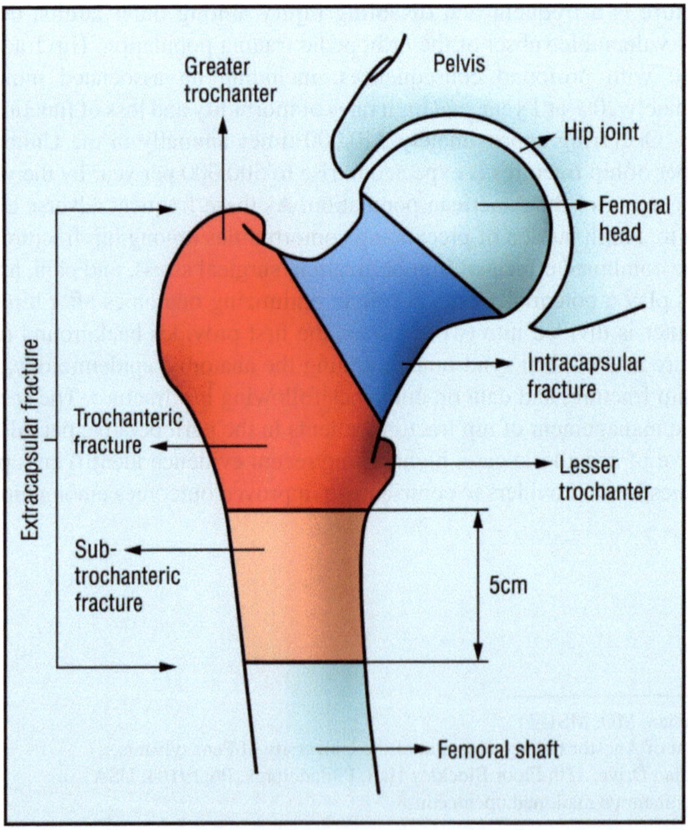

Fig. 22.1 Anatomic locations of hip fractures in adults. Reproduced from (Hip fracture, Parker and Johansen 2006) with permission from BMJ Publishing Group Ltd

while intertrochanteric and subtrochanteric fractures are classified as *extracapsular.* Femoral neck and intertrochanteric fractures occur at approximately equal rates in the population and account for over 90% of hip fractures, with subtrochanteric fractures accounting for the remainder of cases.

Incidence of Hip Fracture

The incidence of hip fracture has been long observed to vary widely from country to country, with age–adjusted rates observed to vary from 39.6 per 100,000 women in Beijing to 274.1 per 100,000 women in Reykjavik between 1990 and 1992. Despite these variations, hip fracture represents a worldwide health problem, occurring approximately 1.6 million times annually, accounting for a high burden of mortality and functional disability. Considering hip fractures along with other fractures commonly associated with osteoporosis, Johnell and Kanis find osteoporotic fractures to account for a greater number of disability–adjusted life years lost worldwide than most common cancers (Fig. 22.2).

In the United States, the frequency of hip fractures makes their prevention and management a crucial concern for public health. Estimates from the late 1990s indicated an annual rate of 340,000 admissions for hip fracture in the USA with $8.5 billion of healthcare expenditures attributable to this injury in 1995. While more recent data from the USA and Canada suggest that efforts at osteoporosis screening and prevention may have contributed to declining incidence of hip fracture among older adults, the absolute frequency and cost of this injury, combined with the aging of the US population, make it an important ongoing public health concern.

Risk Factors

In healthy individuals, the anatomy of the proximal femur serves as a strong conduit for stress transfer from the pelvis to the femoral shaft; as a result, the minority of hip fractures occurring in individuals under 50 years of age or without osteoporosis typically result from high–impact trauma, such as a motor vehicle collision. In contrast, the vast majority of operative hip fractures occur as a result of low–impact traumatic injury, such as a fall from standing in the setting of reduced bone strength, with high rates of osteopenia and osteoporosis among hip fracture patients. The World Health Organization's FRAX tool (http://shef.ac.uk/FRAX) allows for country–specific prediction of 10–year hip fracture risk based on multiple patient factors (Box 22.1).

Beyond these factors, historical data and recent epidemiologic research have identified a range of physical, cognitive, and socioeconomic factors associated with hip fracture. Among controls of similar age, institutionalized adults have been observed to experience a threefold increase in rates of hip fracture. Among

Box 22.1 Risk Factors for Hip Fracture

- Decreased bone mineral density
- Increasing age
- Female sex
- Caucasian race
- Prior fragility fracture
- Parental history of hip fracture
- Current tobacco use
- History of long–term glucocorticoid use
- Rheumatoid arthritis
- Daily alcohol consumption of 3 or more drinks

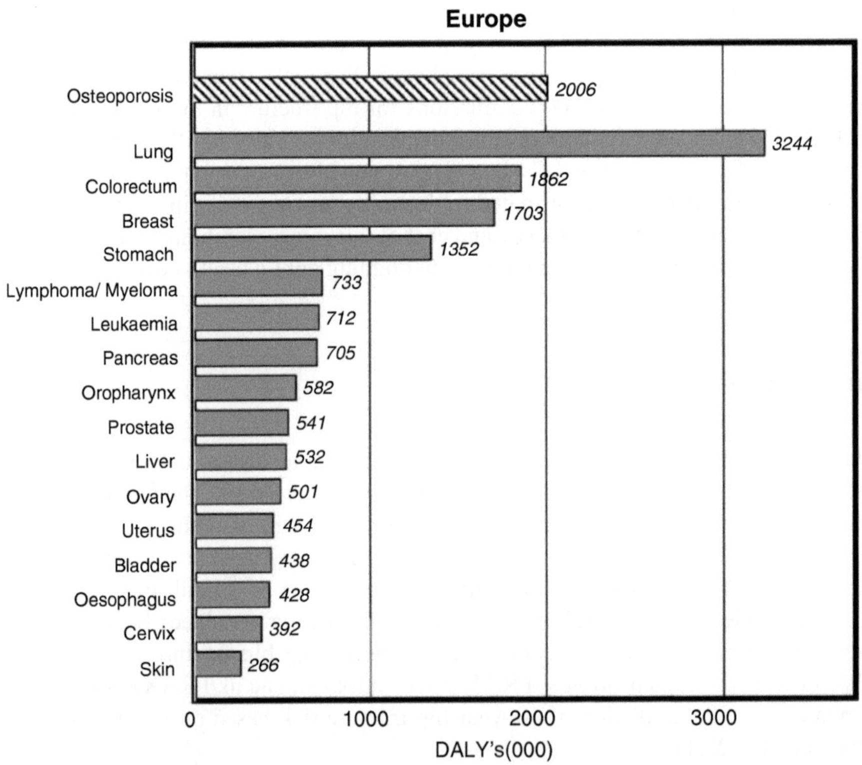

Fig. 22.2 Disability–adjusted life years (DALY's) lost due to osteoporosis and to different neoplastic disorders in Europe. With kind permission from Springer Science+Business Media: Osteoporosis International. An estimate of the worldwide prevalence and disability associated with osteoporotic fractures. O. Johnell. 2006; 17(12)

community–dwelling adults, Wilson and colleagues (2006) recently observed health insurance status, educational level, physical disability, and decreased cognitive functioning to be independent predictors of fracture risk.

Outcomes Following Hip Fracture

Prevalence of Comorbidities Among Patients with Hip Fracture

Patients experiencing hip fracture are characterized by a high rate of medical comorbidities that increase the risk of complications in the perioperative period. Observing a cohort of 2,806 patients admitted over 4 years to a single institution in the United Kingdom, Roche and colleagues found 35% of all hip fracture patients to have one comorbidity, 17% to have two or more comorbidities, and 7% to have three or more comorbidities, with the most common conditions being cardiovascular disease (24%), chronic obstructive pulmonary disease (COPD) (14%), and cerebrovascular disease (13%). A subsequent report by McLaughlin and colleagues of a cohort of 571 hip fracture patients admitted to hospitals in New York found a similarly high rate of comorbidities among hip fracture patients, reporting dementia in 23%, COPD in 14%, congestive heart failure in 16%, and diabetes mellitus in 18%.

Inpatient Complications

The high rate of comorbidities among hip fracture patients increases the risk of postoperative complications. At least one complication occurred in 20% of patients in Roche's 4–year cohort, with the most common adverse events being pulmonary infection (9%), heart failure (5%), and urinary tract infection (4%). In addition to these complications of hip fracture, postoperative delirium represents an important and frequent adverse event following hip fracture, occurring at an overall rate of approximately 20%, with an increased incidence among patients with baseline cognitive impairment. Recent data has highlighted the adverse consequences of delirium among hip fracture patients, which has been found to contribute to increased hospital length of stay, functional disability, morbidity, and mortality.

Mortality

Patients experiencing hip fracture are at high risk for postoperative mortality (Table 22.1). In a recent meta–analysis of 23 studies published between 1957 and 2009 examining the magnitude and duration of excess mortality after hip fracture, Haetjens and collaborators found the relative hazard for all–cause mortality in the first 3 months after hip fracture to be 5.75 (95% confidence interval 4.94, 6.67) in

Table 22.1 Risk–adjusted mortality following hip fracture in US Medicare beneficiaries, by sex, 2005

	30 days	180 days	360 days[a]
Women (%)	5.2	14.3	21.9
95% confidence interval	4.9–5.4	13.9–14.7	21.4–22.4
Men (%)	9.3	22.9	32.5
95% confidence interval	8.8–9.9	22.1–23.8	31.5–33.5

[a]Estimates based on 2004 data for 360–day mortality
Summarized data from: Brauer CA, Coca–Perraillon M, Cutler DM, Rosen AB. Incidence and mortality of hip fractures in the United States. JAMA. 2009;302(14):1573–1579

women and 7.95 (95% confidence interval 6.13, 10.30) in men. While the relative hazard of death declined over time in both men and women, the authors find mortality rates to remain elevated above controls even after 10 years in both groups.

Beyond the overall incidence of death after hip fracture, recent analyses of US Medicare data by Brauer and colleagues suggest that inconsistent advances have been made in hip fracture mortality over the past decade. Examining 30–, 180–, and 360–day mortality, Brauer and colleagues note an overall decrease in mortality after hip fracture between 1986 and 2004, with 30–day mortality falling from 5.9 to 5.2% among women and from 11.9 to 9.3% among men; nonetheless, the majority of these changes were accounted for by advances made between 1986 and 1995, with minimal improvement in mortality occurring between 1996 and 2005.

Multiple risk factors for mortality have been identified, including male sex, pre–fracture nursing home residence, dementia, increasing burden of comorbidities, severity of illness on presentation, and need for assistance in pre–fracture ambulation. Importantly, principal causes of mortality of hip fracture are medical, rather than surgical, in nature, as cardiac, pulmonary, and infectious events constitute the majority of causes of death both during and after hospitalization in this population. In a retrospective cohort of 8,930 patients, Lawrence and colleagues found pronounced increases in 30–day and 1–year mortality among patients experiencing selected postoperative complications. Observing an overall 4% inpatient mortality after repair, they found inpatient mortality among patients experiencing cardiac and/or pulmonary complications to range from 11 to 33%.

Functional Outcomes

Among survivors of hip fracture, recovery of functional independence following fracture repair is often incomplete, adding to the large public health burden of this injury. Seminal work by Magaziner and colleagues observed functional outcomes in a cohort of 674 patients admitted to eight hospitals in Baltimore, Maryland, between 1990 and 1991 and examined recovery from hip fracture in eight areas of function, observing a high incidence of new dependency in a range of physical activities among patients with pre–fracture independence in these areas, ranging in incidence from 20.3% for putting on pants to 89.9% for climbing five stairs. More recently, Hannan and colleagues observed a high degree of post–fracture disability in a cohort of 571 patients admitted to hospitals in the New York metropolitan area between 1997 and 1998, with 12.8% needing total assistance for ambulation at 6 months. Risk factors for impairment in ambulation following hip fracture identified by Hannan and collaborators included pre–fracture limitations in locomotion, increasing medical comorbidities, increasing severity of illness on presentation, increasing age, male sex, nursing home residence, dementia, and pre–fracture need for assistance at home.

Perioperative Management of Hip Fractures

Preface: Understanding the Importance of a Coordinated Approach to Care for Hip Fracture

The combination of chronic medical conditions, acute trauma, and complications of hospitalization and surgery places hip fracture patients at distinctly elevated risk of adverse outcomes. As a result, a coordinated, multidisciplinary approach to perioperative care may be required to optimize the chances for recovery of an individual patient. Structured inpatient guidelines or clinical pathways for hip fracture care indicate that rates of key hospital complications, including delirium, pneumonia, urinary tract infection, and deep venous thrombosis, may be reduced through adoption of a standardized approach to care for hip fracture patients. While local hospital resources and culture may dictate the ultimate shape of any such approach, a collaborative effort involving perspectives from anesthesiology, nursing, orthopedic surgery, internal medicine, geriatrics, nutrition, and physical therapy, based on clinical research, has the potential to improve hip fracture outcomes. While we review below recent evidence–based practices for anesthetic care, perioperative efforts to optimize outcomes following hip fracture repair should ideally fit within a broader, multidisciplinary approach to care for these complex patients.

Patient Selection for Operative Repair

Due to the high risk of mortality, pain, and loss of function associated with an unrepaired hip fracture in an older adult, operative repair is now considered the standard of care for all types of hip fracture in developed nations, with few contraindications (Box 22.2).

In the limited subset of patients treated nonoperatively, a course of bed rest is indicated to minimize fracture movement and promote fracture healing. Skeletal traction may also be used to improve fracture alignment, restore fracture length,

Box 22.2 Contraindications to Operative Repair for Hip Fracture

- A moribund patient
- Patient refusal
- Late presentation of a fracture that has already begun to heal
- No chance of functional recovery due to severe debilitating illnesses or syndromes

Summarization of data from: British Orthopaedic Association. The Care of Patients With Fragility Fractures. In: C. Currie (Eds.) Available from http://www.nhfd.co.uk/. 2007.

reduce deformity, and decrease muscle spasms. In the general population, nonoperative management of lower extremity fractures with skeletal traction is associated with fracture malunion, limb shortening, skin and respiratory complications, and prolonged hospitalization. In the elderly population, the morbidity of prolonged bed rest is even greater, resulting in severe deconditioning, frequent pulmonary complications, and decubitus ulcers.

Given the generally poor results associated with nonoperative treatment and the improvements in surgical treatment options, anesthetic techniques, and postoperative management, surgical treatment of hip fractures in the elderly population has become the standard of care, with general goals of restoring functional anatomy, allowing for early mobilization, and promoting fracture healing. In defining the goals of surgery, the patient's age, preexisting medical comorbidities, current medical condition, and previous level of function must be considered in conjunction with the patient's desires and risks associated with surgery. Beyond these concerns, variations in the anatomy, biomechanics, and healing potential between intracapsular (e.g., femoral neck) and extracapsular (e.g., intertrochanteric and subtrochanteric) hip fractures determine the distinct surgical approaches to each type. It is important to understand which surgical treatment is being proposed as this will impact patient positioning, duration of anesthesia, blood loss, length of surgery, and postoperative pain.

Surgical Approaches to Intracapsular Hip Fractures

The degree of fracture displacement is the primary determinant of the choice of surgical treatment for a femoral neck fracture in an elderly patient. In addition to fracture configuration and bone quality, however, the patient's medical comorbidities, activity level, and cognitive status must all be considered when determining the best treatment option. Overall, in situ screw fixation is favored for non–displaced fractures, allowing for preservation of native bone and offering a minimally invasive method of fracture stabilization. The procedure involves placement of multiple screws into the femoral neck under fluoroscopic guidance through small skin

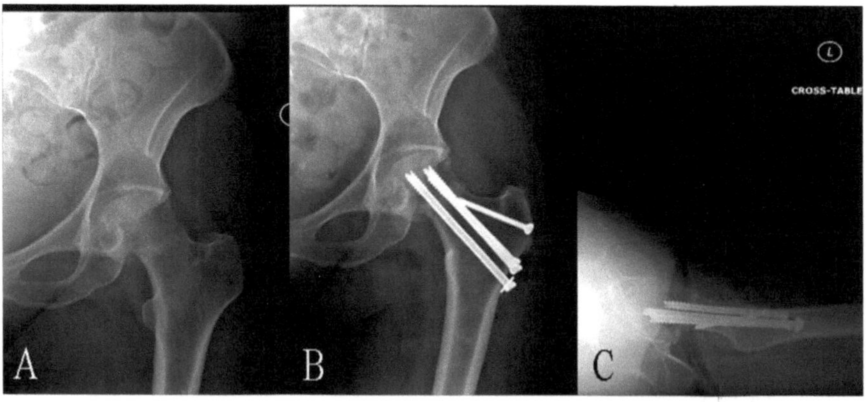

Fig. 22.3 (**a**) Anteroposterior (AP) radiograph showing a non–displaced femoral neck fracture treated with percutaneous pin fixation. (**b**) and (**c**) showing postoperative radiographs in the AP and lateral projections, respectively

incisions over the lateral thigh. The screws begin in the lateral femoral cortex, cross the fracture site, and terminate in the subchondral bone of the femoral head (Fig. 22.3). Surgical time and blood loss are often minimal.

In the geriatric patient with a displaced femoral neck fracture, hip arthroplasty is typically indicated. Total hip arthroplasty is more commonly reserved for the active, ambulatory elder with good cognitive function, as this group of patients will place higher demands on the hip while adhering to standard mobility precautions to prevent dislocation. Due to the durability of current implants and surgical techniques, patients undergoing hip arthroplasty may allow for immediate postoperative weight bearing and rehabilitation (Fig. 22.4), and offers improved outcomes compared to internal fixation. A randomized study comparing total hip arthroplasty to internal fixation in patients over 70 years of age with minimal cognitive deficits who lived and ambulated independently prior to fracture revealed that patients who underwent total hip arthroplasty had a 4% complication rate and a 4% reoperation rate compared to 42% and 47%, respectively, in the internal fixation group. Alternately, among geriatric patients that have concomitant dementia, hemiarthroplasty may be chosen to allow for immediate postoperative weight bearing with a low chance of dislocation. Arthroplasty and hemiarthroplasty may both be done in the lateral or supine position and are associated with greater blood loss than is percutaneous fixation.

Finally, among patients undergoing hemiarthroplasty, repair fixation may be improved by use of cementing techniques. Despite this, however, cementing has been demonstrated to increase the risk of intraoperative medical complications and death, likely due to embolization of the bone marrow contents during cement placement and hypotension associated with release of the cement monomer release. As a result, the rate of intraoperative sudden death during arthroplasty for a femoral neck fracture is estimated to be 1 in 500, making the use of cement a decision to be based on the patient's perceived functional demands as well as overall health and the coexistence of medical problems.

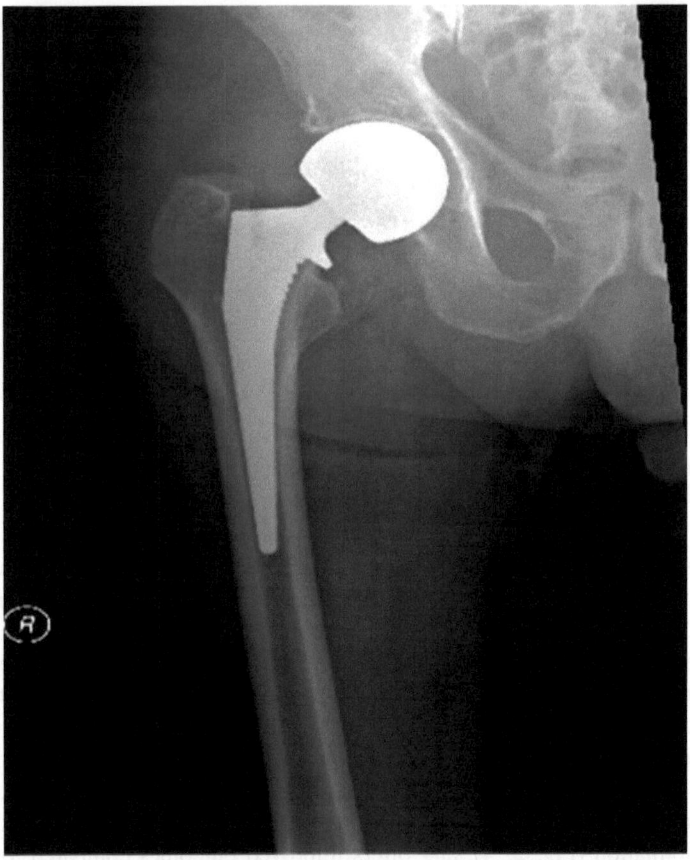

Fig. 22.4 A right hip hemiarthroplasty seen on an AP radiograph, with replacement of the femoral head and neck. The acetabulum is left intact. No cement was used for this procedure

Surgical Approach to Extracapsular Hip Fractures

Similar to femoral neck fractures, multiple surgical options exist for the treatment of extracapsular hip fractures. Once again, operative treatment is the standard of care except in the situation of severe medical comorbidity. Currently, the sliding hip screw and the intramedullary hip screw are the most commonly used surgical constructs, providing stable fracture fixation while allowing the patient to begin early mobilization and weight bearing. Surgical fixation of an intertrochanteric fracture is no different from any other geriatric hip fracture—the surgeon must consider not only fracture pattern but also the patient's age, medical condition, and pre–injury functional status.

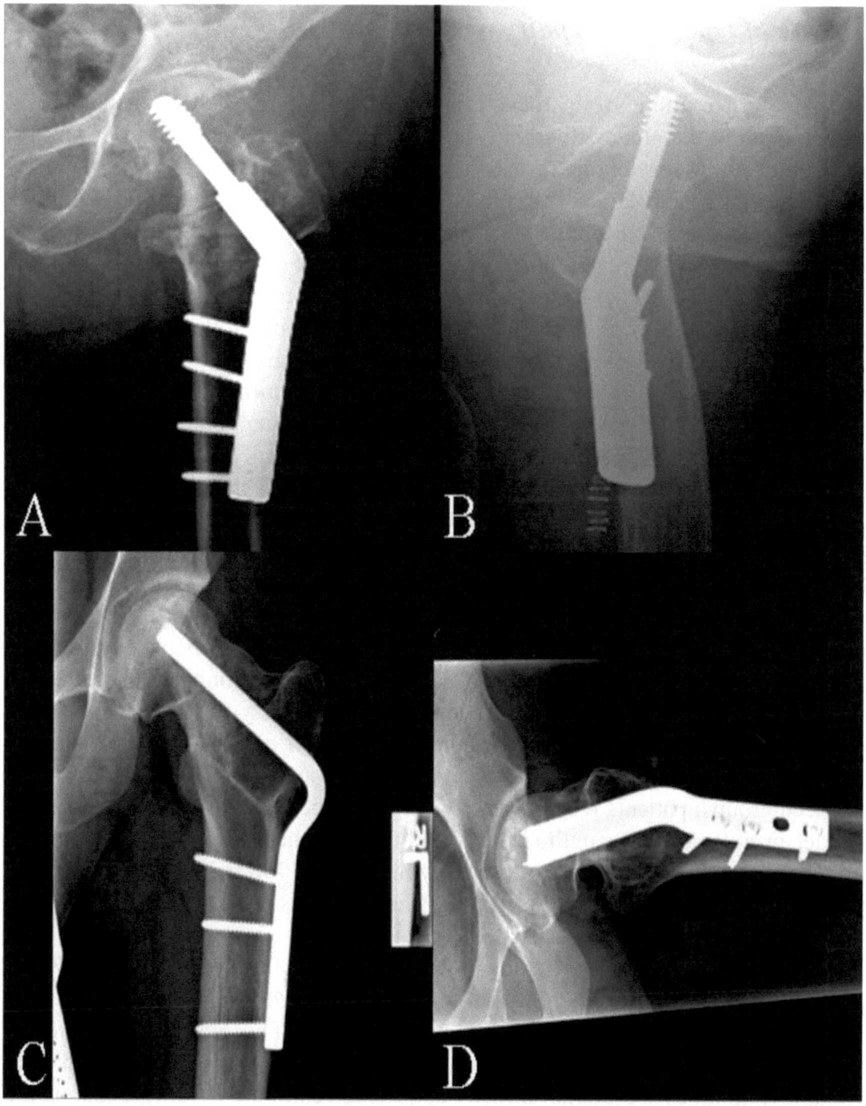

Fig. 22.5 AP and lateral radiographs of an intertrochanteric fracture treated with a dynamic hip screw (**a** and **b**) and a fixed–angle blade plate (**c** and **d**)

Commonly referred to as a compression hip screw or a dynamic hip screw (DHS), sliding hip screws allow for controlled, dynamic compression at the fracture site. This device simultaneously maintains alignment and enhances compression at the fracture site. Sliding hip screws are placed through a lateral incision over the femur. Screw fixation is used to secure the plate portion of the construct to the femoral shaft (Fig. 22.5). Depending on the degree of soft tissue dissection, blood loss can vary from minimal (less than 50 cc) to significant.

Timing of Operative Repair

The appropriate timing of operative repair for hip fracture has been the subject of examination in the clinical literature for over 2 decades. While delays in surgical repair may allow for volume resuscitation, preoperative evaluation, and optimization of preoperative risk factors, prolonged delays may result in increased complications of hospitalization among hip fracture patients due to extended periods of immobilization and pain, potentially increasing the risk of deep venous thrombosis, pneumonia, pressure ulcer formation, and urinary tract infection.

Efforts to assess clear differences in patient outcomes following hip fracture attributable to early versus delayed repair have been difficult to demonstrate in clinical research due to the inability to conduct randomized controlled trials of surgical timing; further, retrospective analyses of the timing of hip fracture care are likely to be subject to confounding due to difficulties in fully controlling for unobserved differences between patients receiving early versus delayed operative therapy. Despite this, recent investigations and large–scale systematic reviews of surgical time for hip fracture argue for operative repair within 48 h among medically stable patients.

A prospective cohort study by Orosz and colleagues of 1,206 hip fracture patients admitted to four hospitals in the New York metropolitan area between 1997 and 1999 used propensity score methods to evaluate outcomes among patients receiving early surgery (up to 24 h after admission), and late surgery (more than 24 h after admission) among patients with a similar likelihood of early surgery was similar. While they found no difference in mortality or functional independence at 6 months between groups, patients receiving early surgery experienced less severe pain and shorter overall hospital length of stay. Additionally, the odds of major complications, such as pneumonia or cardiac arrhythmia, were lower in the early–surgery group in a subgroup analysis of medically stable patients (odds ratio, 0.26; 95% CI, 0.07–0.95).

A more recent retrospective study by McGuire and colleagues examining 18,209 patients admitted for hip fracture between 1995 and 1996 evaluated differences in survival between patients receiving surgery within 48 h of hospital admission versus those undergoing surgery 48 h or more following presentations. Using instrumental variable techniques to account for likely unobserved confounders differentiating the early–surgery and late–surgery groups, the authors found a 15% increased risk of mortality at 30 days among the late–surgery group ($p=0.047$).

While a recent meta–analysis by Shiga and colleagues of 16 studies published between 1992 and 2007 argues for still greater mortality reductions associated with surgical repair within 48 h of admission, the precise relationship between early surgery and perioperative outcomes remains unresolved. Nonetheless, expert opinion increasingly supports surgical repair of hip fracture among medically stable patients during the first 48 h of the hospital stay. For the consulting anesthesia provider, such evidence should highlight the importance of minimizing delays in evaluation and optimization prior to surgery to increase the likelihood of completion of surgical repair within a time frame that may provide the best chances of survival and functional recovery. In the absence of concurrent acute medical emergencies, delays in operative care for diagnostic procedures that will not change anesthetic management should be avoided to optimize patient outcomes.

Preoperative Evaluation and Optimization

Preoperative management of the hip fracture patient presents unique challenges of balancing the needs to stabilize acute medical illnesses and optimize chronic medical conditions with a need for expedient operative repair to improve outcomes. Given the high burden of comorbid illness present in this population, a thorough assessment of existing chronic diseases and current medications should be carried out, and existing illnesses managed as directed by consensus guidelines were available.

Beyond chronic illnesses, hip fracture patients may present with a range of acute conditions potentially representing the cause of a fall. These may include, but are not limited to, a novel cerebrovascular accident or transient ischemic attack, community–acquired pneumonia, myocardial infarction, novel arrhythmia, exacerbation of congestive heart failure, acute hypoglycemia, or urinary tract infection. As a result, the preoperative history and physical should seek to elucidate signs and symptoms consistent with a dangerous process underlying a fall, including loss of consciousness, shortness of breath, chest pain, palpitations, altered mental status, or focal neurologic deficits. As outlined by the American College of Cardiology/American Heart Association guidelines for preoperative cardiovascular evaluation and management, identification of a life–threatening process underlying an admitting diagnosis of hip fracture warrants immediate management and stabilization prior to surgery.

Preoperative Analgesia

Recent clinical research has lent emphasis to the potential for anesthesia providers to influence hip fracture outcomes through involvement in pain management during the preoperative period. While parenteral analgesia using opiate medications remains a common approach to preoperative pain management for hip fracture, a growing body of evidence suggests the potential for regional and neuraxial pain management techniques to provide improved analgesia.

In a systematic review of nerve blocks for analgesia in hip fractures, Parker and colleagues identified nine studies conducted between 1995 and 2007 examining analgesia achieved with nerve blocks administered at the time of hospital admission, with the majority of these examining femoral nerve blocks. The studies reviewed varied in protocol designs and outcomes measured and provide limited insight into differences in clinical end points such as mortality, associated with preoperative nerve blocks for hip fracture patients. However, overall, preoperative nerve blockade was associated with statistically significant reductions in reported pain levels and in the quantity of parenteral or oral analgesics required for pain control, arguing for the use of preoperative nerve blocks as an element of preoperative pain management for hip fracture care.

Preoperative epidural analgesia for hip fracture has been examined in two studies, with equivocal results regarding preoperative pain control. Nonetheless, both suggest the potential for neuraxial analgesia, initiated at time of hospital admission, to reduce the rate of adverse cardiac events among hip fracture patients. Matot and colleagues randomized 77 patients to preoperative analgesic regimens of intramuscular meperidine (1 mg/kg, every 6 h) versus a continuous infusion of epidural bupivacaine (0.5%; 45 mg/24 h) and methadone (16 mg/24 h). While the two groups did not differ in pain scores following initiation of analgesia, investigators observed a greater incidence of preoperative adverse cardiac events in the control versus intervention group (20.5% vs. 0%, $p=0.01$). Epidural analgesia was continued into the postoperative period for the intervention group, but no difference was observed in the rate of intraoperative or postoperative adverse cardiac events between groups.

In a smaller study, Scheinin and colleagues randomized 55 patients to an epidural infusion of 0.01% bupivacaine with 10 mcg/mL of fentanyl (3–5 mL/h) versus intramuscular oxycodone (0.1–0.15 mg/kg every 6 h), initiated at the time of hospital presentation. While they observed no significant differences in the overall rates of myocardial ischemia between groups, as measured by continuous ECG (Holter) monitor, control patients experienced significantly more intraoperative ischemic episodes than did intervention patients (26.7% vs. 0%, $p=0.005$).

While these two studies require further confirmation in additional clinical trials, they provide a preliminary argument that epidural techniques for analgesia may reduce the rates of perioperative cardiac events among hip fracture patients. Nonetheless, the ability of any such reductions, if truly achievable in clinical practice, to yield benefits in survival or functional recovery for hip fracture patients remains unknown.

Intraoperative Management

Monitoring and Intravenous Access

Monitoring approaches for the hip fracture patient are dictated by choice of anesthetic technique, preexisting patient comorbidities, and cardiopulmonary function of the patient at the time of presentation. At a minimum, monitors should include five–lead electrocardiography, intermittent noninvasive blood pressure measurement, pulse oximetry, and, if general endotracheal anesthesia is planned, capnography.

In the presence of severe known cardiovascular disease, such as critical aortic stenosis, or flow–limiting coronary artery disease, invasive hemodynamic monitoring should be considered. As approximately 50% of hip fracture patients may require transfusion in the perioperative period intravenous access, potentially including central venous access should be established prior to incision. In patients with extracapsular hip fractures or are undergoing total hip replacement, the risk of blood loss is increased, and additional intravenous access, with or without invasive hemodynamic monitors, should be considered for these patients.

Choice of Anesthetic Technique

Common approaches to anesthesia for hip fracture include general anesthesia (either through an endotracheal tube or, where appropriate, via a supraglottic airway) and neuraxial anesthesia (via spinal or epidural). The optimal approach to anesthesia for hip fracture remains a source of controversy among experts. Potential complications of general anesthesia include medication reactions, difficulty in establishing or maintaining a patent airway, respiratory depression, and aspiration of gastric contents. In contrast, regional techniques have the potential for intraoperative hypotension potentially compromising cardiac or cerebral blood flow and carry a risk of an inadequate or failed block, balanced against the potential to reduce the incidence of deep venous thrombosis among hip fracture patients.

Despite the differences in potential complications of these two techniques, clinical research has not yielded definitive answers regarding differences in survival for patients receiving regional versus general anesthesia. In a prospective cohort study of 9,245 patients undergoing surgery for hip fracture between 1983 and 1993, O'Hara and colleagues examined differences in mortality among patients receiving regional and general anesthesia. After adjustment for confounders, the authors observed a nonsignificant increase in the odds of death at 30 days among the 65.8% of patients who received general anesthesia (odds ratio 1.08, 95% CI 0.84–1.38). No differences were found between groups in the adjusted odds of 7–day mortality, myocardial infarction, congestive heart failure, pneumonia, or postoperative change in mental status.

Despite these negative findings, O'Hara's study remains difficult to interpret in terms of clinical decision–making for hip fracture care. It was carefully conducted based on detailed chart review data and used multivariate analyses to control for a range of potential confounders. Yet the greater prevalence of key medical comorbidities, higher American Society of Anesthesiologists Physical Status classification scores, and age over 80 among patients receiving regional anesthesia raise concern for potential unobserved differences between groups that may have prevented detection of a true difference in outcomes between groups attributable to one or the other treatment.

While randomized clinical trials can alleviate such selection effects by random assignment of individuals to clinical treatments, methodological limitations of available studies, heterogeneity in outcomes examined, and changes in anesthetic practice over time make it difficult to reach definitive conclusions regarding the advantage of one technique over another. Indeed, a recent meta–analysis identified 22 such trials conducted between 1977 and 2003 concluded that insufficient evidence existed to rule out clinically important differences between regional and general anesthesia. While regional anesthesia appeared to decrease the relative risk of delirium after hip fracture (pooled RR 0.50, 95% CI 0.26–0.95), the authors find insufficient evidence to draw conclusions regarding the relationship between anesthetic technique and mortality after hip fracture.

In the absence of definitive clinical evidence supporting one technique over another, decisions regarding the use of regional versus general anesthesia for hip fracture should be based on clinical evaluation of the individual patient, as well as consideration of practical concerns that may vary between institutions. Given the widespread use of pharmacologic thromboprophylaxis, decisions regarding the use of neuraxial techniques must be made within the context of local approaches to anticoagulation management and consideration of the risks of epidural hematoma formation in a given patient. Lastly, the choice of anesthetic technique should optimally incorporate a discussion of patient and family preferences for care following a careful discussion, where possible, of potential risks and benefits of each approach.

Management of Sedation During Regional Anesthesia

For patients receiving regional anesthesia for hip fracture repair, recent clinical evidence suggests that a targeted sedation strategy may offer pronounced benefits in reducing delirium among hip fracture patients. Sieber and colleagues (2010) conducted a well–designed trial of sedation management in hip fracture surgery, randomizing 114 patients, all receiving spinal anesthesia for hip fracture repair, to a regimen of "deep" or "light" propofol sedation, titrated to a Bispectral Index (BIS) monitor score of 50 or 80, respectively, with a maximum of 2 mg of midazolam for sedation during block placement in each group. Observing a reduced rate of delirium in the "light" sedation group (11/57 patients, 19%) versus the "deep" sedation group (23/57 patients, 40%), the authors find that one case of delirium could be prevented for every 4.7 patients managed with a "light" sedation regimen. While these results require confirmation in further clinical trials, they offer a suggestion that careful titration of sedation during regional anesthesia for hip fracture may contribute to improved short–term outcomes.

Transfusion Management

The optimal hemoglobin level at which to initiate transfusion therapy is an important, unresolved clinical issue throughout perioperative medicine. While hemotherapy may be necessary to preserve oxygen delivery to vital tissues in the presence of acute anemia, its risks, including the potential for infection, transfusion–related lung injury, immunosuppression, alloimmunization, and acute and delayed hemolytic transfusion reactions, make determination of the optimal hemoglobin target a complex task. Hip fracture patients present a population in which balancing the risks and benefits of blood transfusion is of heightened complexity due to the advanced age and high burden of medical comorbidity in this population. Indeed, while a higher transfusion target, in theory, may optimize cerebral oxygen delivery and lessen the risk of postoperative altered mental status, the increased intravascular volume associated with transfusion may pose added risks in the presence of coexisting heart failure. Current opinion is divided regarding the safety of transfusion thresholds below 10 mg/dL for patients with known cardiovascular disease, as may be the case with many hip fracture patients. Further, few prior trials have evaluated the relationship between blood transfusion and functional recovery, an outcome of particular relevance to hip fracture patients.

Extensive clinical research has examined the optimal "trigger" hemoglobin level for transfusion initiation in hip fracture patients. In a retrospective cohort study of 8,787 hip fracture patients treated between 1983 and 1993, Carson and colleagues examined postoperative mortality associated with transfusion of red blood cells across a range of trigger hemoglobin levels. Forty two percent of all patients received a transfusion, with 55.6% of patients with a hemoglobin level between 8.0 and 10.0 g/dL receiving a transfusion and 90.5% of all patients with a hemoglobin level below 8.0 g/dL receiving a transfusion. After adjustment for trigger hemoglobin level, 30–day and 90–day mortality did not differ between patients receiving pre–or postoperative transfusions and those who did not. Notably, the high percentage of patients receiving a transfusion for hemoglobin below 8.0 g/dL precluded firm conclusions regarding transfusion triggers below this level.

Further investigations of the optimal hemoglobin transfusion level are ongoing; Carson and colleagues have recently completed a large, randomized clinical trial of transfusion triggers in postoperative hip fracture patients. This trial, the transfusion trigger trial for functional outcomes in cardiovascular patients undergoing surgical hip fracture repair (FOCUS), enrolled 2,016 hip fracture patients at 47 North American medical centers with initial postoperative hemoglobin levels below 10.0 g/dL, evidence of prior cardiac risk factors (e.g., hypertension, diabetes, prior myocardial infarction) and no evidence of active bleeding. Patients were assigned to one of two transfusion strategies: (1) symptomatic transfusion, defined as transfusion for symptoms attributable to anemia (e.g., dyspnea, chest pain, altered mental status) or for a hemoglobin level below 8.0 g/dL or (2) transfusion, in 1 unit quantities, as necessary to keep the hemoglobin level above 10.0 g/dL.

Data collection for the full trial has been completed, with the principal results made publically available in abstract form in 2009. These preliminary results suggest no difference between groups transfused according to the symptomatic or threshold strategy. Mean hemoglobin prior to transfusion was 9.2 (SD 0.5) in the threshold group and 7.9 (SD 0.5) in the symptomatic group; median number of units transfused was two for the threshold group (interquartile range: 1, 2) and zero for the symptomatic group (interquartile range: 0, 1). Outcomes did not differ between groups, with an odds ratio for death or inability to walk at 60 days of 1.03 (95% CI 0.85, 1.23) and an odds ratio for death at 60 days of 1.19 (95% CI 0.76, 1.86) for the threshold group versus the symptomatic group.

While these results remain preliminary and have yet to appear in full publication, the findings of the FOCUS trial are thus likely to argue for equivalence between use of a threshold hemoglobin of 8.0 mg/dL to one aiming for a 10 mg/dL transfusion target. Such work is likely to lend support for the safety of transfusion thresholds below 10 mg/dL in hip fracture patients with known cardiovascular risk factors from both the perspective of patient survival and recovery of functional independence.

Postoperative Care

After surgery, regardless of type of fracture or type of surgery performed, all patients undergo a regimented and rigorous rehabilitation process. Patients are allowed to weight bear as tolerated on the injured extremity without concern for displacing or disrupting the surgical fixation. It was found by Koval and his colleagues that patients after hip fracture surgery (both femoral neck and intertrochanteric hip fractures) who were allowed to weight bear as tolerated self–limited the amount of weight placed on their extremity. The rehabilitation process after surgery is a multidisciplinary effort involving orthopedists, geriatricians, rehabilitation specialists, anesthesiologists, physiotherapists, and occupational therapists. The recommended protocol consists of early standing and progression to ambulation. The first postoperative day should involve standing and unrestricted weight bearing on both lower extremities with the use of an assist device (walker, cane, crutches). As walking ability improves, over the course of the next several postoperative days, the assist device should be adjusted by the physical therapist.

Pain Management

Adequate management of pain in the postoperative period represents a crucial determinant of postoperative mobilization and outcomes following hip fracture in which anesthesia providers have the potential to contribute to improved outcomes for hip fracture patients. Examining a prospective cohort of 411 hip fracture patients admitted to New York area hospitals between 1997 and 1998, Morrison and colleagues examined the association between postoperative pain scores and a range of in–hospital and 6 month outcomes. Patients with higher pain scores at rest had longer hospital length of stay ($p=0.03$), were more likely to have physical therapy sessions missed or shortened ($p=0.002$), were less likely to walk by postoperative day three ($p=0.001$), and had significantly lower locomotion ability at 6 months ($p=0.02$).

In a separate analysis, Morrison and colleagues examined risk factors for development of postoperative delirium within a similar cohort. Along with preoperative cognitive impairment, hemodynamic instability, and heart failure, receipt of analgesia of less than 10 mg of intravenous morphine sulfate equivalents per day was an independent risk factor for delirium (relative risk: 5.4, 95% CI 2.4–12.3), as was treatment with meperidine for analgesia (relative risk: 2.4, 95% CI 1.3–4.5). Among patients without preoperative cognitive impairment, severe pain was associated with a profound increase in the risk of delirium (relative risk: 9.0, 95% CI 1.8–45.2), further arguing for the importance of adequate postoperative pain control to improving hip fracture outcomes.

As highlighted by the findings of Morrison and colleagues, the approach to analgesia for hip fracture patients should account both for the need to control pain and the risk of adverse effects attributable to treatment. Importantly, in selecting among parenteral analgesics, meperidine is likely to carry risks of postoperative alterations in mental status and should be avoided as a primary analgesic for hip fracture patients in favor of analgesics carrying lower risks of neurologic dysfunction, such as morphine, hydromorphone, or oxycodone.

The use of neuraxial, rather than parenteral approaches to postoperative analgesia among hip fracture patients, remains a subject of ongoing inquiry. In a randomized, double–blind, placebo–controlled trial, 55 patients received preoperative analgesia and intraoperative anesthesia via an epidural catheter; following surgery, patients in the intervention arm received a continuous epidural infusion of 0.125% bupivacaine and 50 mcg/mL morphine (4 mL/h), while control patients received an epidural infusion of 0.9% saline. Nurse–controlled parenteral analgesia with morphine sulfate was made available to all patients. Intervention patients reported consistently lower pain scores at rest, with knee or hip flexion, with transfer from supine to sitting, and on walking, with no significant differences in rates of nausea and vomiting between groups. While definitive conclusions regarding the risks and benefits of epidural analgesia following hip fracture repair will require further data from larger clinical trials, this work argues that epidural analgesia may offer improved advantages over nurse–controlled parenteral analgesia following hip fracture repair.

Conclusions

Hip fracture represents a common, morbid, and potentially disabling injury among older adults. Due to the frequent nature of postoperative complications among hip fracture patients and the profound consequences that such complications may have for long–term outcomes, high–quality perioperative care is a crucial element in optimizing the chances for functional recovery following surgery for hip fracture repair. Anesthesiologists and other perioperative care providers may potentially contribute to such improved outcomes through reliance on evidence–based practices for hip fracture care, ideally within the framework of a multidisciplinary, structured approach to the inpatient management of this condition.

Key Points

- Hip fracture is a frequent and disabling injury resulting in a high worldwide burden of disability and excess mortality.
- Morbidity and mortality following hip fracture are high, attributable primarily to infectious, cardiac, and pulmonary complications occurring in the postoperative period.
- Surgical repair is indicated for all types of hip fracture; among medically stable patients, early operative repair (within 24–48 h of admission) may maximize chances of functional recovery.
- A coordinated, multidisciplinary approach to hospital care for hip fracture, including standardized recommendations for preoperative, intraoperative, and postoperative care may promote improved hospital outcomes among hip fracture patients.
- Adequate pre– and postoperative pain control may reduce the rate of inpatient complications among older adults with hip fracture; regional anesthetic techniques, including femoral nerve blockade or epidural analgesia, may offer benefits over parenteral analgesia.
- Clinical evidence is equivocal regarding a mortality benefit of a particular anesthetic technique; neuraxial anesthesia, potentially employing a targeted approach to sedation management, may result in a lower incidence of postoperative cognitive dysfunction in the postoperative period.

Suggested Reading

Beaupre LA, Cinats JG, Senthilselvan A, Lier D, Jones CA, Scharfenberger A, et al. Reduced morbidity for elderly patients with a hip fracture after implementation of a perioperative evidence–based clinical pathway. Qual Saf Health Care. 2006;15(5):375–79.

Beaupre LA, Jones CA, Saunders LD, Johnston DW, Buckingham J, Majumdar SR. Best practices for elderly hip fracture patients. A systematic overview of the evidence. J Gen Intern Med. 2005;20(11):1019–25.

Bhandari M, Devereaux PJ, Tornetta P, 3rd, Swiontkowski MF, Berry DJ, Haidukewych G, Schemitsch EH, Hanson BP, Koval K, Dirschl D, Leece P, Keel M, Petrisor B, Heetveld M, Guyatt GH: Operative management of displaced femoral neck fractures in elderly patients. An international survey. J Bone Joint Surg Am. 2005;87(9):2122–30.

Blackman DK, Kamimoto LA, Smith SM. Overview: surveillance for selected public health indicators affecting older adults—United States. MMWR CDC Surveill Summ. 1999;48(8):1–6.

Blomfeldt R, Tornkvist H, Ponzer S, Soderqvist A, Tidermark J: Comparison of internal fixation with total hip replacement for displaced femoral neck fractures. Randomized, controlled trial performed at four years. J Bone Joint Surg Am. 2005; 87(8):1680–8.

Brauer CA, Coca–Perraillon M, Cutler DM, Rosen AB. Incidence and mortality of hip fractures in the United States. JAMA. 2009;302(14):1573–79.

British Orthopaedic Association. The Care of Patients With Fragility Fractures. In: C. Currie (Eds.) Available from http://www.nhfd.co.uk/. 2007.

Carson JL, Duff A, Berlin JA, Lawrence VA, Poses RM, Huber EC, et al. Perioperative blood transfusion and postoperative mortality. JAMA. 1998;279(3):199–205.

Carson JL, Terrin ML, Magaziner J, Chaitman BR, Apple FS, Heck DA, et al. Transfusion trigger trial for functional outcomes in cardiovascular patients undergoing surgical hip fracture repair (FOCUS). Transfusion. 2006;46(12):2192–206.

Carson JL, Terrin ML, Magaziner J, Sanders D, Cook DR, Hildebrand K. Transfusion Trigger Trial for Functional Outcomes in Cardiovascular Patients Undergoing Surgical Hip Fracture Repair (FOCUS): The Principal Results (Abstract). Blood (American Society of Hematology Annual Meeting Abstracts). 2009;114(Abstract 6).

Fisher AA, Davis MW, Rubenach SE, Sivakumaran S, Smith PN, Budge MM: Outcomes for older patients with hip fractures: the impact of orthopedic and geriatric medicine cocare. J Orthop Trauma. 2006;20(3):172–8;discussion 179–80.

Fleisher LA, Beckman JA, Brown KA, Calkins H, Chaikof E, Fleischmann KE, et al. ACC/AHA 2007 guidelines on perioperative cardiovascular evaluation and care for noncardiac surgery: executive summary: a report of the American College of Cardiology/American Heart Association Task Force on Practice Guidelines (Writing Committee to Revise the 2002 Guidelines on Perioperative Cardiovascular Evaluation for Noncardiac Surgery). Anesth Analg. 2008;106(3):685–712.

Foss NB, Kristensen MT, Kristensen BB, Jensen PS. Kehlet H. Effect of postoperative epidural analgesia on rehabilitation and pain after hip fracture surgery: a randomized, double–blind, placebo–controlled trial. Anesthesiology. 2005;102(6):1197–204.

Halbert J, Crotty M, Whitehead C, Cameron I, Kurrle S, Graham S, Handoll H, Finnegan T, Jones T, Foley A, Shanahan M: Multi–disciplinary rehabilitation after hip fracture is associated with improved outcome: A systematic review. J Rehabil Med. 2007;39(7):507–12.

Hannan EL, Magaziner J, Wang JJ, Eastwood EA, Silberzweig SB, Gilbert M, et al. Mortality and locomotion 6 months after hospitalization for hip fracture: risk factors and risk–adjusted hospital outcomes. JAMA. 2001;285(21):2736–742.

Iorio R, Healy WL, Lemos DW, Appleby D, Lucchesi CA, Saleh KJ. Displaced femoral neck fractures in the elderly: outcomes and cost effectiveness. Clin Orthop Relat Res. 2001(383):229–42.

Johnell O, Kanis JA. An estimate of the worldwide prevalence and disability associated with osteoporotic fractures. Osteoporos Int. 2006;17(12):1726–733.

Kanis JA, Oden A, Johansson H, Borgstrom F, Strom O, McCloskey E. FRAX and its applications to clinical practice. Bone. 2009;44(5):734–43.

Koval KJ, Zuckerman JD. Hip Fractures: A Practical Guide to Management. New York: Springer. 2000.

Lawrence VA, Hilsenbeck SG, Noveck H, Poses RM, Carson JL. Medical complications and outcomes after hip fracture repair. Arch Intern Med. 2002;162(18):2053–57.

Magaziner J, Hawkes W, Hebel JR, Zimmerman SI, Fox KM, Dolan M, et al. Recovery from hip fracture in eight areas of function. J Gerontol A Biol Sci Med Sci. 2000;55(9):M498–507.

Marcantonio ER, Flacker JM, Wright RJ, Resnick NM. Reducing delirium after hip fracture: a randomized trial. Journal of the American Geriatrics Society. 2001;(5):516–522. Retrieved from http://www.mrw.interscience.wiley.com/cochrane/clcentral/articles/295/CN–00348295/frame.html.

Matot I, Oppenheim–Eden A, Ratrot R, Baranova J, Davidson E, Eylon S, et al. Preoperative cardiac events in elderly patients with hip fracture randomized to epidural or conventional analgesia. Anesthesiology. 2003;98(1):156–63.

McGuire KJ, Bernstein J, Polsky D, Silber JH. The 2004 Marshall Urist award: delays until surgery after hip fracture increases mortality. Clin Orthop Relat Res. 2004;(428):294–301.

Morrison RS, Magaziner J, Gilbert M, Koval KJ, McLaughlin MA, Orosz G, et al. Relationship between pain and opioid analgesics on the development of delirium following hip fracture. J Gerontol A Biol Sci Med Sci. 2003;58(1):76–81.

Morrison RS, Magaziner J, McLaughlin MA, Orosz G, Silberzweig SB, Koval KJ, et al. The impact of post–operative pain on outcomes following hip fracture. Pain. 2003;103(3):303–11.

Neuman MD, Archan S, Karlawish JH, Schwartz JS, Fleisher LA.The relationship between short-term mortality and quality of care for hip fracture: a meta-analysis of clinical pathways for hip fracture. J Am Geriatr Soc. 2009;57(11):2046–2054.

O'Hara DA, Duff A, Berlin JA, Poses RM, Lawrence VA, Huber EC, et al. The effect of anesthetic technique on postoperative outcomes in hip fracture repair. Anesthesiology. 2000;92(4):947–957.

Orosz GM, Magaziner J, Hannan EL, Morrison RS, Koval K, Gilbert M, et al. Association of timing of surgery for hip fracture and patient outcomes. JAMA. 2004;291(14):1738–1743.

Parker M, Johansen A. Hip fracture. BMJ. 2006;333(7557):27–30.

Parker MJ, Griffiths R, Appadu BN. Nerve blocks (subcostal, lateral cutaneous, femoral, triple, psoas) for hip fractures. Cochrane Database Syst Rev. 2002;(1):CD001159.

Parker MJ, Handoll HH, Griffiths R. Anaesthesia for hip fracture surgery in adults. Cochrane Database Syst Rev. 2004;(4):CD000521.

Scheini H, Virtanen T, Kentala E, Uotila P, Laitio T, Hartiala J, et al. Epidural infusion of bupivacaine and fentanyl reduces perioperative myocardial ischaemia in elderly patients with hip fracture—a randomized controlled trial. Acta Anaesthesiol Scand. 2000;44(9):1061–1070.

Schwartz AV, Kelsey JL, Maggi S, Tuttleman M, Ho SC, Jonsson PV, et al. International variation in the incidence of hip fractures: cross–national project on osteoporosis for the World Health Organization Program for Research on Aging. Osteoporos Int. 1999;9(3):242–253.

Shiga T, Wajima Z, Ohe Y. Is operative delay associated with increased mortality of hip fracture patients? Systematic review, meta–analysis, and meta–regression. Can J Anaesth. 2008;55(3):146–154.

Sieber FE, Zakriya KJ, Gottschalk A, Blute MR, Lee HB, Rosenberg PB, et al. Sedation depth during spinal anesthesia and the development of postoperative delirium in elderly patients undergoing hip fracture repair. Mayo Clin Proc. 2010;85(1):18–26.

Wilson RT, Chase GA, Chrischilles EA, Wallace RB. Hip fracture risk among community–dwelling elderly people in the United States: a prospective study of physical, cognitive, and socioeconomic indicators. Am J Public Health. 2006;96(7):1210–1218.

Zuckerman JD, Sakales SR, Fabian DR, Frankel VH. Hip fractures in geriatric patients. Results of an interdisciplinary hospital care program. Clin Orthop Relat Res. 1992;274:213–225.

Zuckerman JD, Skovron ML, Koval KJ, Aharonoff G, Frankel VH. Postoperative complications and mortality associated with operative delay in older patients who have a fracture of the hip. J Bone Joint Surg Am. 1995;77(10):1551–6.

Chapter 23
Polypharmacy and Medicines to Avoid

Lale E. Odekon

Introduction

The number of individuals surviving past age 65 is increasing globally and the likelihood of suffering from chronic diseases is also rising as the demographics shift. Since even a single medical condition may require multiple medications, it is not surprising that each additional disease significantly increases the risk for polypharmacy–related adverse drug reactions (ADRs) and morbidity. This is especially so when each comorbidity requires the care of a different specialist as is frequently seen in the aged population.

The relevance of polypharmacy for anesthesiologists must be recognized—greater than 30% of individuals older than 65 will undergo at least one surgical procedure during the remainder of their lifetime. Thus, anesthesiologists, as perioperative physicians, are in a pivotal position to review the patients' medications for potentially avoidable interactions and polypharmacy–related events.

Medication Use

As noted above aging is associated with increasing comorbidities, and an analysis of Medicare beneficiaries in the USA revealed that greater than three–fourths of this group of older patients suffered from one or more chronic diseases. Each new complaint or disease beyond the index disease can add a prescription and/or the addition of nonprescription drugs and herbal products, thereby significantly increasing the risk of ADRs (Tables 23.1 and 23.2). The risk of an ADR is compounded by the fact

L.E. Odekon, MD, PhD (✉)
Anesthesiology and Critical Care Medicine, Johns Hopkins Bayview Medical Center,
4940 Eastern Avenue, A577, Baltimore, MD 21224, USA
e–mail: laleodekon@earthlink.net

S.R. Barnett (ed.), *Manual of Geriatric Anesthesia*, DOI 10.1007/978-1-4614-3888-5_23,

Table 23.1 Common medication groups frequently implicated in ADRs

Medication groups
Cardiovascular drugs
Anticholinergics
Antidepressants
Antibiotics
Diuretics
Hypoglicemic agents
Opioids
Anticoagulants (Warfarin)

Table 23.2 Common types of ADR's

Adverse drug reactions
Altered blood pressure control
Mental status changes
Electrolyte disturbances
Hemorrhagic events

that in studies conducted leading to FDA drug approval, the participants selected are generally free of disease except one for which treatment is sought and are typically younger than 65 years of age.

Polypharmacy

Polypharmacy is defined as ingesting five or more prescription drugs at one time. Practitioners taking care of elderly individuals need to consider that even with a lower number of prescription drugs, polypharmacy may present with over–the–counter drug or herbal medicine use. Of the potential drug interactions, drug–drug, drug–disease, and drug–herbal product are the most relevant in the perioperative setting. Examples of drug–drug interactions include antihypertensives and vasodilators (ACE inhibitors and an induction agent) causing excessive hypotension; and quinidine and barbiturate use decreasing the effectiveness of the antiarrhythmic. During the pre–anesthetic assessment, it is important to enquire specifically about medications recently started as these may have changed from the time of the initial interview or the last procedure.

Polypharmacy may impact an individual in multiple ways—one example is the impact on the underlying enzyme systems. Concurrent use of medications which inhibit/induce hepatic cytochrome P450 isoenzymes or modulate the efflux transporter P–glycoprotein, or alter glomerular filtration rate (GFR) may result in an adverse drug reaction. Some examples include:

1. Patients on digoxin who are started on clarithromycin presenting with digoxin toxicity.
2. Patients on cyclosporine and repaglinide presenting with hypoglycemia.
3. Patients on ACEI, presenting with hyperkalemia following the addition of spironolactone.

Age and Polypharmacy

Age itself is not regarded as a risk factor for ADRs. Instead multiple comorbidities, the polypharmacy that these comorbidities necessitate, and the pharmacokinetic and pharmacodynamic changes found with advancing years most likely account for the increased ADRs in the geriatric population. With these considerations in mind in 1991, Beers and coauthors developed criteria to distinguish medications whose potential risk outweighed their benefits when used in geriatric patients. The initial tool that was devised for use in nursing homes was revised and updated to apply to geriatric patients in general (Table 23.3. 2002 Criteria for Potentially Inappropriate Medication use in Older Adults: Independent of diagnosis or Condition). More recently the same authors provided a consensus opinion on "preferred" medications in the elderly for central nervous system (CNS) pathologies. In 2012, at the time this chapter went into publication the American Geriatrics Society published its latest updated Beers Criteria, removing drugs no longer in use and incorporating newer drugs introduced since 2002.The reader is encouraged to consult the Journal of American Geriatrics Society, 2012.

The perioperative period presents an ideal checkpoint to evaluate the appropriateness of the patient's medications to determine if therapeutic end–points are met. In addition to the Beers Criteria, the anesthesiologist may be assisted in ruling out potential ADRs by use of a computerized decision support system, electronic data systems, and a multidisciplinary team approach. The ideal future state might be one that employs an automated system based on appropriate software with a designated supervising pharmacist who will provide a cross–referenced (e.g., surgical medication list vs. anesthesiology medication list) safety check. Until that state is achieved, it is the anesthesiologist who must remain the gatekeepers and strive to ensure that perioperative patients are on appropriate medications with minimal opportunity for adverse drug–drug or drug–disease interactions.

Implications of Aging for Pharmacokinetics and Pharmacodynamics

Pharmacokinetics

The elderly population is heterogeneous with respect to:

1. Fitness or frailty
2. The extent of physiologic reserve available; and
3. The response to medication, particularly to those with a low therapeutic index (Table 23.4).

Therefore, each new medication introduced, whether in a physician's office or in the perioperative setting, needs to be started at a low dose and titrated slowly to desired effect, taking into consideration reliable, anticipated changes in several key organ systems. These are briefly reviewed below.

Table 23.3 2002 criteria for potentially inappropriate medication use in older adults: independent of diagnoses or conditions

Drug	Concern	Severity rating (high or low)
Propoxyphene (Darvon) and combination products (Darvon with ASA, Darvon–N, and Darvocet–N)	Offers few analgesic advantages over acetaminophen, yet has the adverse effects of other narcotic drugs	Low
Indomethacin (Indocin and Indocin SR)	Of all available nonsteroidal anti–inflammatory drugs, this drug produces the most CNS adverse effects	High
Pentazocine (Talwin)	Narcotic analgesic that causes more CNS adverse effects, including confusion and hallucinations, more commonly than other narcotic drugs. Additionally, it is mixed agonist and antagonist	High
Trimethobenzamide (Tigan)	One of the least effective antiemetic drugs, yet it can cause extrapyramidal adverse effects	High
Muscle relaxants and antispasmodics: methocarbamol (Robaxin), carisoprodol (Soma), clorozoxazone (Paraflex), metaxalone (Skelaxin), cyclobenzaprine (Flexeril), and oxybutynin (Ditropan). Do not consider the extended–release Ditropan XL	Most muscle relaxants and antispasmodic drugs are poorly tolerated by elderly patients, since these cause anticholinergic adverse effects, sedation, and weakness. Additionally, their effectiveness at doses tolerated by elderly patients is questionable	High
Flurazepam (Dalmane)	This benzodiazepine hypnotic has an extremely long half–life in elderly patients (often days), producing prolonged sedation and increasing the incidence of falls and fracture. Medium– or short–acting benzodiazepines are preferable	High
Amitriptyline (Elavil), chlordiazepoxide–amitriptyline (Limbitrol), and perphenazine–amitriptyline (Triavil)	Because of its strong anticholinergic and sedation properties, amitriptyline is rarely the antidepressant of choice for elderly patients	High
Amitryptyline (Sinequan)	Because of its strong anticholinergic and sedation properties, amitryptyline is rarely the antidepressant of choice for elderly patients	High
Meprobamate (Miltown and Equanif)	This is a highly addictive and sedating anxiolytic. Those using meprobamate for prolonged periods may become addicted and may need to be withdrawn slowly	High
Doses of short–acting benzodiazepines: doses greater than Iorazepam (Ativan) e mg; oxazepam (Serax), 60 mg; alprazolam (Xanax), 2 mg; temazepam (Restoril), 15 mg; and triazolam (Halcion), 0.25 mg	Because of increased sensitivity to benzodiazepines in elderly patients smaller doses may be effective as well as safer. Total daily doses should rarely exceed the suggested maximums	High

Long–acting benzodiazepoxide (Librium), chlordiazepoxide–amitriptyline (Limbitrol) clidinium–chlordiazepoxide (Librax), diazepam (Valium), quazepam (Doral), halazepam (Paxipam) and chlorazepate (Tranxene)	These drugs have a long half–life in elderly patients (often several days), producing prolonged sedation and increasing the risk of falls and fractures. Short– and intermediate–acting benzodiazepines are preferred if a benzodiazepine is required	High
Disopyramide (Norpace and Norpace CR)	Of all antiarrhythmic drugs, this is the most potent negative inotrope and therefore may induce heart failure in elderly patients. It is also strong anticholinergic. Other antiarrhythmic drugs should be used	High
Digoxin (Lanoxin) (should not exceed >0.125 mg/d except when treating atrial arrhythmias)	Decreased renal clearance may lead to increased risk of toxic effects	Low
Short–acting dipyridamole (Persantine). Do not consider the long–acting dipyridamole (which has better properties than the short–acting in older adults) except with patients with artificial heart valves	May cause orthostatic hypotension	Low
Methyldopa (Aldomet) and methyldopa–hydrochlorothiazide (Aldoril)	May cause bradycardia and exacerbate depression in elderly patients	High
Reserpine at doses > 0.25 mg	May induce depression, impotence, sedation, and orthostatic hypotension	Low
Chlorpropamide (Diabinese)	It has prolonged half–life in elderly patients and could cause prolonged hypoglycemia. Additionally, it is the only oral hypoglycemic agent that cause SIADH	High
Gastrointestinal antispasmodic drugs: dicyclomine (Bentyl), hyoscyamine (Levsin and Levsinex), propantheline (Pro–Banthine), belladonna alkaloids (Donnatal and others), and clidinium–chlordiazepoxide (Librax)	GI antispasmodic drugs are highly anticholinergic and have uncertain effectiveness. These drugs should be avoided (especially for long–term use)	High
Anticholinergics and antihistamines: chlorpheniramine (Chlor–Trimeton), diphenhydramine (Benadryl), hydroxyzine (Vistaril and Atarax), cyproheptadine (Periactin), promethazine (Phenergan), tripelennamine, dexchlorpheniramine (Polaramine)	All nonprescription and many prescription antihistamines may have potent anticholinergic properties. Nonanticholinergic antihistamines are preferred in elderly patients when treating allergic reactions	High
Diphenhydramine (Benadryl)	May cause confusion and sedation. Should not be used as a hypnotic, and when used to treat emergency allergic reactions, it should be used in the smallest possible dose	High

(continued)

Table 23.3 (continued)

Drug	Concern	Severity rating (high or low)
Ergot mesyloids (Hydergine) and cyclandelate (Cyclospasmol)	Have not been shown to be effective in the doses studied	Low
Ferrous sulfate >325 mg/d	Doses >325 mg/d do not dramatically increase the amount absorbed but greatly increase the incidence of constipation	Low
All barbiturates (except phenobarbital) except when used to control seizures	Are highly addictive and cause more adverse effects than most sedative or hypnotic drugs in elderly patients	High
Meperidine (Demerol)	Not an effective oral analgesic in doses commonly used. May cause confusion and has many disadvantages to other narcotic drugs	High
Ticlopidine (Ticlid)	Has been shown to be no better than aspirin in preventing clotting and may be considerably more toxic. Safer, more effective alternatives exist	High
Ketorolac (Toradol)	Immediate and long–term use should be avoided in older persons, since a significant number have asymptomatic GI pathologic conditions	High
Amphetamines and anorexic agents	These drugs have potential for causing dependence, hypertension, angina, and myocardial infarction	High
Long–term use of full–dosage, longer half–life, non–COX–selective NSAIDs: naproxen (Naprosyn, Avaprox, and Aleve), oxaprozin (Daypro), and piroxicam (Feldene)	Have the potential to produce GI bleeding, renal failure, high blood pressure, and heart failure	High
Daily fluoxetine (Prozac)	Long half–life of drug and risk of producing excessive CNS stimulation, sleep disturbances, and increasing agitation. Safer alternatives exist	High
Long–term use of stimulant laxatives: bisacodyl (Dulcolax), cascara sagrada, and Neoloid except in the presence of opiate analgesic use	May exacerbate bowel dysfunction	High
Amiodarone (Cordarone)	Associated with QT interval problems and risk of provoking torsades de pointes. Lack efficacy in older adults	High
Orphenadrine (Norflex)	Causes more sedation and anticholinergic adverse effects than safer alternatives	High
Guanethidine (Ismelin)	May cause orthostatic hypotension. Safer alternatives exist	High
Guanadrel (Hylorel)	May cause orthostatic hypotension	High
Cyclandelate (Cyclospasmol)	Lack of efficacy	Low

Isoxsuprine (Vasodilan)	Lack of efficacy	Low
Nitrofurantoin (Macrodantin)	Potential for renal impairment. Safer alternatives available	High
Doxazosin (Cardura)	Potential for hypotension, dry mouth, and urinary problems	Low
Methyltestosterone (Android, Virilon, and Testrad)	Potential for prostatic hypertrophy and cardiac problems	High
Thioridazine (Mellaril)	Greater potential for CNS and extrapyramidal adverse effects	High
Mesoridazine (Serentil)	CNS and extrapyramidal and adverse effects	High
Short–acting nifedipine (Procardia and Adalat)	Potential for hypotension and constipation	High
Clonidine (Catapres)	Potential for orthostatic hypotension and CNS adverse effects	Low
Mineral oil	Potential for aspiration and adverse effects. Safer alternatives available	High
Cimetidine (Tagamet)	CNS adverse effects including confusion	Low
Ethacrynic acid (Edecrin)	Potential for hypertension and fluid imbalances. Safer alternatives available	Low
Desiccated thyroid	Concerns about cardiac effects. Safer alternatives available	High
Amphetamines (excluding methylphenidate hydrochloride and anorexics)	CNS stimulant adverse effects	High
Estrogens only (oral)	Evidence of the carcinogenic (breast and endometrial cancer) potential of these agents and lack of cardioprotective effect in older women	Low

Reprinted with permission from Archives of Internal Medicine. 2003;163:2716–2724.

Table 23.4 Drugs with narrow therapeutic indices

Medication
Digoxin
Calcium channel blockers
Anti–arrhythmic
Tri cyclic antidepressants
Central acting analgesics
Warfarin
Phenytoin
Theophylline

With a decrease in liver mass and perfusion, medications eliminated by first–pass effect (e.g., propranolol, labetalol, lidocaine, fentanyl, remifentanil) may have increased levels. Alternatively, pro–drugs requiring activation in the liver (e.g., enalapril) may have decreased bioavailability. Cytochrome P450 mediates phase I reactions (oxidation, reduction, and hydrolysis) that may be impaired secondary to reduction in liver mass and blood flow. Phase II metabolism (glucuronidation) remains largely unaffected.

Renal mass is decreased by 25–30% with age and renal blood flow decreases by 1% each year starting in the fourth decade of life. However the drop in glomerular filtration rate (GFR) with age may not be as steep as previously believed, but due to decreased muscle mass in the elderly, the serum creatinine may not reliably reflect GFR. In elderly patients, when using the Cockroft–Gault formula to estimate GFR, the patient's body habitus (e.g., edema, obesity, or cachexia) can decrease the accuracy of the estimation. Ultimately whether due to aging itself or comorbidities a lower than normal GFR may be a risk factor for ADR especially when water–soluble drugs are prescribed. Most renally excreted drugs with narrow therapeutic indexes (e.g., digoxin, aminoglycosides, lithium) will need to have their dosages readjusted in the elderly.

Absorption and Distribution

In the absence of gastric mucosal atrophy or an *H. pylori* infection, gastric acid secretion remains relatively stable with advanced age. Some slowing of transit through and active transport across the gastrointestinal tract may be present; however, this has not been shown to be clinically significant.

Body composition changes with age in favor of fat versus total body water and lean body mass. As a consequence, the distribution of lipophilic drugs such as diazepam may increase and their half–life may be extended. On the other hand, plasma concentration of polar drugs such as digoxin may be higher as a consequence of contracted total body water. This necessitates lowering the loading dose for such drugs as digoxin.

In healthy elderly individuals, serum albumin concentrations do not change significantly. However, an age–related change in the binding potential of plasma proteins may be clinically relevant for drugs with a small volume of distribution and therapeutic index, such as warfarin. Other highly protein–bound medications (e.g., nonsteroidal anti–inflammatory agents, diclofenac, solifenacin) do not appear to be affected.

Pharmacodynamics

In general geriatric patients frequently exhibit altered sensitivity/tolerance to medications. The change in drug effect may be secondary to:

1. Altered receptor structure (affinity)
2. Altered receptor abundance
3. Changes in second messenger downstream from the receptor
4. A defect in the counterbalancing mechanisms.

Of all the age–associated alterations in pharmacodynamics, those pertaining to the cardiovascular system and the central nervous system appear to be the most crucial for an elderly patient undergoing anesthesia for a surgical procedure. Attenuation of heart rate response to isoproterenol is an example of an altered β–adrenergic cardiovascular response: in contrast response to α–adrenergic agents appears to be maintained. An increased central sensitivity to the anticholinergic effects of antidepressants or drugs with strong anticholinergic properties such as diphenhydramine is an example of age–related central nervous system responses.

Adverse Drugs Reactions

ADRs are among the top six causes of death in the United States, and the incidence has not changed in the last three decades. A drug–drug interaction in which the second drug could alter the absorption, distribution, or metabolism of the index drug and thus leads to a higher/lower serum concentration of that drug would be an example of a pharmacokinetic interaction. The isoenzymes of hepatic cytochrome P450 are a frequent intersection point for such interaction. Tables 23.5 and 23.6 list clinically relevant examples. A pharmacodynamic interaction, on the other hand, occurs when a drug enhances or diminishes the intended or unwanted effect of another drug, as with TCAs causing a decline in the cognitive capacity of a patient on cholinesterase inhibitors for Alzheimer's dementia.

Genetic Polymorphism

Our expanding knowledge base of genetic polymorphism has revolutionized our understanding of pharmacotherapy, for example beta blockade responsiveness and selective opioid metabolism. It is conceivable that in the future it may be possible to

Table 23.5 Drugs metabolized by cytochrome P–450 enzymes

Enzyme	Substrates	
CYP1A2	Antidepressants	[a]Amitriptyline HCl, [a]clomipramine HCl, [a]desipramine HCl, [a]imipramine HCl
	Antipsychotics	[a]Clozapine, [a]haloperidol
	Benzodiazepines	Chlordiazepoxide, diazepam
	Other	Caffeine, propranolol, tacrine HCl, [a]theophylline, R–warfarin[a]
CYP2C9	Antidepressants	[a]Amitriptyline, [a]clomipramine, [a]imipramine
	Other	Diazepam, losartan potassium, omeprazole, [a]phenytoin, [a]S–warfarin
CYP2C19	Antidepressants	Citalopram
	Amitriptyline	
CYP2D6	Analgesics	Codeine, dextromethorphan, fentanyl, hydrocodone, meperidine HCl, methadone HCl, morphine sulfate, oxycodone HCl
	Antiarrhythmics	Flecainide acetate, [a]mexiletine, [a]propafenone HCl
	Antidepressants	Fluoxetine HCl, fluvoxamine maleate, [a]hydroxybupropion, [a]paroxetine HCl trazodone HCl, venlafaxine, [a]tricyclic antidepressants
	Antipsychotics	Chlorpromazine HCl, [a]haloperidol, [a]perphenazine, [a]risperidone, [a]thioridazine HCl
	Beta blockers	Bisoprolol fumarate, labetalol HCl, metoprolol, pindolol, propranolol, timolol maleate
CYP344	Analgesics	Acetaminophen, alfentanil HCl, codeine, dextromethorphan,
	Antiarrhythmics	Disopyramide, lidocaine HCl, quinidine
	Anticonvulsants	[a]Carbamazepine, [a]ethosuximide
	Antidepressants	[a]Citalopram, desipramine, nefazodone HCl, sertraline HCl, trazodone
	Antifungal drugs	Itraconazole, ketoconazole
	Antihistamines	Loratadine
	Benzodiazepines	Alprazolam, clonazepam, midazolam HCl, triazolam
	Calcium channel blockers	Amlodipine, felodipine, isradipine, mibefradil, verapamil HCl
	Chemotherapeutics	Busulfan, [a]doxorubicin HCl, [a]etoposide, [a]paclitaxel, tamoxifen citrate, [a]vinblastine sulfate, [a]vincristine sulfate
	Cholesterol–lowering drugs	[a]Atorvastatin calcium, [a]fluvastatin sodium, [a]lovastatin, [a]pravastatin sodium, [a]simvastatin
	Immunosuppressants	Cyclosporine, tacrolimus
	Macrolide antibiotics	Clarithromycin, erythromycin, troleandomycin
	Steroids	Estradiol, cortisol, methylprednisolone, prednisone, testosterone
	Other	[a]Cisapride, [a]rifampin, R–warfarin

[a]Has low therapeutic–to–toxic ratio; thus, combination with antidepressants that might significantly inhibit its metabolism should be undertaken with extreme caution or avoided if possible.

Table 23.6 Inhibitors of cytochrome P–450 enzymes

Enyzme	Inhibitors	
CYP1A2	Antibiotics	Ciprofloxacin, clarithromycin, erythromycin, levofloxacin, norfloxacin
	Antidepressants	Citalopram, [a]fluoxetine HCl, [a]fluvoxamine maleate, [a]mirtazapine, [a]paroxetine HCl, [a]sertraline HCl
	Other	Cimetidine, grapefruit juice, ketoconazole
CYP2C9	Antidepressants	Fluoxetine, [a]fluvoxamine, [a]paroxetine, [a]sertraline
	Other	Amiodarone HCl, chloramphenicol, fluconazole, omeprazole
CYP2C19	Antidepressants	Fluoxetine, fluvoxamine, [a]paroxetine, [a]sertraline
	Other	Fluconazole, omeprazole
CYP2D6	Antiarrhythmics	Amiodarone, propafenone HCl, quinidine
	Antidepressants	Clomipramine HCl, desipramine HCl, [a]desmethylcitalopram, fluoxetine, S–norfluoxetine, [a]fluvoxamine, [a]mirtazapine, paroxetine, sertraline, [a]venlafaxine
	Antipsychotics	Fluphenazine, haloperidol
	Other	Cimetidine
CYP3A4	Antiarrhythmics	Amiodarone
	Antibiotics/antibacterials	Clarithromycin, erythromycin, metronidazole, norfloxacin, troleandomycin
	Antidepressants	[a]Fluoxetine, fluvoxamine, [a]mirtazapine, nefazodone HCl, [a]paroxetine, [a]sertraline
	Antifungal drugs	Fluconazole, ketoconazole, itraconazole
	Other	Grapefruit juice, quinine

[a]Weak Inhibitor

Reprinted with permission from Cadieux RJ. Antidepressant drug interactions in the elderly. Postgrad Med. 1999;106:231–249. Postgraduate Medicine is a registered trademark of JTE Multimedia, LLC 1235 Westlakes Drive, Suite 320, Berywn, PA 19312 (610) 889–3730.

identify patients that may be more susceptible to developing polypharmacy ADRs based on their inherent metabolic capabilities.

Studies have shown that single nucleotide polymorphisms of β–2 adrenergic receptors determine whether β–adrenergic antagonism will be effective in treatment of myocardial ischemia. Most importantly, significant data have emerged on the polymorphism of metabolic enzymes of the cytochrome P450 family, which mediate the metabolism of 40–50% of all medications. CYP2D6 is one isoenzyme of this family. Genetic polymorphism of this enzyme results in poor metabolizers and ultra-rapid metabolizers. Antidepressants are metabolized by this enzyme, as is tramadol, a μ–receptor agonist, an SSRI, and an SNRI. Paroxetine (an antidepressant) will inhibit this enzyme, and individuals who are genetically poor metabolizers may have diminished pain relief as a consequence. On the other hand, genetically ultra-rapid metabolizers may experience opioid–related adverse effects with reasonable tramadol doses as well as with codeine administration.

This is an evolving area and it is possible in the future that underlying genetics may influence choices of certain medications.

Perioperative Considerations in Geriatric Patients with Chronic Conditions

By 2020 nearly 50% percent of Americans are expected to have at least one chronic condition (an estimated 157 million individuals). Of these, one–half will have multiple chronic conditions. By grouping conditions by major diagnostic category (MDC) according to the organ system involved, it was possible to identify 16 major groups of disease. Using this categorization; cardiovascular disease had a prevalence of 58%, followed by endocrine/metabolic/nutritional (43%), musculoskeletal (25%), eye (20%), respiratory (15%), and mental (15%) diseases. For the purposes of the study, even though within each group there were several different conditions, each group was treated as one. Comorbidity was cited only if another group of MDC's was involved. This was based on the premise that an individual, with conditions in more than one MDC was more likely to see more than one kind of specialist, thus increasing the risk of a lapse in coordinated care and ADRs. In each of the above five MDCs, the percentage of individuals with four or more conditions was nearly 50%. The following sections will review selectively the more frequently encountered relevant drug interactions.

Cardiovascular Medications

Hypertension (HTN), coronary artery disease (CAD), and congestive heart failure (CHF) are commonly encountered diagnoses in persons older than 65 years. Angiotensin–converting enzyme inhibitors (ACEIs) or angiotensin type–1 receptor blockers (ARBs), β–adrenergic receptor blockers (BBs), diuretics, and statins are frequently prescribed medications in this setting, and multiple large clinical trials have shown the combination of such drugs to be beneficial in heart failure. However, the combination and frequency of these drugs may also result in adverse interactions. Examples include ACEIs, which are known to also inhibit bradykinins. These have been shown to be associated with prolonged and occasionally refractory hypotension upon induction of anesthesia. This appears to be partially related to the timing of the last dose, and if ACEIs/ARBs are administered within 10 h of induction of anesthesia, or if the patient is on concomitant diuretic therapy, the likelihood intraoperatively of hypotensive episodes increases. Given the likelihood of hypotension, most authors agree that ACEIs/ARBs should be held for 10 h before surgery. Alternatively, if the patient is dependent on this medication, empirically one might consider administering one–half of the usual dose before surgery.

Some drug combinations can be unfavorable and a combination of an ACEI and spironolactone may lead to *hyperkalemia,* the extent of which depends on the patient's renal function and the dose of spironolactone. Carvedilol (a nonselective β–adrenergic blocker), spironolactone (an aldosterone antagonist), and ACEIs/ARBs have all also been associated with induction of hyperkalemia. It is recommended that when these are used in combination, serum potassium levels should to be monitored periodically even if spironolactone is prescribed at a low dose of 25 mg/day.

Digoxin, because of its pharmacologic properties and narrow therapeutic range, is another cardiovascular drug frequently involved in ADRs, especially when combined with loop/thiazide diuretics, beta blockers, atorvastatin, or simvastatin. Diuretic–induced hypokalemia or hypomagnesemia may enhance the inhibitory effects of cardiac glycosides on Na+/K+–ATPase. Use of beta blockers may inhibit the P–glycoprotein–mediated transport of digoxin, though the clinical significance of this remains undetermined. The same mechanism is proposed as a theoretical mechanism whereby statins may increase digoxin levels.

Antiarrhythmics such as amiodarone, diltiazem, and verapamil are inhibitors of hepatic P450 enzymes, especially CYP3A4. These enzymes are responsible for metabolizing statins. The concurrent use of these two classes of medications may increase *myotoxicity* and hence the risk of rhabdomyolysis.

Psychotropic Medications

With advancing age, the use of medications for dementia, depression, psychosis, and Parkinson's disease increases. Medications for these conditions are also commonly implicated in ADRs. Some studies have suggested that they may also increase the risk of postoperative delirium and agitation. Of the multiple risk factors for delirium, it is possible that polypharmacy may be amenable to intervention in the perioperative setting. A review of the some pertinent drug–drug and drug–disease reactions encountered is presented below (See also chapters 24 and 25).

Antidepressants

TCAs are heterocyclic compounds used in treatment of depression since 1950s. More recently the use of TCAs has been extended to cover neuropathic pain (NP), post–traumatic stress disorder, fibromyalgia, and smoking cessation. Side effects include increased heart rate, slowed cardiac conduction, and orthostatic hypotension in addition anticholinergic effects might interfere with treatment for Alzheimer's Dementia. If a TCA is needed, the medication with the least anticholinergic effects (desipramine, nortriptyline) should be chosen. It is prudent to initiate treatment with the lowest possible dose and then titrate to effect with close supervision of the blood pressure.

Elderly surgical patients are frequently prescribed antidepressants or antipsychotics (e.g., haloperidol, risperidol), which may prolong the Q–T interval. If these drugs are present in the perioperative patient, volatile anesthetics like sevoflurane or antibiotics such as erythromycin may have additive effects in prolonging Q–T interval. The clinical significance of these interactions is not clear.

Monoamine oxidase Inhibitors (MAOIs) alleviate depression by inhibiting the enzymes that metabolize neurotransmitters leading to an increase in the available levels of, for example serotonin, norepinephrine, and occasionally dopamine. Except for moclobemide, a reversible selective inhibitor of MAO–A, MAOIs cause irreversible inhibition of the enzyme and consequently the effects can last 30 days, with some new enzyme generated two weeks after discontinuation. Patients on these medications have heightened sensitivity to vasopressors, in particular to indirect–acting sympathomimetics such as ephedrine. It is safest to avoid hypotension but if treatment is needed, gradual titration of a direct–acting $\alpha 1$–agonist such as phenylephrine is preferred. Other drugs not to be used with MAOIs are meperidine, selective serotonin reuptake inhibitors (SSRIs), and selective norepinephrine reuptake inhibitors (SNRIs).

Meperidine

Meperidine is an opioid with anticholinergic effects that might cause postoperative delirium. The same effect will result in tachycardia, which is not well tolerated in the elderly. Additionally, it has negative inotropic effects, with resultant decreased cardiac output. In elderly patients with diminished renal function, both meperidine and its metabolite normeperidine may accumulate with repeated doses and cause seizures. In individuals on MAOI treatment, administration of meperidine can give rise to a serotonergic crisis (see below). If absolutely necessary for treatment of postoperative shivering, a single dose of 12.5 mg is admissible.

SSRI and SNRIs

SSRIs inhibit neuronal uptake of serotonin and elevate mood; they do not have anticholinergic effects. However, their use with other medications that inhibit serotonin uptake (MAOIs, tramadol, weight–reducing agents, triptans) may lead to potentially lethal serotonergic crisis. This syndrome is characterized by agitation, tremor, tachycardia, hypertension, and sweating. If serotonergic crisis occurs it is treated by discontinuing the offending medication, administering cyproheptadine to block serotonin production, and prescribing benzodiazepines for agitation and seizures.

SNRIs (venlafaxine and duloxetine) inhibit the uptake of norepinephrine and thus ameliorate depression symptoms or neuropathic pain. Both are associated with increases in blood pressure and should be used with caution if at all in patients with poorly controlled hypertension or those with significant left ventricular dysfunction.

Dementia

Recent research has suggested that the cognitive decline seen in patients with Alzheimer's disease (AD) may be attenuated by use of cholinesterase inhibitors (rivastigmine, donepezil). A side effect of these drugs is the development of significant bradycardia, and they may also prolong the effect of muscle relaxants metabolized by cholinesterases. At this point many of these reactions are reported as case reports and the clinical significance of these reactions is not fully understood. Another consideration in these patients is drug combinations. It is possible that the benefit derived from the cholinesterase inhibitors treatment may actually be counteracted if medications with anticholinergic effects are such as diphenhydramine (Table 23.3).

Antiparkinson Medication

Levodopa provides the missing dopamine in patients suffering from Parkinson's disease. Because of its short life, it is usually combined with carbidopa to inhibit its metabolism and thus prolong its effect. It is preferable to continue these medications in the perioperative period to avoid an increase in rigidity that may interfere with ventilation efforts. Attempts to treat perioperative nausea and vomiting should avoid dopamine antagonists such as metoclopramide and the phenothiazine prochlorperazine.

Neuropathic Pain (NP) in the Elderly

With the graying of the population, the incidence of NP is on the rise. Diabetes, stoke, degenerative diseases of the spine, and herpes zoster are among the more common causes of NP. Medications most frequently used to treat NP are TCAs, gabapentinoids (gabapentin and pregabalin), and SNRIs (duloxetine, venlafaxine). These patients are most likely to have comorbidities such as hypertension or CAD and to receive treatment for them. With more than one specialist involved in their care (e.g., a cardiologist and a chronic pain specialist), the opportunity for ADRs is high.

Cardiovascular Concerns in Elderly Patients Treated for NP

The cardiovascular effects of TCAs (orthostatic hypotension, slowed cardiac conduction, increased heart rate) were previously mentioned. The other groups of drugs used to treat NP also have adverse effects on the cardiovascular system. The SNRIs cause hypertension and increase the risk of arrhythmias. Transient CHF seen in association with pregabalin use resolves if this medication is discontinued. Use of pregabalin in patients on ACEI therapy increases the likelihood of angioedema. Histamine–releasing opioids such as morphine may also cause adverse cardiovascular effects in the elderly. Methadone, especially in the presence of hypokalemia, structural cardiac disease, or genetic predisposition may result in torsades de pointes. It is recommended that providers obtain an electrocardiogram within one month of the start of methadone treatment, especially if the dose is greater than 100 mg/day.

Polypharmacy in Oncology Patients

In older patients with cancer, as in the general geriatric patient, the anesthesiologist will encounter individuals with multiple comorbid conditions. Polypharmacy and its risk for ADRs are compounded in this population under treatment with highly toxic antineoplastic drugs. As part of their treatment, oncologic patients may be prescribed drugs that are otherwise advisable to avoid. One study found that cimetidine, a well–known inhibitor of cytochrome CYP3, may interfere with taxane metabolism. Cimetidine also inhibits the metabolism of metoprolol, propranolol, and labetalol. In a patient taking both, cimetidine and beta–blocker, concentration of the latter will increase with potential hemodynamic consequences. On the other hand verapamil, frequently prescribed for cardiovascular comorbidities, is a substrate for CYP3A, thereby potentially contributing to toxicity of paclitaxel, another antineoplastic agent.

Bleeding Complications Secondary to Drug Interactions

Warfarin is frequently implicated in drug–related hospital admissions most commonly gastrointestinal tract hemorrhage. As cardiovascular conditions rise in geriatric patients, potential interactions with other commonly administrated drugs become more common. Many antibiotics (e.g., ciprofloxacin, clarithromycin, erythromycin, metronidazole, trimethropin–sulfamethoxazole) increase the risk of bleeding if coadministered with warfarin. The potential mechanism for this includes inhibition of hepatic metabolism of warfarin. Other drug–drug interactions to consider to avoid hemorrhagic events would be coadministration of warfarin with any of the following: cimetidine, lovastatin, acetaminophen, aspirin, NSAID, or saw palmetto.

Conclusion

Avoidable ADRs are a significant health problem. Polypharmacy is unlikely to cease to exit. As healthcare professionals, our responsibility is to raise awareness of the problem, educate the healthcare force and patients, and strive to develop fail–safe methods to screen for potential adverse drug–drug interactions (Table 23.7).

Table 23.7 Drugs to avoid in the elderly

Drugs to avoid	
Opioids	Propoxyphene, tramadol, methadone, meperidine
Benzodiazepines	Long acting benzodiazepines, e.g., diazepam
Antidepresants	Tricyclic antidepresants, fluoxetine
H2 blockers	Cimetidine may inhibits cytochrome CYP3
NSAIDS	Substitute by acetaminophen or COX–2 inhibitor

Key Points

- Individuals 65 years of age or older have a high probability of suffering from a cardiovascular, endocrine, CNS diseases for which multiple medications are prescribed by more than one specialist.
- Polypharmacy defined as taking more than five drugs at one time increases the likelihood of ADRs.
- At least one–third of individuals older than 65 years of age will present for surgery.
- In the perioperative period, anesthesiologists have the opportunity to review all medications (prescribed, OTC, herbal) the patient is ingesting for their potential to cause an adverse reaction or to diminish the compensatory reserve of a patient undergoing surgery and anesthesia. The most recently added medications are frequently implicated in ADRs.
- If patient is on ACEI/ACB, consider giving the last dose no sooner than 10 h prior to administration of anesthesia.
- If possible refrain from using medications with anticholinergic properties. If needed one with the weakest anticholinergic properties is advisable.
- When the patient is on more than one drug that is a substrate of cytochrome P450 isoenzymes, or when a drug known to inhibit cytochrome isoenzymes is necessary for the patient, consider adjusting dosages of each and increase vigilance for untoward effects.

Acknowledgment The author wishes to thank Andrea Gomez, MD and Mary-Rita Blute, RN for their assitance during the preparation of this chapter.

Suggested Reading

Ament PW, Bertolino JG, Liszewski JL. Clinically significant drug interactions. Am Fam Physician. 2000;61:1745–1754.

Argoff CE. Clinical implications of opioid pharmacogenetics. Clin J Pain. 2010;26:S16–S20.

Barnett, SR. Polypharmacy and perioperative medications in the elderly. Anesthesiol Clin. 2009;27(3):377–389.

Budnitz DS, Pollock DA, Weidenback KN, et al. National surveillance of emergency department visits for outpatients adverse drug events. JAMA. 2006;296:1858–1866.

Cadieux RJ. Antidepressant drug interactions in the elderly. Postgrad Med. 1999;106:231–249.

Carnahan RM, Lund BC, Perry PJ, et al. The concurrent use of anticholinergics and cholinesterase inhibitors; rare event or common practice? J Am Geriatr Soc. 2004;52:2082–2087.

Confere T, Sprung J, Kumar MM, et al. Angiotensin system inhibitors in a general surgical population. Anesth Analg. 2005;100:636–644.

de Abajo FJ, Garcia–Rodriguez LA. Risk of upper gastrointestinal track bleeding associated with selective serotonin reuptake inhibitors and venlafaxine, therapy: interaction with non–steroidal anti–inflammatory drugs and effect of acid–suppressing agents. Arch Gen Psychiatry. 2008;65;795–803.

Egger SS, Rätz Bravo AE, Hess L, et al. Age-related differences in the prevalance of potential drug-drug interactions in ambulatory dyslipidemic patients treated with statins. Drugs Aging. 2007;24:429–40.

Fick DM, Cooper JW, Wade WE, Waller JL, Mc. Lean JR, Beers MH. Updating the Beers criteria for potentially inappropriate medication use in older adults. Arch Intern Med. 2003;163: 2716–2724.

Heaver JF. Polypharmacy. In: Sieber, FE, ed. Geriatric anesthesia. The McGraw–Hill Companies, Inc; 2007:163–172.

Haanpaa ML, Gourlay GK, Kent JL. Treatment considerations for patients with neuropathic pain, and other medical comorbidities. Mayo Clin Proc. 2010;85:S15–S28.

Hayes BD, Klein–Schwartz W, Barrueto F. Polypharmacy and the geriatric patient. Clin Geriatr Med. 2007;23:371–390.

Inonye SK. Delirium in older persons. N Engl.J.Med. 2006;354:1157–1165.

Jaillon P, Simon T. Genetic polymorphism of beta–adrenergic receptors and mortality in ischemic heart disease. Therapie. 2007;62:1–7.

Johnson EM, Whyte E, Mulsant BH, et al. Cardiovascular changes associated with venlafaxine in the treatment of late–life depression. Am J Geriatr Psychiatry. 2006;14:796–802.

Jones PM, Soderman RM. Intraoperative bradycardia in a patient with Alzheimer's disease treated with two cholinesterase inhibitors. Anaesthesia. 2007;62:109–204.

Kleinsasser A, Loeckinger A, Lindner KH et al. Reversing sevofluorane–associated Q–Tc prolongation by changing to propofol. Anesthesia. 2001;56:248–250.

Lyrica(Pregabalin)[package insert].New York, NY:Pfizer;2006.

Moitra V, Diaz G, Sladen RN. Monitoring hepatic function. In Fleisher LA, cons.ed: Anesthesiology Clin: monitoring. WB. Saunders Inc. 2006;24:857–880.

Pats MT, Costa–Lima B, Monette J, et al. Medications problems in older, newly diagnosed cancer patients in Canada; how common are they? Drugs Aging. 2009;26(6):519–536.

Qato DM, Alexander GC, Conti RM, et al. Use of prescription and over the counter medications and dietary supplements among older adults in the United States. JAMA. 2008;300:2867–78.

SFINX drug interactions. http://www.terveysportti.fi/sfinx/.

Shi S, Morihe K, Klotz U. The clinical implications of ageing for rational drug therapy. Eur J Clin Pharmacol. 2008;64:183–199.

Sokol KC, Knudsen JF, Li MM. Polypharmacy in older oncology patients and the need for an interdisciplinary approach to side effect management. J Clin Pharm Ther. 2007;32:169–175.

Stefanacci RC, Cavallaro E, Beers MH, et al. Developing explicit positive Beers criteria for preferred central nervous system medications in older adults. Consult Pharm. 2009;24:601–610.

Steinman MA, Landfeld CS, Rosenthal GE, et al. Polipharmacy and prescribing quality in older people. J Am Geriatr Soc. 2006;54:1516–1523.

Chapter 24
Dementia and Neurologic Syndromes: Distinctions Between Alzheimer's, Vascular Dementia, and Parkinson's

Aaron LacKamp

Overview

Age-associated neurologic disease can be an important determinant of functional outcome after surgery. Neurologic diseases in the elderly encompass many divergent conditions such as Alzheimer's disease, Parkinson's disease with dementia, cerebrovascular disease, and neurologic effects of other systemic disease. The common elements among the dementias are cognitive decline and a secondary impairment in functional outcome. Any stressor, including surgery and anesthesia, can potentially cause acute deterioration in cognition and function.

It is important to identify pre-existing neurologic deficits and establish the patient's baseline prior to surgery and anesthesia. Proper preoperative examination can reduce frustration and unnecessary testing when trying to distinguish between preoperative diagnoses and new findings after emergence from anesthesia. Furthermore some neurologic conditions may require specific management such as Parkinson's disease. Additionally, neurologic disease may increase the risk of specific complications that may affect functional recovery in both the short-term and long-term. Optimum recovery of function after an operation requires the interplay between cognitive and physical health, and both must be maximized for full functional recovery.

Dementia is the most common age related neurologic illness. The prevalence of dementia will increase and also continues to grow in the Western population. Dementia is increasingly recognized as a predictor of poor outcome and morbidity after surgery. For these reasons, awareness of dementia and its effect on an anesthetic is the first step toward reducing morbidity and functional impairment in this vulnerable population.

A. LacKamp, MD (✉)
Department of Anesthesiology and Critical Care Medicine, The Johns Hopkins Hospital and Johns Hopkins Bayview Medical Center, Office A576, 4940 Eastern Ave, Baltimore, MD 21224, USA
e-mail: alackam1@jhmi.edu

S.R. Barnett (ed.), *Manual of Geriatric Anesthesia*, DOI 10.1007/978-1-4614-3888-5_24,

History

Routine preoperative questioning should include a review of common neurologic symptoms in all elderly patients. In older frail patients and those with known neurological disease, there should be direct questioning about motor weakness, sensory changes, numbness, visual deficits or blindness, and hearing loss. Further in-depth questioning should follow if there is suspicion of additional deficits. Common important findings are the presence of dysphagia in Parkinson's or cerebrovascular disease, and the extent of the functional limitations in the impaired patient including their ambulatory status, the extent of self-care, hygiene, and typical activity level.

In general, when age-associated neurologic disease is suspected an additional brief neurologic history should be obtained. This should include any previous diagnoses and their duration. Pre-existing deficits should be noted including those of a progressive or recurrent nature. Details about exacerbations of symptoms and any known causes, such as "off" symptoms of Parkinson's, are important and may help assess the severity of illness or what to expect postoperatively. Reviewing the current neurologic medications, reactions to prior medications, and deciding which medications will be needed on the day of surgery is an important part of the history.

Dementia is more than memory impairment alone. Dementia as defined in the DSM IV includes memory deficits compared to the previous baseline, additional cognitive deficits, and impairment in social or occupational functioning. Without functional impairment, deficits would be described as mild cognitive impairment. Table 24.1 lists criteria for dementia adapted for this reference.

The brief nature of the anesthesiologist's preoperative interview necessitates an efficient appraisal of the patient's cognitive state. Several clues may be present during the interview that should prompt further questioning or prompt simple bedside testing. Table 24.2 lists early signs of dementia.

Recognizing dementia requires attention to subtle elements of history from the patient and family. The onset of cognitive impairment is usually insidious and patients can develop surprisingly profound deficits that may not have been recognized by caregivers. Patients with moderate to severe cognitive deficits may be functioning well in their familiar living environment but fail to adapt to stressful environments and subsequently decompensate postoperatively or in the hospital. History taking to uncover symptoms of dementia should therefore take into account

Table 24.1 Dementia criteria

Multiple cognitive impairments:

- Memory impairment (either new or previously learned information)
- One of the following cognitive impairments:
  1. Aphasia (language disturbance)
  2. Apraxia (impaired skilled motor skills despite intact motor function)
  3. Agnosia (impaired recognition of familiar objects with intact sensory function)
  4. Executive dysfunction (impaired planning, initiating, organizing, sequencing, or abstraction)
- The deficits impair social or occupational functioning

Table 24.2 Early signs and symptoms of dementia

Sign/Symptom	Example
Forgetfulness	Commonly manifested as short-term memory loss for recently learned names, appointments, purpose of activities, points of conversation, and completed tasks or errands. An individual may repeat questions or requests. The degree of forgetfulness begins to interfere with daily activities and responsibilities
Disorientation	Episodic confusion regarding the exact day, date, or location
Impaired performance on daily tasks	Difficulty performing everyday tasks, such as preparing meals, running household appliances, cleaning, and hygiene (e.g., bathing, toileting, brushing teeth)
Impaired language	Increasing difficulty with selecting and using words. Sentences may become simpler or fragmented
Impaired recognition	Diminished ability to remember or identify familiar faces, objects, sounds, and locations
Impaired abstract thinking	Diminished ability to think clearly about issues, to discuss complex issues and to make logical connections between them, or to comprehend fully things that were previously understood
Impaired judgment	Impairment in the ability to organize and plan and to make appropriate decisions or selections among several possibilities. A person may act in ways that were previously deemed uncharacteristic or inappropriate
Changes in mood or behavior	Increased irritability, loss of emotional control, abusive or inappropriate language, loss of pleasure in particular activities, and apathetic attitudes
Changes in personality	Subtle changes including becoming less sociable, more self-centered, suspicious, fearful, or bothered by others, and reactions to everyday stress may be out of proportion

Adapted from Agronin ed. Alzheimer disease and other dementias: a practical guide. 2nd edn. Table 2.1

the high incidence of denial on the part of the patients and their families. Anosognosia is the pathological lack of insight into one's illness that is often exhibited by demented patients. This may result in anger and frustration on the part of the patient when they are unable to perform simple tasks or tests as expected. The diagnosis of dementia will ultimately be based upon the accumulated weight of specific associated signs and symptoms more than on a direct admission of cognitive decline on the part of the patient.

Exam

An important part of the neurologic examination for the anesthesiologist is the general first impression of the status of the patient. This may range from awake, alert and oriented, lucid and coherent, to disheveled, fidgety, confused, babbling, or even obtunded or comatose. This general impression will be of paramount importance upon anesthetic emergence and in the postoperative period as it will help distinguish new neurologic changes vs. baseline condition. The general impression should include assessment of attention, speech and thought content, and the results of this initial assessment may prompt further examination.

When prompted by history or exam findings, a general motor examination is aimed at rapidly identifying and quantifying any focal weakness. Facial muscle assessments should be included in patients with a history of stroke. Weakness in limbs should be noted as twitch monitors for neuromuscular blockade should not be placed on areas of motor deficit as they may underestimate the degree of blockade.

Positioning concerns may prompt other neurologic examinations. A detailed sensory examination is usually not necessary unless pre-existing deficits could potentially be confused with new deficits caused by positioning or a regional technique involving the affected area is planned. Contractures and immobility may also be present especially in frail or bedridden elderly. If contractures are detected, the safe range of motion should be demonstrated by the awake patient prior to positioning. The airway examination should include assessment of cervical radiculopathy/myelopathy or the potential for neck instability. Spinal cord injuries should include the level of injury as lesions above T6 have increased risk of autonomic dysreflexia.

When dementia is suspected, it is possible to perform simple screening tests to confirm the presence of possible dementia. The MMSE (mini-mental status examination) is a well recognized screening tool for dementia. The MMSE could be conducted in entirety if time permits, however for the anesthesia preoperative examination selected elements may be adequate and more time efficient. For example delayed recall of three words, or the clock-drawing test can be administered together or separately as an abbreviated exam. This approach has been a useful practical tool. See Table 24.3. MMSE See Table 24.4. Dementia subtypes

The definitive diagnosis of dementia will require formal neuropsychiatric testing and a subtype of dementia is assigned based on formal testing and neuroimaging. This type of work-up is clearly beyond the scope of the preoperative evaluation. The subtype of dementia is often considered a presumptive diagnosis because the gold standard for diagnosis of Alzheimer's disease, the most common dementia, is postmortem pathology.

Certain symptoms and findings on neurologic exam may point to specific dementia types, for example extrapyramidal symptoms are often self-evident and may suggest a Parkinsonian syndrome such as from medication side effects, Parkinson's disease or other rarer illnesses such as supranuclear bulbar palsy. The tremor of true Parkinson's disease is most pronounced when the patient is at rest. It often involves the hands, mouth, and head, and is classically described as a "pill-rolling" tremor of the fingers. The frequency is 4–6 times per second. Parkinsonism includes bradykinesia (sluggish movement) and muscle rigidity. Characteristic Parkinsonian findings include the mask-like facial expression from rigidity, "cogwheel" rigidity of the bicep on passive movement of the elbow, and a shuffling gate. When encountering a patient with Parkinson's symptoms the anesthetist should focus on certain elements of the history for example previous respiratory events, postural hypotension,

Table 24.3 Bedside neuropsychiatric examination

Memory	Immediate: repetition of three objects (MMSE)
	Recent: recall of three objects (MMSE)
	Remote: recall of past events
Aphasia	Comprehension: ability to follow simple commands (MMSE and CDT)
	Expressive: repetition of "no ifs, ands, or buts" (MMSE)
	Listen for missed or mispronounced words, or nonsensical words
	Naming (anomia): ask patient to identify common objects (MMSE)
Apraxia	Constructional: ability to copy pentagons on MMSE, clockface on CDT, or simple objects (outline of a cross or a key)
	Ideomotor: ability to demonstrate how to comb hair, brush teeth, or hammer a nail
Agnosia	Prosopagnosia: impaired recognition of familiar faces (e.g. family)
	Astereognosis: impaired recognition of familiar objects via tactile exploration
	Finger agnosia: ask patient to identify finger by touch
Executive Function	Ability to plan and sequence steps of making clock (CDT)
	Ability to reproduce rhythm with finger tapped out by the examiner
	Ability to mimic sequence using same hand (a) slap fist on table, (b) open fist and slap side of hand on table, (c) slap palm on table
Function	IADLs (Instrumental activities of daily living) require higher cognitive function than ADLs and are less dependent on physical factors. Four IADL score: ask caregiver whether the patient needs assistance in these areas: (a) money management, (b) medication management, (c) telephone use, and (d) traveling. Suspect dementia with increased need for assistance

Table 24.4 Neurologic findings and associated dementia types

Neurologic finding	Associated dementias
Extrapyramidal symptoms	Dementia with Lewy bodies, subcortical dementias
Gait disturbances	Normal pressure hydrocephalus, vascular dementia, Parkinson's disease, subcortical dementia, dementia with Lewy bodies, alcohol-induced dementia, tertiary syphilis, multiple system atrophy, multiple sclerosis
Hemiparesis	Vascular dementia due to large-vessel infarct
Frontal release signs	Frontal lobe dementia, other dementias in later stages
Myoclonus	HIV-associated dementia, Creuzfeldt-Jacob disease, uremic encephalopathy, late-stage Alzheimer's disease
Peripheral neuropathy	Vitamin B12 deficiency, hypothyroidism, alcohol-induced dementia, heavy metal poisoning, uremic encephalopathy, HIV-associated dementia
Gaze paralysis	Progressive supranuclear palsy, brainstem tumor
Pseudobulbar palsy (involuntary emotional expression)	HIV-associated dementia, progressive supranuclear palsy, vascular dementia, multiple sclerosis, amyotrophic lateral sclerosis, Parkinson's disease
Focal signs	Brain injury, vascular dementia, multiple sclerosis, corticoganglionic basal degeneration

or difficulty swallowing and any aspiration events. These patients can be very sensitive to opioids and labile blood pressure is frequently encountered.

Parkinsonian movements should be distinguished from dyskinesias which are large abnormal involuntary muscle movements. Dyskinesias can be seen as a side effect of anti-Parkinson's therapy. The movements are usually a "peak-dose" effect when the CNS concentrations of drug are highest. The dyskinesias may become a limiting factor in symptomatic treatment of Parkinson's requiring shortening of the dose intervals to maintain levels within a narrowing therapeutic window. Other unrelated extrapyramidal signs include dystonia, tardive dyskinesia from antipsychotics, and restless leg syndrome. These types of involuntary movements may influence the choice of anesthetic especially if the patient needs to be immobile for the procedure.

Testing: Acute Delirium Versus Dementia

In contrast to dementia, delirium is characterized by fluctuating attentiveness and deficits. There are many potential causes of delirium, and dementia is a risk factor for postoperative delirium. Pain is a major contributor to delirium, and may be very difficult to evaluate in patients with advanced dementia or neurologic diseases that impair communication such as a prior cerebrovascular accident. Although not always considered, acute alcohol intoxication or withdrawal must be considered as a cause of delirium in older patients. Hypothyroidism, hyponatremia, hypercalcemia, and uremia are metabolic causes of reversible cognitive deficits. Testing for these metabolic causes should be performed if suspicion exists of reversible deficits. The classic descriptions of the hypoxic patient developing agitation and the hypercapneic patient developing progressive somnolence should also be considered.

General Anesthetic Management in Patients with Neurodegenerative Disorders

Premedication

Patients with pre-existing neurologic diseases are often more sensitive to the effects of sedative medications and opioids. The need for preoperative sedation in patients with significant neurological diseases should be carefully evaluated, and anxiolytic doses of midazolam should be decreased and titrated cautiously. Low dose propofol infusions may be advantageous for procedural sedation. Sedatives with anticholinergic properties such as scopolamine and diphenhydramine should be avoided as they have been shown to lead to delirium.

Pain should be treated appropriately and opiates should not be withheld. Pain is a major factor in the development of delirium and non-opioid analgesics and regional analgesia should be encouraged when no specific contraindication exists.

Dysphagia is a common problem with demented and neurologically impaired patients and can increase the risk of aspiration. Dementia associated with Parkinson's disease, Pseudobulbar palsy, and prior cerebrovascular accidents are particularly likely to be associated with dysphagia. Dysphagias in this population may not be detected preoperatively unless the anesthetist has heightened suspicion based on a history of stroke, dysarthria, or significantly depressed cognitive level. Chronic aspiration may be unrecognized and a careful pulmonary examination is advised prior to administration of anesthesia. Premedication may be appropriate with proton pump inhibitor, and non-particulate antacids may be used if sedation is minimal. Metoclopramide, a dopaminergic antagonist, is specifically contraindicated in Parkinson's disease.

In the perioperative period it is important to ensure that routine medications for Parkinson's disease are continued and that there is minimal interruption in regular dosing. There is a narrow therapeutic window for dopamine agonists with advanced Parkinson's disease and these patients require frequent doses. Parkinson's patients who miss doses of levodopa are at a higher risk of pulmonary complications.

Intraoperative

Optimum care of the patient with neurodegenerative disease is centered on avoiding known complications or exacerbation of neurologic conditions. The ideal anesthetic should have a short duration of effect with minimal side effects. There is no evidence that a single anesthetic agent or combination is superior to another and it may be beneficial to employ as few agents as possible and to use short-acting drugs whenever possible. Regional anesthesia may offer advantages to certain patients and can also reduce exposure to general anesthetic medications. Regional anesthesia does not eliminate the risk of postoperative cognitive dysfunction or delirium in elderly patients. Regional anesthesia can reduce recovery times for patients, and it can allow for early resumption of oral Parkinson's medications and fewer missed doses in selected surgeries. It is particularly important to document any pre-existing neurological deficits in patients in whom a regional technique is to be offered, so there is no confusion about a potential postoperative injury.

Postoperative

Postoperative concerns are centered on rapidly facilitating return to a maximally functional state. Postoperative pain should be treated aggressively as pain is a major contributor to delirium and impaired function. Early mobility and early activity should be encouraged, and overall the risk of postoperative complications is probably greater in patients with neurologic diseases and dementia such as found in Parkinson's patients and those with Alzheimer's disease.

Behavioral Emergencies

Perioperative behavioral problems may occur more frequently in demented patients. When behavioral emergencies occur, a multimodal approach should be employed beginning with non-pharmacologic interventions. Preoperatively or in the recovery room, it is usually beneficial to involve the family early with a behavioral problem patient. The family may help in allaying the patient's fears, help orient the patient to their current settings, and help identify any unmet needs the patient may have.

For demented or delirious patients who are loud or who exhibit repetitive screaming or disruptive behavior, it is important to try to identify any unmet needs. The first step is always to ensure adequate oxygenation and perfusion. In the recovery room common nonlife threatening causes of delirium include pain, urinary retention, disorientation, sleep deprivation, and social isolation from routine caregivers. Environmental modifications and positive reinforcement and reassurance may help reduce unwanted behavior. A quiet, soothing environment can help soothe an agitated and combative patient. If possible re-establishing normal day–night cycles can be helpful for disoriented patients, and it is important to try to limit disruptions in sleep. Simple interventions such as returning eye glasses and hearing aids, providing access to a clock, calendar, and being able to look out a window, or seeing a loved-one or photos can be beneficial.

Agitation is best addressed by a caregiver who displays a consoling manner. Paranoia is a common symptom in demented patients and this may require a caregiver who is non-confrontational but who can display empathy for the patient's fears. When a patient becomes verbally abusive, support and encouragement must be given to the nursing staff caring for these patients as well. Dangerous or physically combative behavior must be addressed quickly for the safety of the nursing staff and of the patient.

Initiating pharmacologic therapy for a dangerously agitated patient in the recovery room does not require a specific psychiatric diagnosis and may be needed to ensure the safety of the patient and nursing staff. Milder forms of agitation may benefit from medical treatment as well after ensuring that the patient's basic needs are met. Prior to administering any sedative, hypoxia should be excluded by routine postoperative monitoring. Alcohol withdrawal should be included in the differential in elderly patients especially if the patient has been hospitalized for a few days prior to surgery. Alcohol intake is frequently missed or under reported in the preoperative interview.

Although lorazepam is frequently the first line agent for agitation in the younger patient, the atypical antipsychotics are preferred in the elderly. Tables 24.5 and 24.6 list the preferred agents and doses for treatment of the behavioral emergency in the

Table 24.5 Treatment of the behavioral emergency

Drug	IM/IV	Oral	Redose
Olanzapine	5–10 mg	5–20 mg	After 2–4 h max 40/day Orthostatic hypotension acutely
Haloperidol	2–10 mg	5–10 mg	q20–30 min redose q6hr with 25% of the maximum required dose Monitor EKG and QTc More extrapyramidal symptoms
Risperidone	–	1–3 mg BID	
Quetiapine	–	12.5–50 mg qhs	
Lorazepam	0.5–3 mg	1–3 mg	Better treatment of aggressive behaviors. Benzodiazepines may be disadvantageous in demented patients

Table 24.6 Agitation in the demented patient

Olanzapine	1.25–5 mg/day PO
Risperidone	0.25–1 mg/day PO
Haloperidol	0.25–0.5 mg qd or bid PO

demented patient and the treatment of agitation or psychosis in the demented patient. In some patients depression may present as agitation and an SSRI (selective serotonin reuptake inhibitor) would be the most appropriate therapy. Tricyclic antidepressants should not be used in demented patients due to the anticholinergic effects.

If the patient has previously been diagnosed with Lewy body dementia, antipsychotic medications such as haloperidol may cause life-threatening dystonia. Atypical antipsychotics may have a milder side effect profile and might be used in small doses. Acetylcholinesterase inhibitors are the preferred agents for agitation in Lewy body dementia, although their efficacy is not as great. Other proposed treatments for agitation have included anticonvulsants, memantine, and melatonin.

Dementia Subtypes

Alzheimer's Disease

Pathology of Alzheimer's Disease

Alzheimer's disease is the most common dementia in the elderly, accounting for 50–60% of all dementia cases and prevalence increases with age. Alzheimer's dementia will affect 5% of individuals over age 65 and up to 50% of individuals over age 85. Age is the most significant risk factor for dementia.

Risk factors for AD (Alzheimer's disease) include age, low educational achievement, female sex after menopause, family history, and apolipoprotein genotype. Apolipoproteins assemble with triglycerides and cholesterol to form VLDL and transport lipids through the bloodstream. The ApoE epsilon-4 allele is associated with the development of AD, but is not thought to be causal of the disease. A single allele of ApoE e4 confers a fourfold increase in risk and a double allele confers a 19-fold increase in risk compared to non-carriers.

The definitive diagnosis of Alzheimer's disease is based on pathology, either autopsy or biopsy. The diagnosis of probable Alzheimer's disease, as distinguished from other dementias, can be reliably made by expert clinical examination, imaging, and neuropsychiatric testing. There can be some overlap with other dementias as the classic pathology of Alzheimer's may coexist alongside the pathologic findings of other dementias.

The pathology found in patients with Alzheimer's disease includes extracellular plaques of amyloid protein, and of intracellular deposits of neurofibrillary tangles in the brain. The amyloid deposition is considered the hallmark of AD, but neurofibrillary tangles may be seen in other diseases as well. Amyloid is a normal byproduct of cellular activity and may be derived from the transport of synaptic vesicles and the release of neurotransmitters. Amyloid originates from the breakdown of an amyloid precursor protein whose exact function is unknown. The most prevalent of these breakdown products is ABeta-40, which appears to be relatively non-toxic. Another breakdown product is less common, but is specifically implicated in the progression of the disease and is called ABeta-42. Normal neural metabolism includes turnover in these polypeptides throughout life; the cause of the transition to toxicity and deposition disorder is unclear.

The toxicity of Abeta-42 occurs after formation of oligomers (specifically dimers and trimers). The oligomers of ABeta-42 are thought to create artificial pores in lipid membranes, alter the activity of protein ion channels, and to cause oxidative stress and mitochondrial failure. The pathologic finding of plaque formation may in fact be a protective mechanism as the amyloid is less toxic after polymerization and deposition into beta-pleated sheets.

Neurofibrillary tangles are a pathologic finding common to a class of neurodegenerative diseases called Tauopathies. The tau protein is an abundant soluble protein that stabilizes microtubules involved in axonal transport. The tau protein is normal in AD but becomes hyperphosphorylated as the disease progresses and loses solubility. This is in contrast to Parkinson's associated dementia and frontotemporal dementia which are associated with tau mutations. The insoluble tau found in AD forms filamentous structures leading to the development of intracellular deposits. The neuronal loss is out of proportion to the amount of neurofibrillary tangles so the neurofibrillary tangles are unlikely to represent the primary pathogenesis of the disease. The abnormal tau protein can be detected in the CSF and may be a biomarker for incipient Alzheimer's disease in patients with a pre-dementia condition called mild cognitive impairment.

The development of Alzheimer's disease has been linked to abnormal calcium homeostasis. Amyloid proteins induce influx of calcium and there is a depletion of endoplasmic reticulum calcium. The neuron experiences increased excitability and possible excitotoxicity. As the disease progresses there is a loss of synapses, and the degree of synapse loss correlates with severity of dementia.

Table 24.7 Pharmacologic concerns

Anticholinergic	Atropine, scopolamine, hyoscyamine, benztropine, dicyclomine, diphenhydramine, TCA's, exacerbate dementia, and delirium
Antihistaminergic	Sedation
Antidopaminergic	Metoclopramide, butyrophenones, phenothiazines, exacerbate Parkinson's symptoms
Antipsychotics	Lewy body dementia results in severe dystonia
Opioids	Parkinsonian patients experience rigidity
Antiparkinsonian	Dose interruption exacerbates symptoms, levodopa causes exaggerated sympathetic response to ketamine
MAOI interactions	Selegiline (MAOI-B) interaction with meperidine. Agitation, muscular rigidity, sweating, and hyperpyrexia
Orthostatic hypotension	TCA's, bromocriptine, levodopa

Treatment of Alzheimer's Disease

There is no cure for Alzheimer's disease: it is a steadily progressive dementia, some even consider it a terminal condition. Some studies suggest that the rate of decline can be temporarily slowed or even briefly reversed with treatment with cholinesterase inhibitors. However after 12 months the disease continues to progress but possibly at a slower rate of decline than without treatment. Treatment may allow patients to remain independent longer, may delay the move to an institutional setting, and may reduce the burden on families.

Adjunctive treatment guidelines include non-pharmacologic therapies. Examples of these treatments are mental stimulation for example through social group interactions, memory training sessions, and music or pet therapy. Further degeneration may be minimized with adequate nutrition, routine vitamin supplementation, minimizing vascular risk factors, and minimizing the risk of falls and detrimental head injury.

The pharmacologic treatment of AD is aimed at correcting the cholinergic-depleted state. Acetylcholinesterase inhibitors are the initial treatment for early Alzheimer's (Table 24.7). Donepezil, rivastigmine, and galantamine each increase the synaptic acetylcholine levels, and each has similar efficacy. Rivastigmine can also be useful in patients with Parkinson's-associated dementia. The common side effects of the cholinesterase inhibitors include increased gastric acid secretion, increased bronchial secretion, and bradycardia and caution is advised in patient with pulmonary disease or active peptic ulcer disease. The cholinesterase inhibitor should be introduced slowly over weeks to months and may need to be stopped or decreased in the patients with active peptic ulcer disease, active pulmonary disease, or symptomatic bradycardias. After the first year of therapy it is normal to observe resumption of the cognitive decline. It is important to continue the cholinesterase inhibitor as tolerated as the rate of decline will be decreased with treatment.

Memantine is a glutamate (NMDA) receptor antagonist with a low affinity for the receptor. With memantine, neurotransmission still occurs but the calcium flux is reduced and there is less potential for excitotoxicity. Memantine is commonly used in conjunction with a cholinesterase inhibitor. The mechanism of action is different from the cholinesterase inhibitors and the drugs have an additive effect. In early disease memantine is added to a cholinesterase inhibitor after the cholinesterase inhibitor has been titrated. In advanced disease the order of introduction is reversed, memantine becomes the first line agent and a cholinesterase inhibitor is then added to it. Common side effects of memantine include sedation, confusion, headache, and constipation.

Anesthetic Management in Alzheimer's Disease

The anesthetic management of Alzheimer's patients should assume reduced cognitive reserve and the greater likelihood of postoperative cognitive impairment. Alzheimer's patients carry a high risk of developing POCD and delirium. The choice of spinal over general anesthesia does not appear to entirely eliminate the risk. In patient with Alzheimer's Disease, cholinesterase inhibitors are used chronically to increase the central acetylcholine and offset the decline in memory and attention. The cholinesterase inhibitors may also inhibit butyrocholinesterase in the serum and this may rarely cause an exaggerated sensitivity to succinylcholine and prolonged blockade. Bradycardia with these medications has also been described, but is uncommon.

As Alzheimer's disease represents a central cholinergic-depleted state and it is important to avoid anticholinergic medications and drugs with anticholinergic side effects. Atropine and scopolamine are tertiary amines and cross the blood brain barrier and can lead to significant delirium. Glycopyrrolate may be preferable when needing an anticholinergic effect as the quaternary ammonium does not allow it to cross the blood brain barrier. Other drugs with significant anticholinergic side effects include promethazine, diphenhydramine, and tricyclic antidepressants. Avoidance of polypharmacy may help reduce the risk of medication side effects by eliminating unnecessary medication exposures and drug interactions. In general, consider lowering the dose of sedating medications and benzodiazepines in particular to avoid excessive postoperative sedation. Good pain control postoperatively may help reduce the risk of delirium. Short-acting anesthetics should be used when practical to allow the patient to resume normal activities to aid in reorienting the patient and to resume home medications sooner.

Vascular Dementia

Vascular dementia is the second most common form of dementia. After a stroke 20–30% of individuals may develop dementia within 3 months. This accounts for 125,000 new cases per year in the United States versus 360,000 new cases for Alzheimer's dementia. The rate of vascular dementia increases 200-fold when aging from 60 to 90 years old.

Table 24.8 Dementia due to medical illness

Cause	Suggestive findings
Drug effects	Atropine, benztropine, dicyclomine, hyoscyamine, scopolamine, divalproate, carbamazepine, phenytoin, chlorpromazine, thioridazine, azathioprine, clonidine, digitalis, disulfiram, lithium, benzodiazepines, barbiturates, tricyclic antidepressants
Alcohol	Malnutrition, confabulation
Vitamin deficiencies	Thiamine, niacin, cobalamin, folate
Toxins	Mercury, lead, manganese, arsenic, Wilson's disease, organophosphates
Infectious disease	Any severe infection may cause deterioration, commonly UTI, specific CNS infections may seed from tooth abscesses, sinus infections, and cardiac vegetations. Consider also bacterial meningitis, abscess, viral encephalitis, HIV-associated dementia complex, spirochetes, fungal infections, parasitic infection, prion disease, and post-infectious inflammation as possible
Neoplasms	Focal neurologic signs, meningiomas may present without focal signs, demyelination may occur after chemotherapy, radiation may cause cognitive decline
Limbic encephalitis	Memory and psychiatric changes associated with small cell lung cancer or Hodgkin's disease
Normal pressure hydrocephalus	Gait disturbance, urinary incontinence, and somnolence
Renal failure	Uremia, BUN >60, asterixis, headache, weakness, lethargy
Liver failure	Alcoholic cirrhosis, chronic hepatitis, signs include confusion, asterixis, ataxia, and hyperreflexia, worsened by interruption in oral neomycin or lactulose therapy
Endocrine disorders	Hypothyroidism, hyperparathyroidism, Cushing syndrome, diabetes
Autoimmune	SLE (CNS involvement in 75%), MS (30% eventually have cognitive impairment)

There is a considerable overlap between vascular dementia and Alzheimer's dementia, as both are age dependent and some patients may show some component of both. The symptoms of vascular dementia are highly variable and will depend on the regions of the brain involved. Compared to Alzheimer's disease, frontal lobe disinhibition is more common with vascular dementia, while verbal long-term memory deficits are less prominent. The risk factors for vascular dementia are the same as those for vascular disease in general: atherosclerosis, hypertension, hyperlipidemia, diabetes mellitus, and smoking. After having a stroke, the risk of developing dementia is related to stroke severity. Worse outcome is associated with left-sided (dominant hemisphere) stroke, infarct volume greater than 50–100 cc, stroke symptoms: dysphagia, gait impairment, and urinary incontinence and stroke complications: seizures and pneumonias.

The treatment of vascular dementia involves minimizing the risk of recurrent stroke. Acetylcholinesterase inhibitors may be used to improve functionality by increasing cholinergic function. The anesthetic management will be the same as for other dementias. Avoid anticholinergics and attempt early functional recovery (Table 24.8).

Parkinson's with Dementia

Parkinson's disease is the second most common neurodegenerative disorder after Alzheimer's disease. Parkinson's disease is primarily a movement disorder although a small proportion of patients (20–30%) will also have concomitant dementia at presentation over the course of the illness 80% of Parkinson patients will develop some cognitive impairment.

The central defect found in Parkinson's disease is a loss of dopaminergic neurons in the substantia nigra of the basal ganglia. The cardinal symptoms are bradykinesia, cogwheel rigidity, resting tremor, shuffling gait, masked face, and postural instability. In more advanced cases patients may develop significant cognitive impairment, hypophonia, drooling, and micrographia.

Anesthetic risk is increased in Parkinson's disease, with the principle risks being of respiratory complications, extended hospitalizations, and increased mortality in hospitalized patients. Parkinson's patients exhibit swallowing difficulty have an increased risk of aspitation and subsequent pneumonia and respiratory failure. Muscular rigidity and weakness can contribute to respiratory insufficiency, especially as anti-Parkinsonian medications may not be able to be given during long anesthetics.

Orthostatic hypotension is common in Parkinson patients. This is often from the autonomic dysfunction that accompanies Parkinson's disease itself and may also represent a side effect of treatment with levodopa. The orthostatic hypotension is principally of postural nature, and hemodynamic instability during anesthetic induction has not been consistently observed even in a patient with significant postural symptoms.

Surgical approaches are being offered more frequently to treat persistent tremors and other Parkinson symptoms. Special considerations are needed during anesthesia for this type of functional neurosurgery. Deep brain stimulator implantation requires the patients to be off their medications and patient may exhibit significant baseline symptoms. During the procedure the obliteration of the resting tremor can be used to indicate proper lead placement and sedation must be used cautiously. Airway accessibility can be an issue during the case and opioids should be used with extreme caution to avoid any potential for apnea.

Anesthetic induction may either exacerbate movement disorders, such as precipitating severe dyskinesias, or may obliterate the normal Parkinson's associated movements. Similarly emergence can be associated with exacerbation of neurological symptoms such as rigidity and tremors.

Drugs with antidopaminergic effects should be avoided including metoclopramide, butyrophenones, and phenothiazines. Treatment of Parkinson's disease with MAOI's has been a source of concern for anesthesiologists, however currently the MAOI-B selective selegiline is most commonly seen in the treatment of Parkinson's disease. MAOi-B drugs have predominant effects on inhibiting breakdown of dopamine and phenethylamine, and carry little risk of serotonin syndrome. However reports of agitation, muscle rigidity, and hyperthermia have been reported after the combination of Selegiline and meperidine and this combination should be avoided. The classic MAOI-A medications inhibit the breakdown of serotonin, epinephrine, norepinephrine, and also dopamine. In these patients extreme caution must be used in treating hypotension with indirect acting adrenergic medications such as ephedrine to avoid precipitating a hypertensive crisis.

It is important to continue anti-Parkinsonian medications until as close to surgery as possible. L-dopa has a short half life (1–3 h) and is only absorbed from the small intestine, and it can be administered through a nasogastic tube patients with significant symptoms and prolonged surgery. The therapeutic window for L-dopa narrow, and similar symptoms may be elicited from both the disease state and from levodopa excess, including hallucinations, cognitive impairment, dysarthria, and orthostatic hypotension. Thus during prolonged surgeries and hospitalizations it is important that dosing schedules are maintained to prevent "off" symptoms while avoiding dopamine excess and subsequent dyskinesias. After a perioperative hiatus it may take several days to normalize levodopa therapy and the MAOi-B inhibitor Selegiline may be a useful as an adjunct agent in this period.

Neuroleptic malignant syndrome can be precipitated perioperatively by abrupt discontinuation of dopaminergic drugs. On rare occasions NMS may occur spontaneously in Parkinson's patients due to insufficient dopamine. There may be a subset of patients at risk for this complication who have low dopamine levels based on CSF studies, and who have concomitant withdrawal of levodopa and COMT inhibitors. Although neuroleptic malignant syndrome classically requires weeks to develop it has been reported to appear acutely in the perioperative period in the Parkinson's patient. Dantrolene has been used in the treatment of Parkinson's related NMS.

Anesthesia for Parkinson's disease

The optimum care for a patient with Parkinson's disease represents an opportunity for the anesthetist to markedly impact the quality of the patients care perioperativley. The anesthetic goal should include preventing the exacerbation of motor symptoms, and preventing respiratory complications such as aspiration and postoperative respiratory failure. Continuing levodopa on the day of surgery is paramount and scheduled doses of levodopa should continue immediately up to the time of surgery and should resume as soon as feasible postoperatively. It is possible to use a nasogastric tube to administer intraoperative doses as they are due, however the benefit of intraoperative enteral drugs must be weighed against the risk of aspiration and the possibility of poor absorption.

Prevention of aspiration requires increased awareness of pharyngeal dysfunction in patients with Parkinson's disease. Prophylaxis with H2 blockers, proton pump inhibitors and non-particulate antacids may be used. Prochlorperazine, promethazine, and especially metoclopramide should not be used in patients with Parkinson's disease. Patients may require modest delays in extubation to ensure airway protection. Postoperative respiratory failure is largely related to exacerbation of motor symptoms. Chest and abdominal rigidity and poor patient positioning due to rigidity may impair good ventilatory mechanics. High dose fentanyl has been associated with pronounced muscle rigidity in Parkinson's patients.

Regional anesthesia may offer significant advantages to patients, however the risk of aspiration must be considered. Autonomic dysfunction and orthostatic hypotension are common, therefore vigilance during spinal administration is warranted. Additionally, sedated patients under regional may not be able to take intraoperative doses of Parkinson's medications safely, but they may be able to resume postoperative doses sooner than after a general anesthetic.

Frontotemporal Dementia

Frontotemporal dementia is characterized by early involvement appearance of behavioral symptoms and language disturbances. Frontotemporal dementia is relatively uncommon and accounts for only 1–5% of individuals with dementia. It is more prevalent among the early onset dementias, accounting for 12–22% of individuals with dementia younger than 65 years of age.

Behavioral disturbances vary widely. They may include oral behaviors, compulsive behaviors, hypersexual behaviors, delusions, inappropriate social behavior, or generalized apathy. Extrapyramidal symptoms can also occur in these patients. Frontal release signs can occur including grasp reflex, rooting reflex, palmo-mental reflex, sustained glabellar reflex, and Babinski's reflex.

Lewy Body Dementia

Dementia with Lewy bodies is an increasingly common diagnosis amongst elderly patients with dementia. Lewy Body Dementia may be difficult to distinguish from other dementias especially vascular type dementia. Characteristic features include a fluctuating course, visual hallucinations, and Parkinsonism symptoms.

The fluctuations may occur over hours to weeks and may be noticed as decreased attention, somnolence, and cognitive decline. Psychotic symptoms are commonly encountered and can be very disturbing for caretakers. In the perioperative period it is important to rule out acute and potentially reversible delirium.

Dementia with Lewy bodies is distinguished from Parkinson's with dementia by the early development of cognitive impairment in the illness. If parkinsonian movement disorder predates the dementia by more than 12 months the disease is more likely Parkinson's with dementia. If the parkinsonism occurred less than 12 months prior to dementia the illness is more likely Lewy body dementia.

A key challenge with Lewy body dementia is the treatment of behavioral disturbances without worsening the Parkinsonian features. Treatment with antipsychotic medications such as haloperidol and prochlorperazine can trigger acute rigidity, confusion, sedation, or catatonia. Acute sensitivity to antipsychotics may be present in up to 50% of Lewie Body patients. Antidepressants that may have anticholinergic activity should also be avoided as there is a cholinergic deficient state similar to Alzheimer's dementia or vascular dementia. In contrast, patients with Parkinson's with dementia do not have the exquisite sensitivity to antipsychotics.

Dementia with Lewy bodies may respond well to acetylcholinesterase inhibitors. Donepezil, rivastigmine, or galantamine may be started at low doses and titration is slower than with Alzheimer's dementia. Acetylcholinesterase inhibitors are the first line agent for mild behavioral disturbances and psychotic symptoms.

Summary

As the population ages anesthesiologists will encounter more patients with advanced neurological diseases and dementia. These patients are challenging to care for during the perioperative period.

Key Points

- Dementia can have many causes. Dementia implies functional impairment in addition to cognitive deficit. A cholinergic-depleted state in the central nervous system may be present in some patients with dementia.
- Parkinson's disease increases perioperative risk. Specific risks include aspiration, respiratory failure, orthostatic hypotension, and postoperative rigidity. The risks related to Parkinsonian "off" symptoms may be lessened by continuing anti-Parkinson's medications preoperatively, immediately postoperatively, and if possible intraoperatively.
- Epidural and regional anesthesia are excellent options for patients with Parkinson's disease in order to enable patients to restart levodopa immediately following surgery. Non-opioid analgesia may lessen sedation and fentanyl associated rigidity.
- Metoclopramide is specifically contraindicated in Parkinson's disease.
- Medications with anticholinergic effects should be avoided in patients with dementia.

Suggested Reading

Agronin ME, Agronin ME. Alzheimer disease and other dementias: a practical guide. 2nd ed. Philadelphia: Wolters Kluwer Health/Lippincott Williams & Wilkins; 2008:350. http://www.loc.gov/catdir/enhancements/fy0714/2007017730-d.html.

Allen MH, Currier GW, Carpenter D, Ross RW, Docherty JP, Expert Consensus Panel for Behavioral Emergencies 2005. The expert consensus guideline series. Treatment of behavioral emergencies 2005. J Psychiatr Pract. 2005;11 Suppl 1:5–108; quiz 110–12.

Antonini A, Abbruzzese G, Barone P, et al. COMT inhibition with tolcapone in the treatment algorithm of patients with Parkinson's disease (PD): relevance for motor and non-motor features. Neuropsychiatr Dis Treat. 2008;4(1):1–9.

Avidan MS, Searleman AC, Storandt M, et al. Long-term cognitive decline in older subjects was not attributable to noncardiac surgery or major illness. Anesthesiology. 2009;111(5):964–970.

Bedford PD. Adverse cerebral effects of anaesthesia on old people. Lancet. 1955;269(6884): 259–263.

Bijker JB, van Klei WA, Vergouwe Y, et al. Intraoperative hypotension and 1-year mortality after noncardiac surgery. Anesthesiology. 2009;111(6):1217–1226.

Bohnen N, Warner MA, Kokmen E, Kurland LT. Early and midlife exposure to anesthesia and age of onset of Alzheimer's disease. Int J Neurosci. 1994;77(3–4):181–185.

Brambrink AM, Evers AS, Avidan MS, et al. Isoflurane-induced neuroapoptosis in the neonatal rhesus macaque brain. Anesthesiology. 2010;112(4):834–841.

Burton DA, Nicholson G, Hall GM. Anaesthesia in elderly patients with neurodegenerative disorders: special considerations. Drugs Aging. 2004;21(4):229–242.

Cohen E, Bieschke J, Perciavalle RM, Kelly JW, Dillin A. Opposing activities protect against age-onset proteotoxicity. Science. 2006;313(5793):1604–1610.

Deogaonkar A, Deogaonkar M, Lee JY, Ebrahim Z, Schubert A. Propofol-induced dyskinesias controlled with dexmedetomidine during deep brain stimulation surgery. Anesthesiology. 2006;104(6):1337–1339.

Deogaonkar M, Subramanian T. Pathophysiological basis of drug-induced dyskinesias in Parkinson's disease. Brain Res Brain Res Rev. 2005;50(1):156–168.

Fodale V, Quattrone D, Trecroci C, Caminiti V, Santamaria LB. Alzheimer's disease and anesthesia: implications for the central cholinergic system. Br J Anaesth. 2006;97(4):445–452.

Gasparini M, Vanacore N, Schiaffini C, et al. A case-control study on Alzheimer's disease and exposure to anesthesia. Neurol Sci. 2002;23(1):11–14.

Johnson T, Monk T, Rasmussen LS, et al. Postoperative cognitive dysfunction in middle-aged patients. Anesthesiology. 2002;96(6):1351–1357.

Kalenka A, Schwarz A. Anaesthesia and Parkinson's disease: how to manage with new therapies? Curr Opin Anaesthesiol. 2009;22(3):419–424.

Kertai MD, Pal N, Palanca BJ, et al. Association of perioperative risk factors and cumulative duration of low bispectral index with intermediate-term mortality after cardiac surgery in the B-Unaware Trial. Anesthesiology. 2010;112(5):1116–1127.

Korczyn AD, Reichmann H, Boroojerdi B, Hack HJ. Rotigotine transdermal system for perioperative administration. J Neural Transm. 2007;114(2):219–221.

Krauss JK, Akeyson EW, Giam P, Jankovic J. Propofol-induced dyskinesias in Parkinson's disease. Anesth Analg. 1996;83(2):420–422.

Kurz A, Perneczky R. Neurobiology of cognitive disorders. Curr Opin Psychiatry. 2009;22(6):546–551.

Lewis MC, Barnett SR. Postoperative delirium: the tryptophan dysregulation model. Med Hypotheses. 2004;63(3):402–406.

Lewitt PA. Levodopa for the treatment of Parkinson's disease. N Engl J Med. 2008;359(23): 2468–2476.

Liang G, Ward C, Peng J, Zhao Y, Huang B, Wei H. Isoflurane causes greater neurodegeneration than an equivalent exposure of sevoflurane in the developing brain of neonatal mice. Anesthesiology. 2010;112(6):1325–1334.

Lin SH, Chen TY, Lin SZ, et al. Subthalamic deep brain stimulation after anesthetic inhalation in Parkinson disease: a preliminary study. J Neurosurg. 2008;109(2):238–244.

Liu SJ, Gasperini R, Foa L, Small DH. Amyloid-beta Decreases Cell-Surface AMPA Receptors by Increasing Intracellular Calcium and Phosphorylation of GluR2. J Alzheimers Dis. 2010.

McDonagh DL, Mathew JP, White WD, et al. Cognitive function after major noncardiac surgery, apolipoprotein E4 genotype, and biomarkers of brain injury. Anesthesiology. 2010;112(4): 852–859.

Moller JT, Cluitmans P, Rasmussen LS, et al. Long-term postoperative cognitive dysfunction in the elderly ISPOCD1 study. ISPOCD investigators. International Study of Post-Operative Cognitive Dysfunction. Lancet. 1998;351(9106):857–861.
Monk TG, Weldon BC, Garvan CW, et al. Predictors of cognitive dysfunction after major noncardiac surgery. Anesthesiology. 2008;108(1):18–30.
Newman S, Stygall J, Hirani S, Shaefi S, Maze M. Postoperative cognitive dysfunction after noncardiac surgery: a systematic review. Anesthesiology. 2007;106(3):572–590.
Nicholson G, Pereira AC, Hall GM. Parkinson's disease and anaesthesia. Br J Anaesth. 2002;89(6): 904–916.
Nutt JG, Chung KA, Holford NH. Dyskinesia and the antiparkinsonian response always temporally coincide: a retrospective study. Neurology. 2010;74(15):1191–1197.
Peleg S, Sananbenesi F, Zovoilis A, et al. Altered histone acetylation is associated with age-dependent memory impairment in mice. Science. 2010;328(5979):753–756.
Price CC, Garvan CW, Monk TG. Type and severity of cognitive decline in older adults after noncardiac surgery. Anesthesiology. 2008;108(1):8–17.
Querfurth HW, LaFerla FM. Alzheimer's disease. N Engl J Med. 2010;362(4):329–344.
Rozet I, Muangman S, Vavilala MS, et al. Clinical experience with dexmedetomidine for implantation of deep brain stimulators in Parkinson's disease. Anesth Analg. 2006;103(5):1224–1228.
Salthouse TA. Implications of within-person variability in cognitive and neuropsychological functioning for the interpretation of change. Neuropsychology. 2007;21(4):401–411.
Schrag A. Entacapone in the treatment of Parkinson's disease. Lancet Neurol. 2005;4(6): 366–370.
Sieber FE, Gottshalk A, Zakriya KJ, Mears SC, Lee H. General anesthesia occurs frequently in elderly patients during propofol-based sedation and spinal anesthesia. J Clin Anesth. 2010;22(3):179–183.
Sieber FE, Zakriya KJ, Gottschalk A, et al. Sedation depth during spinal anesthesia and the development of postoperative delirium in elderly patients undergoing hip fracture repair. Mayo Clin Proc. 2010;85(1):18–26.
Small DH. Dysregulation of calcium homeostasis in Alzheimer's disease. Neurochem Res. 2009;34(10):1824–1829.
Small DH, Gasperini R, Vincent AJ, Hung AC, Foa L. The role of Abeta-induced calcium dysregulation in the pathogenesis of Alzheimer's disease. J Alzheimers Dis. 2009;16(2):225–233.
Stotz M, Thummler D, Schurch M, Renggli JC, Urwyler A, Pargger H. Fulminant neuroleptic malignant syndrome after perioperative withdrawal of antiParkinsonian medication. Br J Anaesth. 2004;93(6):868–871.
Tabet N, Howard R. Non-pharmacological interventions in the prevention of delirium. Age Ageing. 2009;38(4):374–379.
Tabet N, Howard R. Pharmacological treatment for the prevention of delirium: review of current evidence. Int J Geriatr Psychiatry. 2009;24(10):1037–1044.
Wei H, Xie Z. Anesthesia, calcium homeostasis and Alzheimer's disease. Curr Alzheimer Res. 2009;6(1):30-35.
Williams-Russo P, Sharrock NE, Mattis S, et al. Randomized trial of hypotensive epidural anesthesia in older adults. Anesthesiology. 1999;91(4):926–935.
Williams-Russo P, Sharrock NE, Mattis S, et al. Randomized trial of hypotensive epidural anesthesia in older adults. Anesthesiology. 1999;91(4):926–935.
Williams-Russo P, Sharrock NE, Mattis S, Szatrowski TP, Charlson ME. Cognitive effects after epidural vs general anesthesia in older adults. A randomized trial. JAMA. 1995;274(1):44–50.
Wu CL, Hsu W, Richman JM, Raja SN. Postoperative cognitive function as an outcome of regional anesthesia and analgesia. Reg Anesth Pain Med. 2004;29(3):257–268.
Yang H, Liang G, Hawkins BJ, Madesh M, Pierwola A, Wei H. Inhalational anesthetics induce cell damage by disruption of intracellular calcium homeostasis with different potencies. Anesthesiology. 2008;109(2):243–250.

Chapter 25
Psychotropic Medications in the Elderly

Jason Strauss

Psychiatric disease and dementia are common in older adults and treatment regimens can be complex. In this chapter, the most frequent psychiatric conditions diagnosed in the elderly as well as the most common treatments for these conditions will be discussed. Notable considerations regarding analgesia, anesthesia, and perioperative issues will also be addressed when indicated.

Depression and Antidepressants

Depression is a significant concern in the geriatric population. More than 10% of community-dwelling elders have depressive symptoms significant enough to warrant clinical intervention, with >4% of women and nearly 3% of men over 65 meeting the Diagnostic and Statistical Manual, Fourth Edition, Text Revised (DSM-IV-TR) criteria for Major Depressive Disorder (MDD) at any given time. The criteria for MDD are listed in Table 25.1. Older adults with clinically significant depression may actually be less likely to meet the criteria for MDD. Older patients tend to present with different symptoms from their younger counterparts including increased irritability, decreased motivation, increased feelings of hopelessness and helplessness, and increased somatic and cognitive complaints (Table 25.2).

Despite increased recognition of the signs and symptoms of depression in the geriatric population, this illness remains woefully undertreated. Only 36% of

J. Strauss, MD (✉)
Department of Psychiatry, Division of Geriatric Psychiatry,
Cambridge Health Alliance, Harvard Medical School,
103 Garland Street, Everett, MA 02149, USA
e-mail: jbstrauss@challiance.org

S.R. Barnett (ed.), *Manual of Geriatric Anesthesia*, DOI 10.1007/978-1-4614-3888-5_25,

Table 25.1 DSM-IV-TR criteria for major depressive disorder

(Must have>5 symptoms including depressed mood for >2 weeks)
• *Depressed Mood*
• Sleep (lack of)
• Interest (lack of)
• Guilt
• Energy (lack of)
• Concentration
• Appetite (lack of)
• Psychomotor retardation
• Suicidal ideation

Table 25.2 Other signs/symptoms of depression in older adults

• Irritability
• Poor motivation/abulia
• Hopelessness/Helplessness
• Somatic complaints
• Increase in cognitive complaints

community-dwelling elderly patients with clinically significant depression are treated with an antidepressant. Of the elderly patients taking antidepressants, 43% are treated with suboptimal doses and 12% are taking potentially hazardous doses.

Suicide is also a significant issue for older adults. Non-Hispanic white men aged 85 and older had a rate of 50 suicide deaths per 100,000 persons, which is higher than any other age group (CDC 2005). Risk factors for suicide in the elderly are: (1) severe or psychotic depression; (2) comorbid alcoholism; (3) recent loss/bereavement; (4) new disability; and (5) sedative/hypnotic use. Fortunately, treatment of depression lowers the overall suicide risk in older individuals.

Most antidepressants work by increasing the available amount of the neurotransmitters implicated in depression including serotonin, norepinephrine, and dopamine. Newer antidepressants such as selective serotonin reuptake inhibitors (SSRIs) have generally supplanted older medications such as tricyclic antidepressants (TCAs) and monoamine oxidase inhibitors (MAOIs) on the basis of improved side-effect profiles. Differences in tolerability between newer and older antidepressants can be especially pronounced in the geriatric population. Conventional wisdom has been that the efficacy of newer antidepressants is pretty much equal, and that the choice of medication should be based primarily on side-effect profile, particularly in older adults.

Selective Serotonin Reuptake Inhibitors

SSRIs have been first-line agents in treating depression since the 1980s. SSRIs inhibit primarily the serotonin transporter, decreasing the reuptake of serotonin back into the presynaptic neuron. Thus, SSRIs increase the amount of serotonin available

Table 25.3 SSRIs in older adults

Drug	Starting dose range	Therapeutic dose range
Citalopram	10–20 mg/day	20–40 mg/day
Escitalopram	5–10 mg/day	10–20 mg/day
Fluoxetine	10–20 mg/day	20–60 mg/day
Fluvoxamine	25–50 mg/day	50–200 mg/day
Paroxetine	5–10 mg/day	20–40 mg/day
Sertraline	12.5–25 mg/day	50–150 mg/day

for binding to target receptors. The six SSRIs are fluoxetine (Prozac), fluvoxamine (Luvox), paroxetine (Paxil), sertraline (Zoloft), citalopram (Celexa), and escitalopram (Lexapro). All are available in generic formulations. Table 25.3 compares the SSRIs and their therapeutic doses in older adults.

In general, SSRIs should be started at the lowest possible dose to maximize tolerability in older patients and then titrated slowly. Sertraline, citalopram, and escitalopram are thought to be the best-tolerated SSRIs in the elderly and should be used first. A significant drawback of these medications is that they take quite a while to work—it requires one to be on a medication for 8–12 weeks at a therapeutic dose to determine whether a trial of an SSRI can be deemed successful or unsuccessful. It can be a challenge for patients, families, and clinicians to endure such a trial.

The most common side effects of SSRIs include GI distress, nausea, constipation, diarrhea, anorexia, and sexual dysfunction. SSRIs may increase the risk of suicide during their first month of use, although afterwards, these agents are clearly helpful in preventing suicide and self-injury. Other adverse effects of SSRIs are more prevalent in older adults and may have implications in the perioperative period. These effects include increased fall risk, increased risk of hyponatremia secondary to SIADH, and increased risk of gastrointestinal bleeding thought to be secondary to anti-platelet effects. The absolute risk of GI bleeding is low in patients using SSRIs and is felt to be comparable to the risk in patients taking similarly non-steroidal anti-inflammatory drugs (NSAIDS) or aspirin.

SSRIs are implicated in serotonin syndrome, caused by an overstimulation of postsynaptic serotonin receptors, leading to mental status changes, neuromuscular signs such as rigidity, tremor, clonus, and hyperreflexia, and autonomic hypersensitivity. Serotonin syndrome is treated by eliminating offending drugs, symptomatic treatment, and supportive care, including treatment of agitation and anxiety when indicated. In some cases, serotonin antagonists such as cyproheptadine may be useful. There is little in the literature comparing treatment of serotonin syndrome in older patients compared with younger adults.

SSRIs may interact with opioid analgesics such as meperidine, fentanyl, pethidine, pentazocine, and tramadol to cause serotonin syndrome. The combination of paroxetine and tramadol may result in sedation and impairment of analgesic action. In addition, midazolam metabolites may inhibit cytochrome P450 3A4, leading to elevated serum levels of SSRIs, particularly long-acting agents such as fluoxetine.

Anesthesiology literature generally supports the continuation of SSRIs during surgery, as abrupt discontinuation can lead to SSRI withdrawal symptoms including dizziness, lethargy, paresthesias, GI complaints, anxiety, and agitation. These symptoms are most pronounced in short-acting SSRIs such as paroxetine.

Other Newer Antidepressants

Venlafaxine (Effexor) and duloxetine (Cymbalta) interfere with both serotonin and noradrenergic reuptake and are collectively called SNRIs. The noradrenergic effects of these medications potentially make them more desirable options if energy and motivation are prominent depressive symptoms in a geriatric patient. Venlafaxine is more serotoninergic at lower doses and increasingly noradrenergic at higher doses, whereas duloxetine has strong affinity for serotonin and norepinephrine regardless of the dosing. As venlafaxine and duloxetine, like paroxetine, have short half-lives compared with other antidepressants, they are likely to cause withdrawal symptoms if abruptly discontinued. Other adverse effects of SNRIs are generally similar to SSRIs and also include dose-related hypertension (more established with venlafaxine than duloxetine).

Bupropion (Wellbutrin) is an antidepressant which increases reuptake of norepinephrine and dopamine. It is also indicated for smoking cessation (brand name: Zyban). Bupropion is an activating agent, making it a good choice for elders struggling with energy, motivation, and appetite. It is a potent inhibitor of cytochrome P450 2D6. Notably, bupropion causes significant fewer GI side effects than SSRIs and SNRIs and does not cause sexual side effects. Bupropion is also the only antidepressant which does not cause syndrome of inappropriate antidiuretic hormone (SIADH). However, bupropion is more likely than other antidepressants to cause or exacerbate anxiety and insomnia. It also lowers the seizure threshold, making it a poor choice in individuals with comorbid alcoholism.

Mirtazapine (Remeron) has a complicated mechanism of action, with primary antidepressant effects felt to be due to increased release of serotonin and norepinephrine through alpha-2 adrenergic antagonism. As mirtazapine is antihistaminic (particularly at low doses), it is felt to be an excellent choice for depressed elders with insomnia and/or anorexia as prominent symptoms. It has few cytochrome P450 interactions. The side effects of mirtazapine include somnolence, increased appetite with weight gain, and hyponatremia secondary to SIADH. Less common adverse effects include orthostasis, increased serum cholesterol and triglycerides, and blood dyscrasias.

Table 25.4 compares dosing of commonly used non-SSRI antidepressants in the geriatric population.

There are little data looking at the use of these antidepressants during the perioperative period. There have been case reports that venlafaxine can cause fentanyl-induced rigidity during emergence from general anesthesia. There is no evidence that venlafaxine-induced hypertension is problematic during the perioperative period. Otherwise, there is no evidence that the above medications cause complica-

Table 25.4 Newer non-SSRI antidepressants in older adults

Drug	Starting dose range	Therapeutic dose range
Bupropion	50–100 mg/day	150–300 mg/day
Duloxetine	20–30 mg/day	30–60 mg/day
Mirtazapine	7.5–15 mg/day	15–30 mg/day
Venlafaxine	37.5–50 mg/day	75–300 mg/day

Table 25.5 Relative severity of side effects of tricyclic antidepressants

Drug	Anticholinergic effects	Sedation	Orthostasis	Cardiac effects	Weight gain
Amitriptyline	++++	++++	++++	+++	++++
Clomipramine	+++	+++	+++	+++	+++
Desipramine	+	+	++	+++	+
Doxepin	+++	++++	+++	++	+++
Imipramine	+++	+++	++++	+++	+++
Nortriptyline	+	++	+	++	++

tions during surgery. Mirtazapine and venlafaxine may interact with tramadol to cause serotonin syndrome.

Tricyclic Antidepressants

TCAs have proven to be effective antidepressants, but their side-effect profiles preclude them from being first-line agents, particularly in the geriatric population. TCAs work by inhibiting the reuptake of serotonin, norepinephrine, and dopamine (leading to antidepressant effects) and binding to muscarinic, histaminergic, and alpha-1 adrenergic receptors (causing unwanted side effects). While prescribing a TCA to an older patient, nortriptyline and desipramine should be considered first, since these are the least anticholinergic of the TCAs.

The prominent side effects of TCAs include orthostatic hypotension, sedation, confusion, dry mouth, constipation, and urinary retention. TCAs can cause cardiac dysrhythmias, most notably ventricular tachycardia, which can progress to ventricular fibrillation and sudden cardiac death. TCAs are contraindicated in patients with ischemic heart disease, as they are proarrhythmic in this population. These cardiac effects make TCAs far more fatal than other antidepressants in case of an overdose. TCAs can also lower the seizure threshold. Table 25.5 compares the relative severity of side effects of TCAs.

Perioperatively, older patients taking TCAs should have close cardiac and hemodynamic monitoring. TCAs can interact with sympathicomimetics to cause a hypertensive crisis. Hypertensive crises may be avoided in patients using TCAs by using indirect-acting sympathetic pressor amines such as neosynephrine. The combination of TCAs and enflurane can lead to induction of seizures. Anticholinergic properties of TCAs induce a post-operative delirium. For elective surgery, when there is adequate time, some practitioners advocate tapering TCAs 2 weeks prior to surgery and obtaining a baseline EKG performed prior to surgery. If tapering is planned it needs to be done in conjunction with the patient's psychiatrist or primary caregiver. If TCAs are stopped abruptly prior to surgery, a patient can experience withdrawal symptoms such as GI symptoms, malaise, sleep disturbance, and vivid dreams. Postoperatively the TCA can be slowly reinstated in geriatric adults.

Monoamine Oxide Inhibitors

MAOIs are rarely prescribed except in cases in which a patient has failed numerous other medication trials. These medications work by blocking monoamine oxidase, the enzyme responsible for the breakdown of serotonin, norepinephrine, and dopamine in the presynaptic neuron. MAOIs are characterized as being either irreversible or reversible. Unfortunately, MAOIs often cause significant orthostasis, particularly in the elderly. They may also cause a hypertensive crisis with intake of tyramine-rich foods, and one must adhere to a strict diet if taking these medications.

MAOIs have extensive interactions with anesthetic agents potentially leading to dangerous, and even lethal pressor, effect. The combination of meperidine and the irreversible MAOI phenelzine can cause significant toxicity including serotonin syndrome. While some suggest that MAOIs should be tapered at least 2 weeks prior to a surgical procedure, many patients are safely maintained on MAOIs perioperatively. MAOIs should never be abruptly withdrawn, as doing so may lead to significant psychiatric symptoms such as hallucinations, paranoid delusions, severe depression, and suicidality. Close psychiatric monitoring is required to determine whether an MAOI should be restarted postoperatively.

Electroconvulsive Therapy (see chapter 19)

The administration of electroconvulsive therapy (ECT) is one of the few places where the worlds of anesthesiology and psychiatry intersect. ECT is always performed with an anesthesiologist present, and common anesthetic agents used in ECT include methohexital, propofol, etomidate, and thiopental. Succinylcholine is usually used for neuromuscular blockade, and atropine or glycopyrrolate may be needed if there is concern that the procedure may induce a parasympathetically mediated bradycardia. ECT is a particularly helpful treatment in older patients with severe melancholic depression resistant to medications and depression with psychotic features. Evidence suggests that ECT is superior to pharmacological treatments with regard to efficacy, but safety and tolerability have not yet been conclusively demonstrated. Confusion and memory complaints are the major concerns in this population.

Antipsychotics

Despite the controversy existing over the use of antipsychotics in older patients, particularly those with dementia, these medications are an important part of a clinician's arsenal when treating geriatric patients in intrapsychic distress.

Antipsychotics are generally categorized as being typical or atypical. Typical antipsychotics are older medications which more classically block D2 receptors. Atypical antipsychotics are more heterogeneous, but in general have greater blockage of 5-HT2 receptors than D2 receptors, accounting for their lower rate of extrapyramidal side effects compared with typical antipsychotics.

Older patients with chronic psychotic disorders such as schizophrenia and schizoaffective disorders benefit from antipsychotic medications, as these medications are helpful in (and FDA approved for) improving symptoms such as hallucinations, delusions, and disorganized thinking. Antipsychotic medications are also front-line, FDA-approved treatments for patients with bipolar disorder. More recently, atypical antipsychotics such as quetiapine (Seroquel), olanzapine (Zyprexa), and aripiperazole (Abilify) have obtained FDA indications as adjunctive agents for treatment-resistant depression.

Use of Antipsychotics in Treating Elderly Patients with Dementia

Atypical antipsychotics in particular are used in an off-label manner in treating problematic behaviors associated with dementia. Empirically, these medications can be helpful in treating agitation directly attributable to psychotic symptoms such as paranoia and hallucinations in the demented elderly, but there is a dearth of good data supporting this. Unfortunately, both atypical and typical antipsychotic medications are also associated with an increased risk of strokes and sudden cardiac death in older patients with dementia. All antipsychotics are also associated with increased risk of mortality, with typical being worse than atypical in this regard. For this reason, atypical antipsychotics should often be thought of first if antipsychotic treatment is seriously considered.

As a whole, antipsychotic medications should be prescribed thoughtfully and judiciously in this population, carefully weighing benefits and risks. If a clinician feels that an antipsychotic is an appropriate treatment, then family members and the patient's health care proxy should be included in the discussion. The goal is to use the lowest possible therapeutic dose for the shortest amount of time.

Table 25.6 Atypical antipsychotics in older adults

Drug	Starting dose range	Therapeutic dose range
Aripiperazole	1–2.5 mg/day	2.5–15 mg/day
Clozapine	6.25–12.5 mg/day	25–400 mg/day
Olanzapine	1.25–2.5 mg/day	2.5–15 mg/day
Quetiapine	6.25–25 mg/day	25–200 mg/day
Risperidone	0.125–0.25 mg/day	0.25–2 mg/day
Ziprasidone	10–20 mg/day	20–80 mg/day

Atypical Antipsychotics

The so-called atypical antipsychotics are risperidone (Risperdal), olanzapine (Zyprexa), quetiapine (Seroquel), aripiperazole (Abilify), ziprasidone (Geodon), and clozapine (Clozaril). Table 25.6 lists the common range of dosages of these medications in geriatric patients as well as their formulations. Therapeutic blood levels of these medications are generally not checked. As a whole, the choice of antipsychotic used in the elderly is based upon side-effect profiles, comorbid medical conditions, and formulations (i.e., availability in sublingual and/or intramuscular forms). Atypical antipsychotics have relatively few significant cytochrome P450 interactions, although olanzapine and clozapine are substrates for cytochrome P450 1A2. Table 25.6 compares the dosing of atypical antipsychotic medications in older adults.

In addition to being associated with increased risk for overall mortality, strokes, and sudden cardiac death, these medications have other potential side effects. All antipsychotics are associated with Qtc prolongation in a dose-dependent and level-dependent manner. EKGs should be checked regularly in patients on antipsychotics, although specific frequency has not yet been established. Of the atypical antipsychotics, ziprasidone is known to have the greatest impact on Qtc interval and is rarely used in the geriatric population.

Olanzapine, clozapine, quetiapine, and risperidone are associated with an increased risk of developing the metabolic syndrome, characterized by abnormalities in three or more of the following: waist circumference, fasting blood glucose, blood pressure, triglycerides, and high-density lipoprotein (HDL) cholesterol. All of these parameters should be monitored at baseline prior to beginning treatment, 3 months following initiation of treatment, and then on a yearly basis, with the exception of blood pressures, which should be checked monthly for 3 months and then annually. This can be a particularly troublesome issue in the elderly, many of whom already have chronic diseases such as diabetes, coronary artery disease, hypertension, and dyslipidemias. Close monitoring and regular communication with primary care physicians is essential in older patients taking atypical antipsychotics. Aripiperazole does not seem to increase the risk for developing metabolic syndrome.

Although most studies indicate that the risk of extrapyramidal side effects (EPS) is lower in atypical antipsychotics than typical antipsychotics, all antipsychotics can increase the risk of symptoms such as akathisia, parkinsonism, and tardive dyskinesia. Older adults may be at greater risk of developing certain EPS compared with their younger counterparts including akathisia and drug-induced parkinsonism. When patients are on these medications, the Abnormal Involuntary Movement Scales (AIMS) should be performed at least every 6 months.

With regard to other potential side effects, in addition to presenting the greatest risk for EPS among atypical antipsychotics, risperidone can also cause elevated prolactin levels (generally with little clinical significance). While quetiapine presents lowest risk for EPS (making it a good choice in patients with Parkinson disease or Lewy body dementia), it is particularly sedating, and its anti-adrenergic effects can lead to orthostasis. Olanzapine and clozapine are anticholinergic and can occasionally cause paradoxical agitation in addition to dry mouth, constipation, and urinary retention. Clozapine can increase the risk of agranulocytosis, and patients on this medication need to have complete blood counts and absolute neutrophil counts drawn regularly. Clozapine should also be given only with extreme caution with benzodiazepines, as this combination can lead to cardiovascular and respiratory depression causing sudden death. Aripiperazole can be activating, leading to increased anxiety and agitation.

Typical Antipsychotics

Typical antipsychotics tend to be used in more specific situations in older adults including acute agitation in delirium and psychotic symptoms which do not respond to atypical antipsychotics. In addition, several typical antipsychotics such as haloperidol (Haldol) and fluphenazine (Prolixin) come in long-acting depot forms, potentially making them viable choices in patients who struggle with treatment adherence. Table 25.7 lists doses of commonly used typical antipsychotic drugs in the geriatric population.

In general, typical antipsychotics are categorized as being high potency, medium potency, and low potency. Higher potency medications such as haloperidol and fluphenazine have greater D2 blockade, leading to increased risk of EPS symptoms. Lower potency typical antipsychotics including chlorpromazine (Thorazine) have less D2 blockade and greater affinity for adrenergic, muscarinic, and histaminic receptors. These medications carry increased risk of adverse effects such as orthostasis, anticholinergic side effects, and sedation. Perphenazine (Trilafon) is a medium potency typical antipsychotic which may have a better side-effect profile in older adults than other agents discussed in this section. Typical antipsychotics do not seem to increase the risk for developing the metabolic syndrome. Table 25.8 compares the side-effect profiles of typical and atypical antipsychotic medications.

Neuroleptic Malignant Syndrome

Neuroleptic malignant syndrome (NMS) is a worrisome adverse effect of antipsychotics and shares many features with malignant hyperthermia (MH), although the

Table 25.7 Selected typical antipsychotics in older adults

Drug	Starting dose range	Therapeutic dose range
Chlorpromazine	6.25–12.5 mg/day	25–100 mg/day
Fluphenazine	0.25–0.5 mg/day	0.5–4 mg/day
Haloperidol	0.25–0.5 mg/day	0.5–4 mg/day
Perphenazine	2–4 mg/day	2–16 mg/day

Table 25.8 Relative severity of side effects of antipsychotic medications

Drug	Sedation	EPS	Anticholinergic effects	Orthostasis	Increased Qtc	Weight gain
Aripiperazole	0	+	Minimal	Minimal	0	Minimal
Clozapine	+++	0	+++	+++	+	+++
Olanzapine	++	Minimal	++	+/++	Minimal	+++
Quetiapine	++	0	+	++	++	++
Risperidone	+	+/++	+	++	++	++
Ziprasidone	+	+	+	+	+++	Minimal
Chlorpromazine	+++	+	+++	+++	++	++
Fluphenazine	+	+++	+	+	++	+
Haloperidol	+	+++	+	+	++	+
Perphenazine	+	++	+	++	++	+

exact relationship between the two is unclear. NMS is characterized by high fever, muscle rigidity, autonomic instability, and fluctuating consciousness, potentially leading to rhabdomyolysis, renal failure, and disseminated intravascular coagulation. CK, WBC count, and liver transaminases are generally markedly elevated in patients with NMS. NMS is less prevalent in geriatric patients compared with their younger counterparts, and typical antipsychotics are more likely to cause NMS than atypical. Treatment of NMS generally includes removing the offending antipsychotic, aggressive hydration, and control of medical issues. If rising CK levels cannot be controlled or if there is extensive rigidity, treatment with bromocriptine or dantrolene may be indicated. It is unclear whether patients with a history of NMS who require anesthesia should be treated with the same precautions as patients susceptible to MH.

Perioperative Considerations with Antipsychotics

With regard to interactions between anesthetics and antipsychotics, this has been looked at much more extensively with typical antipsychotic compared with atypical. Low-potency antipsychotics such as chlorpromazine and thioridazine can interact with atropine or scopolamine to cause extensive central and peripheral anticholinergic effects and with sympathomimetic agents such as epinephrine to cause alpha adrenergic effects such as vasodilatation and hypotension. Halogenated inhalation anesthetics may interact with antipsychotics leading to

Table 25.9 DSM-IV-TR criteria for a manic episode

A distinct period of abnormally and persistently elevated, expansive or irritable mood, lasting at least 1 week (or any duration if hospitalization is necessary)
During the period of mood disturbance, three (or more) of the following symptoms have persisted (four if the mood is only irritable) and have been present to a significant degree:
1. Inflated self-esteem or grandiosity
2. Decreased need for sleep (e.g., feels rested after only 3 h of sleep)
3. More talkative than usual or pressure to keep talking
4. Flight of ideas or subjective experience that thoughts are racing
5. Distractibility (i.e., attention too easily drawn to unimportant or irrelevant external stimuli)
6. Increase in goal-directed activity (at work, at school, or sexually) or psychomotor agitation
7. Excessive involvement in pleasurable activities that have a high potential for painful consequences (e.g., engaging in unrestrained buying sprees, sexual indiscretions, or foolish business investments)

hypotension. Finally, typical antipsychotics may potentiate the effects of narcotic analgesics.

Given the potential adverse effects of antipsychotics, patients taking these medications should have extensive perioperative evaluation and cardiac and hemodynamic monitoring.

There are little data to guide how antipsychotics should be used prior to anesthesia in geriatric patients. Use of antipsychotics during the perioperative period can make patients more susceptible to the hypotensive effects of anesthetics, but discontinuation of antipsychotics can exacerbate psychosis and agitation post-operatively. Kudoh et al. (2005) found that chronic schizophrenic patients (of all ages) who discontinued antipsychotics 72 h prior to surgery were more than twice as likely to develop post-operative confusion than patients who continued antipsychotics during this period (31 versus 14%). Notably, the same study found that the frequency of arrhythmias and hypotension did not differ between the two groups (16 versus 18%). Since it is likely that benefits of continuing antipsychotics outweigh risks, it is recommended by Huyse et al. (2006) that these medications be continued during the perioperative period.

Mood Stabilizers

Older patients with bipolar disorder account for 5–19% of acute care visits at geriatric psychiatry services. Patients with bipolar disorder can present in varying ways, either in acute mania, hypomania, depression, or in a mixed state with both manic and depressive symptoms. Table 25.9 lists the DSM-IV-TR Criteria for a manic episode. While many of these patients have had lifelong history of fluctuating mood symptoms, it is not uncommon for older individuals to have their first manic episode later in life. Late onset mania is thought to potentially have a vascular etiology. Manic symptoms in older adults can also have a medical etiology such as a brain mass, medication effects, or hyperthyroidism (called secondary mania).

Table 25.10 Mood stabilizers in older adults

Drug	Starting dose range	Therapeutic dose range	Therapeutic blood level
Carbamazepine	200 mg/day	200–800 mg/day	4–8 mcg/mL
Lamotrigine	12.5–25 mg/day	50–300 mg/day	N/A
Lithium	75–150 mg/day	150–1,800 mg/day	0.5–1.0 mEq/L
Oxcarbazepine	150–300 mg/day	300–1,200 mg/day	N/A
Valproate	125–250 mg/day	250–1,500 mg/day	65–90 mcg/mL

As symptoms of mania can be distressing to patients, family members, and caretakers, effective psychopharmacological management is essential. However, when choosing an agent in an older adult with bipolar disorder, it is essential to consider tolerability, side-effect profile, and potential interactions with other medications in addition to efficacy.

In general, lithium and the anticonvulsant valproate (Depakote) are first-line treatments for bipolar mania in older adults. Atypical antipsychotics such as quetiapine, olanzapine, risperidone, and aripiperazole are also useful treatments in this setting, although, as described, their use can lead to significant effects. Lithium and lamotrigine (Lamictal) should be considered first in geriatric patients with bipolar disorder who present with depressive symptoms. Second-line treatments to be considered include carbamazepine (Tegretol) and oxcarbazepine (Trileptal). Benzodiazepines (see below) can be effective adjunctive treatments in patients with bipolar disorder, although they should be used carefully given their side-effect profile. Table 25.10 compares commonly used mood stabilizers in older adults.

Lithium

Lithium is an effective treatment of bipolar disorder in older adults, although its exact mechanism of action remains unclear. Lithium may also be neuroprotective in older adults. Aging leads to decreases in total body water and increases in adipose tissue and this can affect the distribution of lithium. Common diseases in older adults such as renal failure and congestive heart failure affect lithium clearance, and fluid shifts secondary to dehydration or infection can rapidly lead to toxicity. Signs of lithium toxicity include ataxia, tremors, diarrhea, weakness, and fatigue. If there is concern about toxicity, for example due to concurrent illnesses or surgery, trough blood levels of lithium can be checked and if desired these can be checked every 3 months. Target lithium serum levels for older patients with acute mania can range from 0.4 to 1.0 mEq/L, with the exact level being determined clinically based upon response and tolerability.

Even in the absence of toxicity, the side effects of lithium can be extensive. These include dizziness, nausea, vomiting, weight gain, tremor, hypothyroidism, hypotension, ataxia, blurred vision, cardiac arrhythmias, and diabetes insipidus. It is recommended that patients taking lithium have their renal function checked every 3 months and thyroid-stimulating hormone (TSH) checked every 6 months. Chronic use of lithium may result in decreased renal concentrating ability which usually resolves upon discontinuation of this agent. In older patients, lithium should be dosed once daily to minimize adverse renal effects. Lithium can interact with neuromuscular-blocking agents such as succinylcholine, affecting the reversal of neuromuscular blockade. More commonly, lithium interacts with medications such as NSAIDs, ACE-inhibitors, and thiazide diuretics, resulting in decreased lithium clearance and lithium toxicity.

Huyse et al. (2006) recommends discontinuation of lithium 72 h prior to a surgical procedure, provided it is not felt that abrupt discontinuation of this agent will lead to acute withdrawal symptoms. Postoperatively, these patients should have fluid status, electrolytes, and hemodynamic status closely monitored. They should also be followed psychiatrically. If patients are medically stable one week postoperatively, then lithium should be restarted to minimize the risk of recurrence of mania or other symptoms of bipolar disorder.

Anticonvulsants

Valproate increases the availability of GABA and down-regulating AMPA GluR1 synaptic expression, although its exact mechanism of action is unclear. Part of valproate's utility in older patients is its availability in many formulations, including intramuscular and intravenous forms, and as sprinkles which can be inconspicuously be added to foods. Valproate is generally well tolerated in older adults, particularly with slow titration. Serum levels of valproate should be checked routinely, and the target levels are determined clinically and generally range from 65 to 90 mcg/mL in geriatric patients with acute mania. As with lithium, valproate levels should be checked every 3 months. As valproate can rarely cause hepatotoxicity (unrelated to dose) and thrombocytopenia, it is recommended that CBC and LFTs be checked every 6 months. More common side effects of valproate include dyspepsia, nausea, vomiting, weight gain, tremor, and muscle weakness.

Lamotrigine blocks presynaptic voltage-sensitive sodium channels which in turn modulates the release of excitatory amino acids glutamate and aspartate. It is generally well tolerated, with most common side effects being headache, dizziness, sedation, nausea, ataxia, blurred vision, and rash. Much more rarely, lamotrigine can cause Stevens–Johnson syndrome or toxic epidermal necrolysis, particularly when the medication is titrated too rapidly. Adding valproate drastically increases the elimination half-life of lamotrigine, increasing the risk of adverse effects.

Carbamazepine is known to inhibit voltage-gated sodium channels. This agent has significant cytochrome P450 interactions and is an inducer of cytochrome P450 3A4 and cytochrome P450 2 C19, decreasing the concentrations of numerous psychotropic and cardiac medications. Initial use of carbamazepine as well as dose increases leads to a phenomenon called autoinduction, in which the metabolism and clearance of carbamazepine itself is stimulated (through cytochrome P450 3A4 induction). Thus, serum levels need to be monitored carefully upon initiation or titration of carbamazepine (1 week after change and then every 3 months) with a target serum level in older patients being 4–8 mcg/mL.

Carbamazepine's side effect profile has caused it to fall out of favor as a preferred agent to treat bipolar disorder, particularly in the geriatric population. Carbamazepine is rarely associated with aplastic anemia (1 in 200,000 patients in the general population). It can also cause significant elevation of LFTs and is occasionally associated with hepatic insufficiency or failure. It is recommended that older patients taking carbamazepine have CBC and LFTs checked every 4–6 months. Carbamazepine can also cause bradycardia and conduction delays, particularly in the AV node and bundle of His' (Steckler 1994), and EKGs should be checked regularly on patients taking this medication. Other adverse effects of carbamazepine include confusion, sedation, dizziness, ataxia, rash, including Stevens–Johnson syndrome, and SIADH. Sodium levels should also be checked periodically in patients taking carbamazepine.

Oxcarbazepine is structurally related to carbamazepine, but is significantly better tolerated because its metabolites are less toxic. Its mechanism of action is thought to be similar to that of carbamazepine. Oxcarbazepine is generally well tolerated with its most notable adverse effect being hyponatremia (25% in older adults). However, this is usually asymptomatic, with only 3.8% of elderly patients needing to discontinue oxcarbazepine secondary to hyponatremia. Sodium levels should be monitored periodically. Other side effects include dizziness, somnolence, fatigue, and GI effects.

Anticonvulsants themselves have analgesic effects and are primary and adjunctive treatments of many types of pain, including headaches and postoperative pain. They appear to have little negative interaction with anesthetic agents, and only carbamazepine is known to prolong the effects of succinylcholine postoperatively. There appear to be few perioperative and postoperative considerations for patients taking anticonvulsant medications.

Medications Used to Treat Dementia

The most common dementias in developed countries are Alzheimer's disease (35%), mixed vascular dementia and Alzheimer's disease (15%), dementia with Lewy bodies (15%), vascular dementia (10%), and frontotemporal dementia (5%). Unfortunately, there are few medications which have been shown to be helpful in interfering with the course of dementia. Two classes of medications which are used are cholinesterase inhibitors and NMDA agonists. At this time, both classes of medications only have FDA approval for treating Alzheimer's disease. Table 25.11 compares the dosing of memory-enhancing medications in the elderly.

Of the four cholinesterase inhibitors available, only three are widely used, as tacrine (Cognex) is almost never used anymore secondary to its hepatotoxic side effects and will not be discussed further. The other medications in this class are

Table 25.11 Memory-enhancing medications in older adults

Drug	Starting dose range	Therapeutic dose range
Donepezil	5 mg/day	10 mg/day
Galantamine	8 mg/day	16–24 mg/day
Memantine	5 mg/day	10–20 mg/day
Rivastigmine	3 mg/day	9–12 mg/day

donepezil (Aricept), galantamine (Razadyne), and rivastigmine (Exelon). These medications have been shown to have similar efficacy in all stages of Alzheimer's dementia. Cholinesterase inhibitors are likely helpful in treating dementia with Lewy bodies as these patients have particularly reduced levels of choline acetyltransferase, the enzyme which catalyzes the synthesis of acetylcholine. The choice with regard to which agent to use has most to do with side effect profile, dosing (donepezil is given once daily, galantamine and rivastigmine are dosed twice daily), and formulation (rivastigmine comes in a patch form). Donepezil and galantamine are metabolized hepatically, while rivastigmine is metabolized by local cholinesterases. The most common side effects of cholinesterase inhibitors are nausea, diarrhea, anorexia, headache, insomnia, and muscle cramping. Vivid dreams are also common in patients taking these medications.

Given that cholinesterase inhibitors increase the concentration of acetylcholine at the sites of neurotransmission, they can theoretically interfere with neuromuscular antagonists. There is at least one case report of a patient taking donepezil experiencing prolonged paralysis post-operatively following a procedure in which succinylcholine was administered.

Memantine (Namenda) is an antagonist at the NMDA receptor, blocking the action of the excitatory neurotransmitter glutamate. Memantine has FDA approval for use in moderate and severe Alzheimer's disease, and the combination of memantine and a cholinesterase inhibitor has been found to be well tolerated and significantly more helpful than placebo in patients with moderate to severe Alzheimer's disease. At least one review study has indicated that memantine can be helpful in patients with vascular dementia. Memantine has little hepatic metabolism. The most common side effects of memantine are dizziness, headache, and constipation. Much less common but more worrisome adverse effects include agitation, hallucinations, and strokes.

As memantine has a similar mechanism of action to analgesics ketamine and dextromethorphan, it is being looked at as an adjunctive agent for postoperative pain management.

Anxiolytics/Sedatives

Anxiety and insomnia are two troublesome issues in geriatric patients, as clinicians struggle with a dearth of effective medications but a wealth of troublesome side effects from the agents that are available.

Table 25.12 Selected benzodiazepine medications in older adults

Drug	Relative potency	Half-life (hours)	Starting dose range	Therapeutic dose range
Alprazolam	1	12–15	0.25–0.5 mg/day	0.25–2 mg/day
Clonazepam	0.5–1	18–50 (plus metabolite half-life of 50–100)	0.25–0.5 mg/day	0.5–2 mg/day
Diazepam	10	20–80	2.5–5 mg/day	2.5–10 mg/day
Lorazepam	2	10–20	0.25–0.5 mg/day	0.5–4 mg/day
Oxazepam	30	5–20	10–20 mg/day	10–45 mg/day

Anxiety

Although the incidence and prevalence of primary anxiety disorders are lower in the geriatric population than in younger patients, anxiety is a very common symptom in older people. Anxiety can either be situation dependent or secondary to another disorder such as dementia. While SSRIs are first-line treatments for anxiety disorders, it takes 8–12 weeks of being on these medications at a therapeutic dose before they are effective. Benzodiazepines, which are $GABA_A$ agonists, are effective medications in treating anxiety and panic attacks in the short term, but they are often prescribed inappropriately in older adults and can have considerable side effects.

When prescribing a benzodiazepine to a geriatric patient, the Beers criteria (1997) suggests that clinicians use the lowest possible therapeutic dose. Benzodiazepines with shorter half-lives should be considered first, as longer acting agents in this class can build up in fatty tissues, leading to toxicity and significant side effects with repeated use. In addition, it is more desirable to use a benzodiazepine which is metabolized via conjugation rather than oxidation, as conjugated agents generally do not have active metabolites. Given these criteria, the first benzodiazepines considered in older patients should be lorazepam (Ativan) and oxazepam (Serax). Other commonly used benzodiazepines in younger patients including clonazepam (Klonopin) and diazepam (Valium) should almost always be avoided in the geriatric population as the combined half lives of the agent and metabolite are generally several days. Table 25.12 compares the doses, potencies, and half-lives of common benzodiazepines used to treat anxiety.

Side effects of benzodiazepines, particularly at excessive doses, include confusion, sedation, increased risk for falls, and increased risk of motor vehicle accidents. These symptoms are often exacerbated in patients who are also taking opioid analgesics. Benzodiazepines should generally be avoided in the context of delirium, as they are likely to cause paradoxical agitation. Insufficient doses of benzodiazepines or doses that are given too far apart can lead to increased anxiety or withdrawal symptoms. Although many patients and clinicians are concerned about benzodiazepine dependence, this is generally not an issue unless there is a previous history of substance dependence or history of medication abuse or misuse. Benzodiazepine medications should always be tapered and not abruptly stopped, as doing so could lead to withdrawal symptoms.

Buspirone (BuSpar) is a non-benzodiazepine anxiolytic which acts as an agonist at the presynaptic 5-HT_{1A} receptor and a partial agonist at the postsynaptic 5-HT_{1A} receptor. Buspirone is generally a well-tolerated medication with dizziness, drowsiness, and headache being the most common side effects. Buspirone is generally less effective in patients who have recently been exposed to benzodiazepine agents. Buspirone has been implicated in the cases of serotonin syndrome.

Insomnia

Insomnia is an all-too-common problem in older adults, particularly in patients with dementia, leading to increased risk of falls, cognitive impairment, poor quality of life, and earlier placement in long-term care facilities, as well as psychiatric concerns such as increased agitation and psychosis. In addition, insomnia is associated with increased caregiver fatigue and distress. Sleep disturbances in patients with Alzheimer's disease may be in part a result of neuronal losses in the suprachiasmatic nucleus, a region in the hypothalamus that regulates sleep and circadian rhythms.

A formal evaluation of insomnia should include a full synopsis of sleep-wakefulness patterns including total sleep time, nighttime sleep onset, frequency and severity of sleep disruptions (i.e., secondary to need to urinate), frequency of daytime naps, and potential movement or breathing difficulties. A clinician should also consider potential medical and psychiatric issues to determine whether they might be contributing to the sleep disturbance. Common contributors to insomnia include restless legs syndrome, sleep apnea, chronic obstructive pulmonary disease, pain syndromes, gastroesophageal reflux disease, delirium, depression, anxiety, and psychosis. General anesthesia can affect sleep by altering circadian rhythms in the days following administration of these agents, potentially leading to post-operative sleep difficulties.

First-line treatment of insomnia should generally be improving sleep hygiene, which includes interventions such as minimizing noise and light, and avoiding late-day alcohol, tobacco, and caffeine. If treating underlying medical and psychiatric issues and improving sleep hygiene do not significantly improve insomnia, then pharmacologic interventions should be considered. When choosing an agent, side-effect profiles should be strongly considered. As is the case in treating other psychiatric issues in older patients, a clinician should consider using the lowest possible dose of a medication for the shortest possible time.

Melatonin, which is produced in the pineal gland and helps to regulate the sleep–wake cycle, is produced in decreased quantities in older adults. While well tolerated, data on the efficacy of melatonin in the geriatric population is mixed. Melatonin is an over-the-counter supplement, and there is no formal regulation or standardization of dosing (doses of up to 6 mg are likely safe), making it difficult to give recommendations around its use. There are limited data on the use of melatonin-agonist ramelteon (Rozerem) in older adults.

Table 25.13 Hypnotic agents in older adults

Drug	Starting dose range	Therapeutic dose range	Side effect profile
Eszopiclone	1–2 mg	1–2 mg	Headache, dizziness, somnolence
Melatonin	0.3–3 mg	1–6 mg	Headaches, nausea, dizziness
Mirtazapine	7.5–15 mg	7.5–15 mg	Somnolence, weight gain
Ramelteon	8 mg	8 mg	Somnolence, dizziness, nausea
Temazepam	7.5 mg	7.5–15 mg	Confusion, dizziness, somnolence, anxiety
Trazodone	12.5–25 mg	100 mg	Orthostasis, somnolence
Zaleplon	5 mg	5–10 mg	Somnolence, dizziness, hallucinations
Zolpidem	2.5–5 mg	2.5–5 mg	Confusion, somnolence, increased fall risk, agitation

Antidepressant medications are often used to treat insomnia. Trazodone (Desyrel) is a serotonin-specific antidepressant which is empirically thought to be useful in treating insomnia in older adults, regardless of whether they have a comorbid depressive disorder. Trazodone can cause orthostatic hypotension related to its weak alpha-adrenergic activity. Mirtazapine (as described above) may be helpful if a patient has comorbid depression, insomnia, and appetite concerns. Low doses of tricyclic antidepressants may be effective, although there are concerns about side effects including orthostasis, cardiac conduction delays, and anticholinergic effects. Nortriptyline 10 mg and Doxepin <10 mg may be viable options if a patient is deemed appropriate for TCA use.

Benzodiazepines such as temazepam (Restoril) and related agents such as zolpidem (Ambien), eszopiclone (Lunesta), and zaleplon (Sonata) may be useful in cases of transient or short-term insomnia. However, their side-effect profiles (listed in greater detail above) preclude them from being first-line agents in the geriatric population. Appropriate doses of these agents are listed in Table 25.13.

Highly anticholinergic medications such as diphenhydramine generally cause too many adverse effects in older adults to be safely used for insomnia in this population.

Conclusion

Psychiatric conditions are common in older patients causing significant suffering in patients and their caregivers. There are multiple medications available to treat many of these illnesses but they can have significant side effects. As the population ages, more patients with dementia and psychiatric disease will be having surgery and procedures and anesthesiologists will benefit from a working knowledge of the various treatment regimens and their potential risks.

Key Points

- Depression is a prevalent and serious disease in older adults which is often ineffectively treated
- Choosing a proper antidepressant should be based on prominent symptoms and side-effect profile
- Despite their side-effect profiles, antipsychotics can be useful treatments in older adults experiencing significant intrapsychic distress
- Clinicians should be vigilant in monitoring cardiac, metabolic, dopaminergic, and other potential adverse effects of antipsychotics
- Cholinesterase inhibitors can be useful in patients with Alzheimer's dementia or dementia with Lewy bodies, but their utility is less certain in patients with vascular dementia
- Benzodiazepines can be helpful for treating anxiety in older adults. Initial trial should be a low dose of a short-acting benzodiazepine
- If an older adult presents with sleep complaints, non-pharmacological interventions such as improving sleep hygiene and addressing relevant medical issues should be tried prior to beginning a trial of a hypnotic medication

Suggested Reading

Alexopoulos GS, Katz IR, Reynolds CF, et al. Pharmacotherapy of depression in older patients:a summary of the expert consensus guidelines. J Psychiatr Pract. 2001;7:361–376.

Alexopoulos GS, Streim JE, Carpenter D, et al. Using antipsychotic agents in older patients. J Clin Psychiatry. 2004;65 (suppl 2):5–104.

American Diabetes Association, American Psychiatric Association, American Association of Clinical Endocrinologist, et al: Consensus development conference of antipsychotic drugs and obesity and diabetes. Diabetes Care. 2004;27:596–601.

Areosa SA, Sherriff F, McHane R. Memantine for dementia. Cochrane Database Syst Rev. 2005;18:CD003154.

Barak Y, Olmer A, Aizenberg D. Antidepressants reduce the risk of suicide among elderly depressed patients. Neuropsychopharmacology. 2006;31:178–181.

Beers MH. Explicit criteria for determining potentially inappropriate medication use by the elderly. Arch Intern Med. 1997;157:1531–1536.

Boyer EW, Shannon M. The serotonin syndrome. N Engl J Med. 2005;352:1112–1120.

Centers for Disease Control and Prevention, National Center for Injury Prevention and Control. Web-based Injury Statistics Query and Reporting System (WISQARS) 2005. www.cdc.gov/ncipc/wisqars. Accessed July 10, 2010.

Chen ST, Altshuler LL, Melnyk KA, et al. Efficacy of lithium vs. valproate in the treatment of mania in the elderly: a retrospective study. J Clin Psychiatry. 1999;60:181–186.

Crowe S, Collins L. Suxamethonium and donepezil:a cause of prolonged paralysis. Anesthesiol. 2003;98:574–575.

Dawson J, Karalliedde L. Drug interactions and the clinical anaesthetist. Eur J Anaesthesiol. 1998;15:172–189.

Dispersyn G, Pain L, Challet E, et al. General anesthetics effects on circadian temporal structure: an update. Chronobiol Int. 2005;25:835–850.

Du J, Gray NA, Galke CA, et al. Modulation of synaptic plasticity by antimanic agents: the role of AMPA glutamate receptor subunit 1 synaptic expression. J Neurosci. 2004;24:6578–6589.

Dunner DL. Safety and tolerability of emerging pharmacological treatments for bipolar disorder. Bipolar Disord. 2005;7:307–325.
Fink M, Taylor MA. Catatonia: A Clinician's Guide to Diagnosis and Treatment. New York, Cambridge University Press;2004.
Flint AJ. Generalised anxiety disorder in elderly patients: epidemiology, diagnosis and treatment options. Drugs Aging. 2005;22:101–114.
Huyse F, Touw D, Strac van Schijndel, et al. Psychotropic drugs and the perioperative period: a proposal for a guideline in elective surgery. Psychosomatics. 2006;47:8–22.
Hybels CF, Blazer DG. Epidemiology of late-life mental disorders. Clin Geriatr Med. 2003;19:663–696.
Jacobson SA, Pies RW, Katz IR, Clinical Manual of Geriatric Psychopharmacology. Arlington (VA): American Psychiatric Publishing;2007.
Jeste DV, Blazer D, Casey D, et al. ACNP White Paper: update on use of antipsychotic drugs in elderly patients with dementia. Neuropsychopharmacology. 2008;33:957–970.
Kudoh A. Perioperative management for chronic schizophrenic patients. Anesth Analg. 2005;101:1867–1872
Kutluay E, McCague K, D'Souza J, et al. Safety and tolerability of oxcarbazepine in elderly patients in epilepsy. Epilepsy Behav. 2003;4:175–180.
Manly DT, Oakley SP, Bloch RM. Electroconvulsive therapy in old-old patients. Am J Geriatr Psychiatry. 2000;8:232–236.
McEvoy GK, Snow EK, Kester L, et al. AHFS Drug Information. Bethesda, MD, American Society of Health-System Pharmacists;2006.
Ray WA, Chung CP, Murray KT, et al. Atypical Antipsychotic Drugs and the Risk of Sudden Cardiac Death: New Engl J Med. 2009;360:25–35.
Reynolds CF 3rd. Recognition and differentiation of elderly depression in the clinical setting. Geriatrics. 1995;50 (supp 1):S6–S15.
Rowe ML, Chuang DM. Lithium neuroprotection: molecular mechanisms and clinical implications. Expert Rev Mol Med. 2004;18:1–18.
Scharf M, Rogowski R, Hill S, et al. Efficacy and safety of doxepin 1 mg, 3 mg, and 6 mg in elderly patients with primary insomnia: a randomized double-blind, placebo-controlled crossover study. J Clin Psychol. 2009;69:1557–1564.
Schneider LS, Tariot PN, Dagerman KS, et al. Effectiveness of atypical antipsychotic drugs in patients with Alzheimer's disease. N Engl J Med. 2006;355:1525–1538.
Steckler TL. Lithium- and carbamazepine-associated sinus node dysfunction: nine-year experience in a psychiatric hospital. J Clin Psychopharmacol. 1994;14:336–339.
Steffens DC, Helms MJ, Krishnan KRR, et al. Prevalence of depression and its treatment in an elderly population: the Cache County study. Arch Gen Psychiatry. 2000;57:601–607.
Stopa EG, Volicer L, Kuo-Leblanc V. Suprachiasmatic nucleus in severe dementia. J Neuropathol Exp Neurol. 1999;58:29–39.
Strauss J. Insomnia in older adults with dementia. Geriatrics and Aging. 2009;12:77–82.
Suzuki M. Role of N-methyl-D-aspartate receptor antagonists in postoperative pain management: Curr Opin Anaesthesiol. 2009;22:618–622.
Tariot PN, Farlow MR, Grossberg GT, et al. Memantine treatment in patients with moderate to severe Alzheimer disease already receiving donepezil: a randomized controlled trial. JAMA. 2004;291:317–324.
Taylor DM. Antipsychotics and QT prolongation. Acta Psychiat Scand. 2003;107:85–93.
Wang PS, Schneeweiss S, Brookhart MA, et al. Suboptimal antidepressant use in the elderly. J Clin Psychopharmacol. 2005a;25:118–126.
Wang PS, Schneeweiss S, Avorn J, et al. Risk of death in elderly users of conventional vs. atypical antipsychotic medications. N Engl J Med. 2005b;353:2335–2341.
Wirshing WC. Movement disorders associated with neuroleptic treatment. J Clin Psychiatry. 2001;62 (suppl 21):15–18.
Young RC. Evidence-based pharmacological treatment of geriatric bipolar disorder. Psychiatr Clin North Am. 2005;28:837–869.

Index

S.R. Barnett (ed.), *Manual of Geriatric Anesthesia*, DOI 10.1007/978-1-4614-3888-5,

J

K

L

O

T

V

MIX
Papier aus verantwortungsvollen Quellen
Paper from responsible sources
FSC® C105338

If you have any concerns about our products,
you can contact us on
ProductSafety@springernature.com

In case Publisher is established outside the EU,
the EU authorized representative is:
Springer Nature Customer Service Center GmbH
Europaplatz 3, 69115 Heidelberg, Germany

Printed by Libri Plureos GmbH
in Hamburg, Germany